Targeted Molecular Imaging in Oncology

Springer
New York
Berlin
Heidelberg
Barcelona
Hong Kong
London
Milan
Paris
Singapore
Tokyo

E. Edmund Kim, MD   David J. Yang, PhD

Departments of Nuclear Medicine and Diagnostic Radiology,
The University of Texas M.D. Anderson Cancer Center,
Houston, Texas

Editors

Targeted Molecular Imaging in Oncology

Foreword by Thomas P. Haynie, MD

With 135 Illustrations

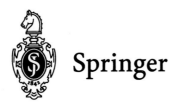 Springer

E. Edmund Kim, MD
David J. Yang, PhD
Departments of Nuclear Medicine and Diagnostic Radiology
The University of Texas M.D. Anderson Cancer Center
Houston, TX 77030
USA

Targeted molecular imaging in oncology / [edited by] E. Edmund Kim, David J. Yang.
    p. ; cm.
  Includes bibliographical references and index.
  ISBN 0-387-95028-1 (h/c : alk. paper)
    1. Cancer—Imaging. I. Kim, E. Edmund. II. Yang, David J.
    [DNLM: 1. Neoplasms—diagnosis. 2. Diagnostic Imaging—methods. 3.
  Radiopharmaceuticals—diagnostic use. QZ 241 T185 2000]
  RC270.3.D53 T37 2000
  616.99′40754—dc21   00-055719

Printed on acid-free paper.

Production coordinated by Chernow Editorial Services, Inc., and managed by Steven Pisano; manufacturing supervised by Joe Quatela.
Typeset by Best-set Typesetter Ltd., Hong Kong.
Printed and bound by Maple-Vail Book Manufacturing Group, York, PA.
Printed in the United States of America.

9 8 7 6 5 4 3 2 1

ISBN 0-387-95028-1   SPIN 10763642

Springer-Verlag   New York Berlin Heidelberg
A member of BertelsmannSpringer Science+Business Media GmbH

This book is dedicated to our wives,
Bo and Carol,
and our children,
Patrick, Sharon, Matthew, and Victor.

Foreword

The beginning of a new millennium is a time for reflection on the progress in medical history that has occurred during the past 1000 years and for contemplation of the future. Among the most important medical developments of the past millennium are the elucidation of human anatomy, physiology, cell structure, and biochemistry. The discovery of antimicrobial agents, the "magic bullets" of Paul Ehrlich, and the development of molecular pharmacotherapy, which Ehrlich called "chemotherapy," extended the magic bullet from infectious diseases to cancer.

In the past century, the development of body imaging, which began in 1895 with Roentgen's discovery of X-rays, has evolved in several directions. The morphological features and function of internal organs have been defined by X-rays, radionuclide tracers, ultrasound, and magnetic resonance. All of these contribute to the visualization of normal and disease processes, the understanding of pathophysiology, and the accuracy of therapy. Improved body imaging, made possible by the introduction of computerized axial tomography by Hounsfield and Cormack, permitted the development of new cancer treatments and more precise determination of disease stage and response through X-ray computed tomography (CT), magnetic resonance imaging (MRI), single photon emission computed tomography (SPECT), and positron emission tomography (PET).

History has shown how laboratory research and advances in medical care are intertwined. As an example, research on how growth factors trigger cell growth and division by binding to specific receptors and activating signals inside the cell has led to treatment with monoclonal antibodies that bind to the receptors, preventing activation of pathways necessary for cancer development and growth. This receptor blockade concept has led to the development of several therapies, currently in clinical trials, some of which are assisted by radiotracers. The challenge to the imaging specialist is to devise methods to noninvasively determine the existence of these receptors and to evaluate the specificity of uptake and the efficiency of blocking substances. From such studies, new diagnostic and therapeutic procedures can emerge.

The elucidation of genetics and advancing knowledge of the immune system are important contributors to our current concepts of molecular biology and medicine. Today, imaging specialists are integrating the work of basic scientists from many areas to advance imaging methods. To do so, they must be knowledgeable, not only about the clinical specialties that they serve, but also about the medical science that they bring to bear on the problem. *Targeted Molecular Imaging in Oncology* seeks to bridge that gap for those interested in exploring this exciting field.

What wonders will be seen in the third millennium? If the past is any guide, quite a few.

THOMAS P. HAYNIE, MD
Professor Emeritus of Nuclear Medicine
The University of Texas M.D. Anderson Cancer Center
Houston, TX

Preface

The practice of medicine is changing and with it a self-conscious realization of its limitation and failure to favorably influence the demography of human disease. In response to a questioning public and a political climate obsessed with cost-effective therapies, thoughtful doctors are increasingly conscious of contemporary high-tech practice. It is a time of revelation in biology, but given the ethos of medicine, the distraction of its practice, and its pastoral demands, the excitement of evolving techniques of molecular biology has neither been generally felt nor appreciated by practitioners. Cancer is viewed as a failure of multiple chemical processes or genetic disease. The care of cancer patients has become a cooperative multidisciplinary endeavor. It is critical for imaging specialists to embrace and participate in a multidisciplinary environment so that they are considered valued and equal partners.

We have put together *Targeted Molecular Imaging in Oncology* emphasizing MRI, MRS, and PET techniques for probing molecular or biochemical processes in cancer diagnosis or management. The major goal of oncologic imaging is to answer specific clinical questions about cancer patients. Given the pace of discovering new information in molecular biology, our desire is to demonstrate how targeted imaging is impinging on oncology practice as well as research and to indicate what lies ahead.

This book is organized into twenty-one chapters. The first four chapters discuss the basic principles of cancer molecular biology, imaging strategies, SPECT, PET, MRI, and MRS. The next twelve chapters deal with radiopharmaceuticals, antibodies, contrast agents and targeted SPECT, PET, and MRI applications. The last five chapters discuss new imaging approaches about angiogenesis, apoptosis/hypoxia, signal transduction/antisense, gene delivery and expression, and optical imaging. None of the chapters can be complete due to continuous evolution of technical development. However, our net has been cast wide to show the extent of molecular imaging in clinical medicine.

The goal of this book is to provide curious oncologists and imaging specialists with a basis to explore the medical potential of targeted molecular imaging for the better management of cancer patients.

E. EDMUND KIM, MD
DAVID J. YANG, PhD

Acknowledgments

We are very appreciative and indebted to Judy S. Bunch for her tremendous efforts to make this book the best of its kind by typing and editing materials. We are also deeply grateful to all our colleagues whom we often harassed for their timely contributions. We wish to thank Dr. Donald Podoloff for his support of our work. Finally, we wish to thank Rob Albano at Springer-Verlag who supported us in the creation and editing of this book.

E. EDMUND KIM, MD
DAVID J. YANG, PhD

Contents

Contributors

TOMIO INOUE, MD
Department of Nuclear Medicine, Gunma University School of Medicine, 3-39-22 Showa-machi, Maebashi 371, Japan

EDWARD F. JACKSON, PhD
Department of Diagnostic Radiology, The University of Texas M.D. Anderson Cancer Center, Houston, TX 77030, USA

ZUXING KAN, MD, PhD
Department of Diagnostic Radiology, The University of Texas M.D. Anderson Cancer Center, Houston, TX 77030, USA

E. EDMUND KIM, MD
Departments of Nuclear Medicine and Diagnostic Radiology, The University of Texas M.D. Anderson Cancer Center, Houston, TX 77030, USA

CHUN LI, PhD
Department of Diagnostic Radiology, The University of Texas M.D. Anderson Cancer Center, Houston, TX 77030, USA

CAROLYN NICHOL, PhD
Department of Diagnostic Radiology, The University of Texas M.D. Anderson Cancer Center, Houston, TX 77030, USA

NOBORU ORIUCHI, MD
Department of Nuclear Medicine, Gunma University of School of Medicine, 3-39-22 Showa-machi, Maebash 371, Japan

JORGE URIBE, PhD
Department of Nuclear Medicine, The University of Texas M.D. Anderson Cancer Center, Houston, TX 77030, USA

FRANKLIN C.L. WONG, MD
Departments of Nuclear Medicine and Neuro-Oncology, The University of Texas M.D. Anderson Cancer Center, Houston, TX 77030, USA

WAI-HOI "GARY" WONG, PHD
Department of Nuclear Medicine, The University of Texas M.D. Anderson
Cancer Center, Houston, TX 77030, USA

KENNETH C. WRIGHT, PHD
Department of Diagnostic Radiology, The University of Texas M.D. Anderson
Cancer Center, Houston, TX 77030, USA

DAVID J. YANG, PHD
Department of Nuclear Medicine, The University of Texas M.D. Anderson
Cancer Center, Houston, TX 77030, USA

1
Principles of Basic Sciences Related to Cancer

E. Edmund Kim and David J. Yang

Cancer Molecular Biology

The evidence that cancer has a genetic basis originates from three observations: first, carcinogens cause DNA mutations; second, tumors frequently display specific chromosomal abnormalities; and third, in rare cancer syndromes, a predisposition to the development of cancer is inherited [1]. Oncogenes are predominantly components of pathways that activate cell division in response to growth factor stimulation. Malignant transformation can be a consequence of mutations that increase their activity or expression. Mutations that inactivate tumor suppressor genes are commonly found in human tumor samples. The role of these genes is to encode proteins that constrain proliferation, in some cases by direct interactions with members of the oncogene family.

The gene is the basic unit of inheritance and determinant of all phenotypes. The DNA of a normal human cell contains approximately 30,000 to 40,000 genes, but only a fraction of these are expressed in any particular cell at any given time [2]. A gene exerts its effects when its DNA is transcribed into a messenger RNA (mRNA), which is in turn translated into a protein. Every gene consists of several functional components. However, there are two major functional units: the promoter and coding regions [3]. The promoter region controls when and in what tissue a gene is expressed. The coding region is the part of the gene that dictates the amino acid sequence of the protein encoded by the gene. DNA is a linear polymer of nucleotides that consists of an invariant portion, a five-carbon deoxyribose sugar with a phosphate group, and a variable portion, the base. Of the four bases, two are purines, adenine (A) and guanine (G), and two are pyrimidines, cytosine (C) and thymine (T). Ordinarily, the nucleotide bases of one strand of DNA interact with those of another strand to make double-stranded DNA. This base pairing is specific, so that A interacts with T, and C interacts with G. In every strand of a DNA polymer, the phosphate substitutions are located between the 5'- and 3'-carbons of the ribose molecules. The genetic code reads in the 5'- to 3'-direction. In double-stranded DNA, the strand that carries the translatable code in the 5'- to 3'-direction is called the sense strand, while its complementary partner is the antisense strand. In the nucleus, DNA is not present as naked nucleic acid; rather, DNA is in close association with a number of accessory proteins, such as the histones, to make the structure called chromatin [4]. The DNA double helix is ordinarily twisted on itself to form a supercoiled structure, which must unwind partially during DNA replication and transcription [5].

Genes can be cut from total genomic DNA using restriction endonucleases that recognize specific nucleotide sequences [6]. Individual genes can be captured and replicated in bulk for detailed analysis. This process is called cloning and employs bacterial plasmids and viruses (phages) as carriers for the cloned genes [7]. Enzymes called DNA ligases join foreign DNA to plasmid or phage vectors, which can then replicate within bacterial cells to create gene libraries [8]. Each colony or plaque represents a different DNA clone. Specific clones containing specific genes can be identified on the basis of their nucleotide sequences, expanded into large-scale cultures, and their recombinant DNA isolated. In this way, new genes are cloned.

Cloned gene fragments are called probes because they are used to probe native DNA or RNA for the gene of interest. A gene probe must contain enough nucleotide sequences so that it will recognize the sequences of its corresponding gene. Recognition occurs by a process called nucleic acid hybridization, in which two pieces of DNA can align themselves by base pairing. Genomic DNA is too large to be analyzed easily in the laboratory, but it can be cut into manageable fragments using restriction endonucleases isolated from bacteria. Electrophoresis through an agarose gel can separate these fragments by size. Pulsed-field gel electrophoresis is a variation of this technique that allows the separation of extremely large DNA molecules. Fragments that carry nucleotide sequences corresponding to a gene of interest can then be detected by Southern blotting [9]. For any given region of DNA, the size and number of restriction fragments may vary among individuals, leading to restriction fragment-length polymorphisms (RFLP), which are exploited both in gene mapping and for cancer diagnostics [10]. If one of the RFLPs present in the heterozygous individual's normal DNA is missing from the tumor cell DNA, the tumor is said to have undergone a reduction to homozygosity. This alteration implies a loss of genetic material from the tumor, specifically the DNA that includes the missing RFLP; this is the hallmark of a tumor suppressor gene [11].

Specific nucleotide changes (mutations) that give rise to stable genetic differences can be determined by DNA sequencing. Two methods are used for sequencing DNA: the chemical modification method and the enzymatic chain-termination method. DNA sequencing has been utilized for the analysis of mutated sequences in the tumor suppressor gene p53 [12]. By amplifying specific fragments of DNA, the polymerase chain reaction (PCR) technol-

ogy permits the detection of specific genes in extremely small amounts of tissue or in tissue that has been fixed for histological analysis [13].

The genetic information in DNA is copied or transcribed into mRNA by the enzyme RNA polymerase II. Before being transported to the cytoplasm, primary transcripts in the nucleus are modified by splicing out introns, adding a 5'-cap, and adding a 3'-poly-(A) tract [14]. Cytoplasmic mRNA can be detected by Northern blotting, by nuclease protection assays, or by modified PCR. Although nuclease protection assays are somewhat more technically demanding than Northern blotting, they are more sensitive and can also provide structural information about mRNA transcripts. A retroviral enzyme called reverse transcriptase can make cDNA copies of mRNA transcripts. These cDNAs can be cloned into cDNA libraries, which are useful for isolating and analyzing expressed genes [15].

The genetic information in DNA is transcribed into RNA, and the information in RNA is ultimately translated into protein. Like DNA and RNA, proteins are directional. The amino and carboxy termini of proteins are specified by the 5'- and 3'-ends, respectively, of the cognate in RNAs. After translation, proteins may require further modification to be fully functional. Proteins can be fractionated by size, using electrophoresis through polyacrylamide gels in the presence of the anionic detergent sodium dodecyl sulfate (SDS). SDS-polyacrylamide gel electrophoresis (PAGE) is an integral component of the analytical techniques of immune precipitation and Western blotting [16]. Automated analyzers can directly determine the amino acid sequence of a protein using vanishingly small amounts of material. The mRNA that encodes a protein can be translated in vitro using cellular extracts of rabbit reticulocytes or wheat germ. The DNA that encodes a protein can be transcribed and the RNA translated in vivo using appropriate vector and host cell combinations in culture [17].

Although there have been dramatic advances in the management of patients with several types of cancer, we are still limited by a lack of selectivity of many drugs when used against common solid tumors. Most anticancer drugs have been identified by screening large numbers of chemicals for their antiproliferative efforts on cells followed by trials on animal tumors. Our rapidly increasing knowledge of the molecular genetics of cancer has led to a new phase in the design of drugs that are designed to selectively counter the abnormal growth process involved [1]. It is likely that cancer diagnosis and screening will become more effective and that the rate of early cancer detection will be increased. Carriers of defined cancer-predisposing mutations can be specifically targeted for early detection and administration of cancer-preventing agents. On the cell surface, growth factor antagonists have been developed that mimic the ligand's binding action but lack its stimulatory activity. Other potential receptor inhibitors include blocking antibodies and tyrosine kinase inhibitors. Within the cytoplasm, molecular modeling of *ras* has led to the development of compounds that stabilize *ras* in the inactive GDP binding site [1]. In the nucleus, the artificial regulation of gene expression is a goal possible by switching genes off or on with informational drugs. Technology that corrects genes deleted during tumor evolution is an attractive prospect. New technology is also having an impact on separation of patients into different prognostic categories. In breast cancer, antibodies that detect the overexpression of c-*erb*-B2 gene product are proving useful as an indicator of breast cancer prognosis. In chronic myeloid leukemia, reagents that can identify the fusion product of c-*abl* gene with *bcr* gene are also proving valuable in monitoring effectiveness of chemotherapy and marrow transplantation [1]. These findings suggest that reagents which detect oncogene mutations and expression may soon become routine tools to guide cancer therapy and to gauge prognosis.

Cancer Biochemistry

The biochemistry of cancer received its real beginning with the work of Otto Warburg, who noted a high production of lactate by tumor slices in the presence of oxygen [18]. It has been pointed out that oxygen, which was consumed by neoplastic cells as effectively as by some normal cells, resulted in an inhibition of the formation of glycolytic end products [19]. The inhibition of glycolysis by oxidative phosphorylation has been called the Pasteur effect. Respiration markedly depends on the availability of intermediates such as adenosine diphosphate (ADP) and inorganic phosphate. Competition for ADP and inorganic phosphate occurs in respiration and glycolysis. Several studies suggested local hypoxia as the underlying cause for the apparent deficiency in respiration of tumors [20]. The hypoglycemic effect may, in part, contribute to the problems associated with cachexia in the tumor-bearing host. Greenstein [21] noted that cancers tended to discard certain enzymes or pathways that were not required for growth processes. The enzymatic profiles of the tumors tended to converge to a common pattern, and the adoption of a similar enzymatic matrix by tumors was a reflection of the increase in growth rate. Van Potter [22] proposed the loss of systems of catabolism as a central feature of tumorigenesis.

A number of the enzymatic changes that are observed in tumors resemble those that are found in fetal systems. A tumor may, in fact, represent a dedifferentiation or retrodifferentiation of mature cells. Hexokinases play a vital role in the utilization of glucose, and phosphofructokinase is a key regulatory enzyme in glycolysis. In hepatocarcinogenesis, a progressive reduction in the activity of glucokinase is noted with a concomitant rise in type I hexokinase [23]. In the normal rapidly proliferating systems, regenerating and fetal liver, as well as in hepatomas, type IV phosphofructokinase was found in much higher amounts than in the normal liver [24]. Terminal deoxynucleotidyl-transferase (TdT) catalyzes the linear polymerization of nucleotides onto a suitable template, and TdT+ cells normally appear in the thymus cortex and bone marrow lymphocytes. TdT+ cells were found in blast cells from patients with acute lymphocytic leukemia [25]. Oncofetal proteins of nonenzyme function are found in a variety of tumors and are often referred to as tumor-specific antigens.

Alpha-fetoprotein (AFP) is the serum protein in early extrauterine development, and elevated serum AFP levels were demonstrated in patients with hepatoma, acute liver toxicity, or partial hepatectomy [26]. Carcinoembryonic antigen (CEA) is a serum glycoprotein that is elevated in patients with digestive, lung, or genitourinary cancer, as well as colitis, cirrhosis, or pancreatitis. The increased CEA level may be the result of its release from the membrane by phospholipase or some defect in the phosphatidylinositol complex [27]. The overproduction of CEA may disrupt the intercellular adhesion forces, resulting in more cell movement, less ordered architecture, and more dedifferentiation [28]. Although neither AFP nor CEA is specific for tumors, they increase diagnostic capability and allow for assessing therapeutic efficacy or recurrence of cancer.

Tumors often exhibit bizarre phenotypic expressions that can have profound effects on the patients. A number of nonendocrine cancer cells can manufacture and secrete ectopic substances including hormones and growth factors that enhance bone resorption and lead to increased levels of serotonin, antidiuretic hormone calcitonin, adrenocorticotrophic hormone (ACTH), prostaglandin, and colony-stimulating-factor osteolytic substance, which may be observed in certain types of cancer [29].

The growth of tumors is often accompanied by a striking loss of weight, anorexia, asthenia, and anemia. Cachexia is a major confounder in the chemotherapy of cancer; an increased gluconeogenesis, enhanced director of glucose from peripheral tissue to the tumor, increased fat oxidation, decrease in body lipids, great expenditure of energy, increased turnover rate of total body protein, and elevation in the catabolism of muscle protein have been observed [30]. Although interleukin 1 (IL-1) has been cast as one of the mediators of cachexia, a greater role falls on the unique polypeptide cachectin or tumor necrosis factor (TNF) [31]. TNF–cachectin is elaborated by tumors and binds to receptors in tissues. The resultant complex causes the suppression of specific mRNA synthesis, which then results in changes in intermediary metabolism to feed tumor cells at the expense of the host.

The naturally occurring polyamines, putrescine, spermidine, and spermine, are ubiquitously distributed throughout the eukaryotes. Cell proliferation and differentiation require their biosynthesis [32]. Suppression of tumor growth has been observed when inhibitors of polyamine synthesis were administered [33]. Ornithine decarboxylase (ODC) is a key regulatory enzyme in the biosynthesis of polyamines and undergoes rapid induction on exposure of cells to stimuli including growth factors, hormones, and tumor promoters. Increased ODC has been found in skin cancers and familial polyposis, and ODC genes located to chromosome 2 have been reported [34]. Cyclic adenosine monophosphate (cAMP) may play an important role in the differentiation of certain cells and is formed from the catalytic action of adenyl cyclase, a membrane-bound enzyme that utilizes ATP as substrate. cAMP is involved in a number of phosphorylation reactions through the action of cAMP-dependent protein kinase, called A-kinase. cAMP levels are modulated by external stimuli, such as growth factors and prostaglandins, and may regulate the rate of cell proliferation [35]. Poly (ADP-ribose) polymerase or synthetase is a chromatin-bound enzyme involved in cell transformation, cell differentiation, and DNA repair [36]. Poly (ADP-ribosylation) is activated by DNA strand breaks. When the damage to DNA is severe, activation of the polymerase persists, leading to a depletion of the intracellular pool of ATP.

The death of cells is neither always abnormal nor always detrimental. Although necrosis ensues at the sites of massive cellular injury, most cells die through a more subtle, noninflammatory, energy-dependent form of cell death called apoptosis [37]. Cells undergoing apoptotic cellular suicide rapidly shrink and lose their normal intracellular contacts and, subsequently, exhibit dense chromatic condensation, nuclear fragmentation, cytoplasmic blebbing, and cellular fragmentation into small apoptotic bodies. Necrosis occurs in acute, nonphysiological injury, and necrotic cells swell and lyse, releasing their cytoplasmic and nuclear contents into the intercellular milieu, thus sparking inflammation. Apoptosis is of critical importance both to the pathogenesis of cancers and to their likelihood of resistance to antineoplastic treatments. The protein p53 induces apoptosis by acting as a transcription factor, activating expression of numerous apoptosis-mediating genes. DNA damage causes the p53 protein to turn on genes, the products of which generate free radicals that damage the mitochondria, whose contents, in turn, leak out into the cytoplasm and activate apoptotic caspases [38]. Mutations in genes that lead to reduced apoptosis are generally associated with poor prognosis. New cancer therapies that aim to induce apoptosis specifically in cancer cells are the source of renewed hope for cures. The role of DNA methylation in the production of cancer has been examined [39]. The methylation occurs exclusively in the 5-position of cytosine and, more specifically, when this cytosine is part of the CpG dinucleotide. Less methylation of the CpG sequences in the AFP gene in hepatoma DNA and hypermethylation of specific regions of human chromosomes in tumor cells have been reported [40].

The production and secretion of proteolytic enzymes by tumors represent old observations. The plasminogen activators are involved in fibrinolysis, tissue remodeling, and some stages of malignancy. They are also participants in a number of steps of metastasis [41]. The extracellular matrix (ECM) is a complex medium that is formed from substances which are secreted by cells. The ECM is important in the regulation of cell proliferation and differentiation as well as in determining the metastatic potential of malignant cells. Many cancer cells secrete proteases, glycosidases, heparanases, and type IV collagenase. The ECM is composed of collagen type I–V, depending on the specific tissue; proteoglycans such as chondroitin sulfate; anchorage proteins such as fibronectin that serve as attachment sites to the matrix; and sometimes elastin. Substantial alterations to the plasma membrane of cells occur in neoplastic transformation. Cell transformation has been shown to alter the gangliosides and neutral glycolipids with a number of tumor systems expressing gangliotriosylceramide (Gg3) [42].

Cancer Immunology

The human immune response has evolved to detect and eliminate foreign substances and organisms. This response is mediated by lymphoreticular cells and their products. Bone marrow is the source of both B lymphocytes, which produce antibodies, and T lymphocytes, which mediate cellular immunity [43]. Mature B cells synthesize and express immunoglobulin (Ig) on their cell surface. After interaction with antigen and T-cell products, different clones of B cells differentiate into one or more plasma cells that produce a single antibody which binds noncovalently to a particular antigen. Ig molecules consist of light (L) and heavy (H) polypeptide chains. Each L and H chain can be divided into an amino-terminal variable (V) region and a carboxyl-terminal constant (C) region. The V region of each H and L chain includes three complementarity-determining regions (CDRs), which contribute to the antigen-binding site and determine the specificity of the antibody. Each H-chain C region (C_H) determines the function and isotype of the antibody; these include IgG-1, IgG-2, IgG-3, IgG-4, IgA-1, IgA-2, IgM, IgD, and IgE. The C_H region permits fixation of complement components, antibody-dependent cell-mediated cytotoxicity, Ig-mediated phagocytosis, and transport across the placenta. T lymphocytes arise in bone marrow and differentiate within the thymus [44]. T cells mediate the cellular response, including delayed hypersensitivity, graft rejection, and regulation of other T cells, B cells, monocytes, and marrow progenitors.

The specificity of interactions with different antigens is mediated by a large family of 90-kDa, cell-surface T-cell receptors (TCR) [45]. Different clones of T cells bearing distinctive TCRs recognize different antigenic peptides. T cells mature under the influence of thymic epithelium. Early thymocytes express CD2 and CD7, and common thymocytes acquire CD1, CD4, and CD8. Mature T cells constitute 70% to 80% of normal peripheral blood lymphocytes, and 30% to 40% of lymph nodes, spleen, and gut-associated lymphoid tissue. Antibody production can be augmented by T-cell help. A small population of lymphocytes lacks the markers associated with mature B or T cells. Non-T or non-B cells can exert both antibody-dependent cell-mediated cytotoxicity (ADCC) and natural killer (NK) activity, destroying tumor cells in the presence or absence of specific IgG antibodies. Monocytes, macrophages, and dendritic cells can present antigens to lymphocytes and secrete cytokines, such as IL-1, IL-6, TNF-α, interferons, prostaglandins, and other monokines that can affect the function of both T and B cells. T cells and monocytes produce a large number of factors that mediate intercellular communication and which include the interleukins and cytokines. Cytokines can interact synergistically and can stimulate the release of a cascade of secondary factors.

The process of malignant transformation is a series of DNA mutations of cancer-related genes. The immune system has the potential to discriminate between the normal and the aberrant self. Thus, the protein products of these mutated DNA segments are potentially immunogenic. It is likely that human tumors are linked to prolonged exposure to low-dose carcinogens. Cytotoxic T (Tc) cells specific for autologous tumor cells have been cultured from the peripheral blood of melanoma patients or from the tumor-infiltrating lymphocytes [46]. There is increasing evidence that nonimmunogenic tumors can stimulate the host immune response by immunological manipulations. T cells are capable of mediating the regression of established tumors when adoptively transferred to the tumor-bearing host [47]. T cells do not recognize a native antigen, but rather interact with peptide fragments derived from protein antigens bound to major histocompatibility complex (MHC) molecules on the cell surface. The two major T-cell subsets recognize short sequences of approximately 10 amino acids, presented on the cell surface by a MHC molecule. CD4$^+$ T-helper (T$_H$) cells recognize antigens presented by the MHC class II molecules on antigen-presenting cells, and CD8$^+$ Tc cells recognize intracellular proteins that are mostly synthesized in the cytoplasm, degraded to small peptides, translocated into the endoplasmic reticulum for insertion into a cleft in the MHC class I molecule, and transported through the Golgi stack for expression on the cell surface [48]. For a tumor to be immunogenic, it needs to present processed antigens as peptides bound to MHC class I or class II molecules.

Early studies demonstrated a decreased cell-mediated immunity in cancer patients. It is likely that the immunological deficit does not contribute significantly to the initial tumor progression, especially in patients with solid tumor, but that it reflects a secondary phenomenon. Tumors might arise not because of a general depression in cell-mediated immunity, but because of a specific inability to react effectively against the antigens on the tumor cells. Transfection of MHC class I genes into murine tumor cells often decreases their ability to grow in immunocompetent hosts [49]. With the exception of hematopoietic cancers, most solid tumors do not express MHC class II antigens, and they cannot directly activate tumor-specific CD4$^+$ T$_H$ cells. It has become clear that, in addition to T-cell receptor signaling, activation of T cells requires other critical costimulatory signals. Tumor cell antigen presentation to T cells in the absence of costimulators may induce peripheral tolerance in tumor-specific T-lymphocyte responses. Selective outgrowth of antigen-negative tumor variants under the pressure of tumor-specific T-cell response has been documented in a variety of tumor systems. Antigen-negative immunoselected variants often express fewer immunodominant antigens that can trigger a Tc cell response [50].

A tumor-bearing host may be immunologically tolerant to some tumor antigens. Tumor cells often express carcinoembryonic antigens (CEA), which are not immunogenic because they are expressed as self-proteins during development. However, tolerance to CEA may be broken by immunization with a recombinant vaccinia virus expressing CEA [51]. Tumors can exert local effects that prevent T-cell immune responses from displaying full efficacy. Transforming growth factor-β has been known to inhibit IL-2-dependent proliferation of T-lymphocytes and a variety of T-cell and macrophage functions. The suppressor T cells have been identified as CD4 cells and appear to need several days to be generated in response to tumor growth. The CD4$^+$ T$_H$ cell population containes two subsets that can be differentiated on the basis of the lymphokines they produce. The T_H 1 cells produce IL-2 and interferon γ (IFN-γ) and induce macrophage activation and delayed-type hypersensitivity responses, whereas T_H 2 cells produce IL-4 and IL-10 and selectively induce B-cell responses. The kinetics of tumor growth may allow for the establishment of progressive tumors before an effective immune response develops. In general, immunologically mediated tumor eradication is at its best when the tumor burden is small.

Both RNA and DNA viruses are implicated in the development of tumors. T-cell immunity against virus-induced tumors follows the rules of antiviral immunity. Any tumor virus protein could serve as a target for T cells, provided that it is processed into peptides and presented by MHC molecules on the surface of antigen-presenting cells. The Epstein–Barr virus is associated with B-cell lymphoma, Hodgkin's lymphoma, and nasopharyngeal carcinoma. Human papilloma virus is associated with most human cervical carcinomas. A protective role of the immune system in controlling the growth of DNA virus-induced tumors is suggested by the high frequency of these tumors in immunodeficient individuals. DNA mutation of cancer-related genes can result in the expression of altered proteins that differ from normal ones by a single amino acid residue. Somatic mutations of *ras* oncogenes occur commonly in 90% of pancreatic adenocarcinoma, 50% of colon adenocarcinoma, and 30% of hepatocellular carcinoma. Antibodies reactive to *ras* were detected in 32% of cancer patients but only 3% of people without cancer [52]. The hallmark of chronic myelogenous leukemia is the translocation of the human c-*abl* proto-oncogene from chromosome 9 to the specific breakpoint (bcr) region on chromosome 22 [53]. A recent report has demonstrated that human Tc cells can be generated against the rearranged bcr-abl fusion peptide, providing hopeful immunotherapy [54]. Some genes such as MAGE and HER-2/neu are silent or expressed at low levels in normal tissue. When these genes are deregulated as a consequence of malignant transformation and are expressed inappropriately, they may behave as tumor antigens and evoke immune responses. Patients with HER-2/neu-positive tumors often demonstrate antibody as well as cellular immunity to HER-2/neu, suggesting that tolerance can be circumvented [55]. A fundamental characteristic of malignant cells is the accumulation of genetic mutations required for malignant transformation or maintenance of malignant phenotype. Missense mutations in the p53 tumor suppressor gene are detected in approximately half of human cancers, and p53-derived peptides may represent ideal targets for cellular immunotherapy [56].

Over the years, two approaches have been utilized for cancer immunotherapy—active and passive immunotherapy. In active immunotherapy, attempts have been made to stimulate endogenous antitumor immunity within the host through the administration of bacterial products, chemically defined immunomodulators, cytokines, and vaccines. In passive immunotherapy, antibodies or lymphoreticular cells (adoptive immunotherapy) have been given to the host, providing exogenous immunity. Interferon and Il-2 have been the major cytokines, and their use in melanoma patients has caused some therapeutic response (10%–30%) [57]. Unfortunately, toxic effects have been associated with repeated high-dose Il-2 infusions. The secretion of cytokines by gene-modified tumor cells may more closely resemble the physiological mode of lymphokine delivery to antigen-presenting cells or lymphocytes for immune activation. Virtually all described cytokine genes, including IL-1, IL-2, IL-3, IL-4, IL-6, IL-7, IL-12, IFN-γ, TNF-α, granulocytic colony-stimulating factor, and granulocyte-macrophage colony-stimulating factor (GM-CSF), have been found to be effective in at least some animal tumor models [58]. Using the human melanoma-associated antigen, p97, expressed on murine K1735-M2 cells, it was demonstrated that immunization with transduced tumor cells expressing the co-stimulation molecule B7 resulted in complete regression of tumors that express the human tumor antigen [59]. The efficacy of cytokine-mediated gene therapy may not necessarily be superior to immunization or immunotherapy. However, combining cytokine gene therapy with other molecules such as MHC, cell adhesion protein, tumor, or foreign antigen may allow optimizing treatment schemes. The identification of genes that encode tumor cell-surface peptides which are recognized by Tc cells has provided another form of active immunization. Vaccination with antigen-presenting cells expressing tumor proteins and peptides may improve the efficacy of active immunotherapy.

Many variations on the use of passively administered antibodies in cancer therapy have been tried. Antitumor antibodies conjugated to toxic molecules, radioisotopes, and drugs have been tried, but the practical application has proven considerably more difficult than anticipated. Radioimmunodetection of melanoma using monoclonal antibodies has shown a reasonable degree of localization in melanoma nodules [60]; however, there is limited sensitivity as well as specificity. Antiidiotypic antibodies have been used in the treatment of B-cell lymphomas, but the approach has not proved successful because surface immunoglobulin expression is not functionally related to the malignant transforming property. Some cell-surface antigens expressed by B-cell lymphomas, such as CD19, CD20, CD22, and CD72, are attractive targets for antibody-mediated radioimmunotherapy, and 14 of 28 patients demonstrated a complete remission of a duration exceeding 16 months [61].

Adoptive immunity is the acquisition of immunity in a naive subject as a result of the administration of immunologically activated lymphoid cells. Tumor-reactive lymphoid cells have to be isolated from cancer patients for T-cell therapy to be feasible. This problem was addressed by the discovery of Il-2, a T-cell growth factor. However, early attempts at growing lymphoid cells in IL-2 resulted in the generation of lymphokine-activated killer (LAK) cells [62]. LAK cells have had therapeutic benefit in some patients, but such effector cells frequently lack several of the most attractive qualities of T cells. Use of T cells for tumor treatment is technically more complicated than the use of LAK cells. Potential tumor-reactive T cells isolated from solid tumors of cancer patients, termed tumor-

infiltrating lymphocytes (TIL), are specific in their reactivity to tumor cells, and 19 of 56 melanoma patients experienced objective tumor response [63]. Antigen recognition by T cells involves receptor occupancy by antigen and leads to the second step of activation, transmembrane signaling, which is mediated by a complex of protein, CD3. Several CD3 proteins have an intracellular polypeptide that is phosphorylated when a T-cell receptor binds with the antigen. Although the reactivity of anti-CD3 to T cells is polyclonal, the antitumor effect mediated by the activated cells is immunologically specific [64]. The method of anti-CD3–IL-2 activation has greatly facilitated the procedure of clinical T-cell immunotherapy because of increased understanding of T-cell responses to human tumors.

Cancer Pathology

A tumor is an abnormal mass of tissue, the growth of which exceeds and is uncoordinated with that of the normal tissues, and persists in the same excessive manner after cessation of the stimuli which evoked the change. Tumors are apparently purposeless; they prey on the host and are virtually autonomous. Solid tumors form a mass that is composed of two compartments: the parenchyma (tumor cells) and the stroma. In epithelial tumors, a basal lamina separates clumps of tumor cells from stroma. Stroma is interposed between malignant cells and normal host tissues, and is essential for tumor growth. Stroma is a product of the host that is induced by tumors. Most tumors require stroma if they are to grow beyond a minimal size of 1 to 2mm [65]. Stroma provides a lifeline that is necessary for tumor growth. The bulk of tumor stroma is composed of interstitial connective tissue. The major components of tumor stroma include structural proteins; interstitial fluid; proteoglycans and glycosaminoglycans; new blood vessels (angiogenesis); interstitial collagens (type I, III, and V); fibron; fibronectin; fibroblasts residing in normal connective tissue; and inflammatory cells derived from the blood. Tumors differ markedly from each other in stromal content, and these differences are primarily quantitative at times and largely qualitative in other cases. The events of tumor stoma generation closely resemble those of wound healing. The initial event is a local increase in vascular permeability, followed by extravascular clotting, fibrin deposition, fibrin proteolysis, and infiltration by inflammatory and connective tissue cells, leading to the development of granulation tissue and finally of dense fibrous connective tissue (desmoplasia in tumors and scar in healed wounds) [66]. Tumor stroma is generally a disorganized and poorly supportive parody of normal connective tissue.

Tumor blood vessels are often poorly differentiated, unevenly spaced; they are unequal to the task of supporting the growth and even the life of rapidly metabolizing tumor cells [67]. The result is irregular blood flow, shifting zones of anoxia, low pH, and coagulative necrosis [68]. The presence of necrosis may be helpful in recognizing malignant tumors and distinguishing them from their benign counterparts. Details of the type and origin of the tumor, its differentiation, level of invasion, the numbers of lymph architecture, the presence or absence of hormone receptors, the activity of specific enzymes, ploidy, and frequency of mitosis and cells in S phase may all be relevant in virtually every pathological assessment of tumor. Tumors not infrequently generate an extensive inflammatory response, and atypical hyperplasia can be very difficult to distinguish from in situ carcinoma [69].

Tumors of epithelial cell origin are termed adenomas or papillomas when benign and carcinomas when malignant. Carcinomas account for approximately 80% of all malignant tumors. Further classification is often on the basis of the type of epithelium present, for example, glandular (adenocarcinoma), squamous (squamous cell carcinoma), or transitional cell (transitional cell carcinoma). Malignant tumors of mesenchymal origin are designated sarcomas, such as liposarcoma, fibrosarcoma, or leiomyosarcoma. A few tumors contain neoplastic cells of more than a single type. Adenoacanthoma contains both squamous cell carcinoma and adenocarcinoma elements. A few tumors such as Wilms' tumor contain neoplastic cells from more than one germ layer. Even within a single organ and within a single type of epithelium, several different types of tumors may arise each with its own special characteristics, prognosis, and response to therapy.

The neoplastic cells that constitute the benign tumor are usually well differentiated, closely resembling the corresponding cells of normal tissue. Benign tumors tend to expand uniformly in all directions, and they cause compression atrophy of surrounding normal tissues that results in the formation of a thin rim of fibrous connective tissue. This enveloping connective tissue rim may serve as a capsule that renders benign tumors discrete, readily palpable, and easily movable. Malignant tumors are characterized primarily by the increased numbers and abnormality of their cells, and commonly exhibit abnormal orientation of both tumor cells and stroma. Cytological features of malignancy include altered polarity; tumor cell enlargement; increased ratio of nuclear to cytoplasmic area; pleomorphism of tumor cells and their nuclei; clumping of nuclear chromatin and distribution of chromatin along the nuclear membrane; enlarged nucleoli; atypical or bizarre mitoses; and tumor giant cells with one or more nuclei. Malignant tumors invariably lack a capsule and often invade lymphatics and veins. Malignant tumor cells are transported by lymph or blood flow to distant sites [70].

Tumor grading (G) has traditionally referred to a pathologist's judgment as to a tumor's degree of differentiation and growth rate, often on a scale of I to III or IV, where III or IV represents the least differentiated, fastest dividing tumors. High-grade tumors are more anaplastic and tend to metastasize sooner. Formal grading systems are less popular today than the early days because of their shortcomings. A different scale is required for each type of tumor, and scoring is not always reproducible. Tumors are typically heterogeneous, and the correlation between histological appearance and biological behavior is seldom perfect. Therefore, many pathologists have abandoned attempts to grade cancers and have adopted a descriptive terminology [71,72]. In addition to making an exact histological diagnosis of cancer, it is essential that the clinical stage be determined before making a decision regarding therapy. The recognized importance of staging has led to a variety of international and national attempts to standardize the staging. To date, no single system has been universally accepted. Stage I by the American Joint Committee on Cancer (AJCC) usually indicates a tumor confined to its primary site of origin; stage II indicates metastases to the regional lymph nodes; and stage III often and stage IV always indicate distant metastatic spread. The TNM system by the Unio Internationale Contra Cankrum (UICC) relies on a statement of tumors extent in terms of the primary tumor (T), presence or absence of node metastases (N), and the presence or absence of distant metastases (M). Size criteria vary for different tumors, but decreasing prognosis is indicated by increasing numbers after the T for lesions of increasing size. The presence or absence of regional spread is usually indicated by variations in the secondary category under N for nodes. Distant metastasis is indicated by adding the subscript 1 following M for metastases. The AJCC recognizes several types of cancer staging schemas. The clinical diagnostic staging represents the extent of the cancer before first definitive treatment. Postsurgical resection-pathological staging provides additional information after operation and is useful in planning adjuvant therapy. Other staging types include surgical evaluative staging based on surgical exploration, retreatment staging (usually after a cancer-free interval), and autopsy staging when the cancer is first diagnosed at autopsy. One of the great deficiencies of the present staging methods is their inability to indicate subclinical, microscopic, metastatic lesions.

It is necessary to recognize that tumors are not static entities. Progression is a tumor's acquisition of increasingly malignant properties over time, such as fast growth rate, anaplasia, loss of hormonal responsiveness, chromosomal aberration, drug resistance, and metastatic potential [73]. Progression is thought to depend on clonal evolution. Cancer is associated with genetic and epigenetic plasticity and probably increased mutation rate [74]. Mutant clones have the greatest capacity for proliferation, for metastasis, and for drug resistance. Many tumors develop over time from individual clones of normal stem cell precursors in a series of distinct steps that include dysplasia, carcinoma in situ, and frank malignancy. Tumors vary considerably in their capacity for further progression. Tumors of bone marrow and lymphoid origin are most likely to undergo further morphological change. Chronic myelogenous leukemia commonly progresses to blast crisis, and chronic lymphocytic leukemia may proceed to a large-cell phase (Richter's syndrome). Solid tumors are less apt to change morphologically.

References

1. Ellis MJC, Sikora K. Molecular biology of cancer. In: Cox TM, Sinclair J, eds. Molecular Biology in Medicine. London: Blackwell Science, 1997:149–171.
2. Lewin N. Genes IV, 4th Ed. Oxford: Oxford University Press, 1990.
3. Atchison ML. Enhancers: mechanisms of action and cell specificity. Annu Rev Cell Biol 1988;4:127–137.
4. Laskey RA, Earnshaw WC. Nucleosome assembly. Nature (Lond) 1980;286:763–768.
5. Wang JC. DNA topoisomerases. Annu Rev Biochem 1985;54:665–671.
6. Smith HO. Nucleotide sequence specificity of restriction endonucleases. Science 1979;205:455–457.
7. Cochran BH, Reffel AC, Stiles CD. Molecular cloning of gene sequences regulated by platelet-derived growth factor. Cell 1983;33:939–943.
8. Maniatis T, Hardison RC, Lacy E, et al. The isolation of structural genes from libraries of eukaryotic DNA. Cell 1978;15:687–692.
9. Southern EM. Detection of specific sequences among DNA fragments separated by gel electrophoresis. J Mol Biol 1975;98:503–508.
10. White R, Woodward S, Leppert M, et al. A closely linked genetic marker for cystic fibrosis. Nature (Lond) 1985;318:382–385.
11. Knudson AG. Hereditary cancer, oncogenes, and antioncogenes. Cancer Res 1985;45:1437–1442.
12. Takahashi T, Nau MM, Chiba I, et al. p53: a frequent target for genetic abnormalities in lung cancer. Science 1989;146:491–493.
13. Saiki RK, Gelfand DH, Stoffel S, et al. Primer-directed enzymatic amplification of DNA with

a thermostable DNA polymerase. Science 1988; 239:487–489.

14. Maniatis T, Reed R. The role of small nuclear ribonucleoprotein particles in pre-mRNA splicing. Nature (Lond) 1987;325:673–679.

15. Efstradiatis A, Kafatos FC, Maniatis T. The primary structure of rabbit β-globin mRNA as determined from cloned cDNA. Cell 1977;10: 571–575.

16. Towbin H, Staehelin T, Gordon J. Electrophoretic transfer of proteins from polyacrylamide gels to nitrocellulose sheets: procedure and some applications. Proc Natl Acad Sci USA 1979;76:4350–4354.

17. Derynck R, Remaut E, Saman E, et al. Expression of human fibroblast interferon gene in *Escherichia coli*. Nature (Lond) 1980;287:193–195.

18. Warburg O. On respiratory impairment in cancer cells. Science 1956;124:269–272.

19. Weinhouse S. Oxidative metabolism of neoplastic tissues. Adv Cancer Res 1955;3:269–273.

20. Shapot VS. Some biochemical aspects of the relationship between the tumor and the host. Adv Cancer Res 1972;15:253–258.

21. Greenstein JP. Some biochemical characteristics of morphologically separable cancers. Cancer Res 1956;16:641–645.

22. Potter VR. Biochemistry of cancer. In: Holland JF, Emil F III, eds. Cancer Medicine, 2nd Ed. Philadelphia: Lea & Febiger, 1982:133–143.

23. Walker PR, Potter VR. Isozyme studies on adult, regenerating precancerous and developing liver in relation to findings in hepatomas. Adv Enzyme Regul 1972;10:339–343.

24. Tomaka T, Inamura K, Ann T, Taniuchi K. Multimolecular forms of pyruvate kinase and phosphofructokinase in normal and cancer tissue. Gann Monogr 1972;13:219–224.

25. Bollum FJ, Chang LMS. Terminal transferase in normal and leukemic cells. Adv Cancer Res 1986;47:37–41.

26. Uriel J. Fetal characteristics of cancer. In: Becker FF, ed. Cancer: A Comprehensive Treatise, Vol. 3. New York: Plenum Press, 1975:21–30.

27. Helfta SA, Hefta LJF, Lee TD, et al. Carcinoembryonic antigen is anchored to membranes by covalent attachment to a glycosylphosphatidylinositol moiety: identification of the ethanolamine linkage site. Proc Natl Acad Sci USA 1988;85:4648–4652.

28. Benchimol S, Fuks A, Jothy S, et al. Carcinoembryonic antigen; a human tumor marker, func-

tions as an intercellular adhesion molecule. Cell 1989;57:327–330.

29. Robertson RP, Baylink DJ, Marini JJ, Adkinson HW. Elevated prostaglandins and suppressed parathyroid hormone associated with certain types of cancer. N Engl J Med 1975;293:1278–1281.

30. Heber D, Chlebowski RT, Ishibashi DE, et al. Abnormalities in glucose and protein metabolism in noncachectic lung cancer patients. Cancer Res 1982;43:4815–4820.

31. Wang AM, Creasey AA, Ladner MB, et al. Molecular cloning of the complementary DNA for human tumor necrosis factor. Science 1985;228:149–152.

32. Tabor CW, Tabor H. Polyamines. Annu Rev Biochem 1984;53:749–752.

33. Luk GD, Baylin SB. ODC as a biologic marker in familial colonic polyposis. N Engl J Med 1984;311:80–83.

34. Dice JF. Molecular determinants of protein half-lives in eukaryotic cells. FASEB J 1987;1:349–354.

35. Bourne HR, DeFranco AL. Signal transduction and intracellular messengers. In: Weinberg RA, ed. Oncogenes and Molecular Origins of Cancer. New York: Cold Spring Harbor Laboratory Press, 1989:79–84.

36. Berger NA. Poly (ADP-ribose) in the cellular response to DNA damage. Radiat Res 1985;101: 4–9.

37. Hetts SW. To die or not to die. An overview of apoptosis and its role in disease. JAMA 1998; 270:300–307.

38. Polyak K, Xia Y, Zweier JL, et al. A model for p53-induced apoptosis. Nature (Lond) 1997;389: 300–305.

39. Jones PA, Buckley JD. The role of DNA methylation in cancer. Adv Cancer Res 1990; 54:1–6.

40. de Bustros A, Nelkin BD, Silverman A, et al. The short arm of chromosome 11 is a hot spot for hypermethylation in human neoplasia. Proc Natl Acad Sci USA 1988;85:5693–5696.

41. Vines RL, Coleman MS, Hutton JJ. Reappearance of terminal deoxynucleotidyl transferase containing cells in rat bone marrow following corticosteroid administration. Blood 1980;56: 501–506.

42. Itakomori S. Aberrant glycosylation in tumors and tumor-associated carbohydrate antigens. Adv Cancer Res 1989;52:259–261.

43. Paul WE (1989) The immune system: basic considerations. In: Paul WE, ed. Fundamental

Immunology, 2nd Ed. New York: Raven Press, 1989:3–18.

44. Hodes RJ. T-cell-mediated regulation: help and suppression. In: Paul WE, ed. Fundamental Immunology, 2nd Ed. New York: Raven Press, 1989:587–596.

45. Weiss A. Structure and function of the T cell antigen receptor. J Clin Invest 1990;86:1015–1021.

46. Celis E, Tsai V, Crimi C. Induction of anti-tumor cytotoxic T lymphocytes in normal humans using primary cultures & synthetic peptide epitopes. Proc Natl Acad Sci USA 1993;91:2105–2109.

47. Shu S, Chou T, Sakai K. Lymphocytes generated by in vivo priming and in vitro sensitization demonstrate therapeutic efficacy against a murine tumor that lacks apparent immuno-genicity. J Immunol 1989;143:746–748.

48. Miller AR, McBride WH, Hunt K, Economou JS. Cytokine-mediated gene therapy for cancer. Ann Surg Oncol 1994;1:436–450.

49. Wallich R, Bulbuc N, Hammerling GJ, Katzar S, Segal S, Feldman M. Abrogation of metastatic properties of tumor cells by de novo expression of H-2K antigens following H-2 gene transfec-tion. Nature (Lond) 1985;3125:301–305.

50. Dudley ME, Roopenian DC. Loss of a unique tumor antigen by cytotoxic T lymphocyte immunoselection from a 3-methylcholanthrene-induced mouse sarcoma reveals secondary unique and share antigens. J Exp Med 1996;184:441–447.

51. McLaughlin JP, Schlom J, Kantor JA, Griener JW. Improved immunotherapy of a recombinant carcinoembryonic antigen vaccinia vaccine when given in combination with interleukin-2. Cancer Res 1996;56:2361–2367.

52. Shu S, Plantz GE, Krauss JC, Chang AE. Tumor immunology. JAMA 1997;278:1972–1981.

53. Canaani E, Marcelle C, Fainstein E. bcr-abl RNA in chronic myelogenous leukemia and lymphocytic leukemia. In: Deisseroth A, Arling-haus RB, eds. Chronic Myelogenous Leukemia: Molecular Approaches to Research and Therapy, Part III. New York: Dekker, 1991:217–240.

54. Bocchia M, Korontsuit T, Xy Q. Specific human cellular immunity to bcr-abl oncogene-derived peptides. Blood 1996;87:3587–3592.

55. Cheever MA, Disis ML, Bernhard H. Immunity to oncogenic proteins. Immunol Rev 1995;145:33–59.

56. Houbiers JGA, Nijman HW, van der Burg SH. In vitro induction of human cytotoxic T lympho-cyte responses against peptides of mutated and wild type p53. Eur J Immunol 1993;23:2072–2077.

57. Rosenberg SA, Lotze M, Yang JC. Experience with the use of high-dose interleukin-2 in the treatment of 652 cancer patients. Ann Surg 1989;210:474–484.

58. Vieweg J, Gilboa E. Consideration for the use of cytokine-secreting tumor cell preparation for cancer treatment. Cancer Invest 1995;13:193–201.

59. Chen L, Ashe S, Brady WA. Costimulation of antitumor immunity by the B7 counter receptor for the T lymphocyte molecule CD 28 and CTLA-4. Cell 1992;71:1093–1102.

60. Murrey J, Rosenbaum MG, Sobol RE. Radioim-muno-imaging in malignant melanoma using In-111 labeled monoclonal antibody. Cancer Res 1985;45:2376–2381.

61. Kaminski MS, Zasadny RK, Francis IR. Iodine-131 anti-B1 radioimmunotherapy for B-cell lymphoma. J Clin Oncol 1996;14:1974–1981.

62. Grimm EA, Robb RJ, Roth JA. Lymphokine-activated killer cell phenomenon. III. Evidence that IL 2 is sufficient for direct activation of peripheral blood into lymphokine-activated killer cells. J Exp Med 1983;158:136.

63. Rosenberg SA, Vannelli JR, Yang JC. Treatment of patients with metastatic melanoma with autologous tumor-infiltrating lymphocytes and interleukin-2. J Natl Cancer Inst 1994;86:1159–1166.

64. Chang AE, Aruga A, Cameron MJ. Adoptive immunotherapy with vaccine-primed lymph node cells secondarily activated with anti-CD3 and IL-2. J Clin Oncol 1997;15:796–807.

65. Folkman J. Tumor angiogenesis. Adv Cancer Res 1985;43:175–180.

66. Senger DR, Connolly DT, van de Water L, et al. Purification and NH$_2$-terminal amino acid sequence of guinea pig tumor-secreted vascular permeability factor. Cancer Res 1990;50:1774–1779.

67. Vaupel P, Kallinowski F, Okunieff P. Blood flow, oxygen and nutrient supply, and metabolic microenvironment of human tumors. A review. Cancer Res 1989;49:6449–6454.

68. Tannock IF, Rotin D. Acid pH in tumors and its potential for therapeutic exploitation. Cancer Res 1989;49:4373–4378.

69. Dupont WD, Page DL. Risk factors for breast cancer in women with proliferative breast disease. N Engl J Med 1985;312:146–149.

70. Schnitt SJ, Silen W, Sadowsky NL, et al. Ductal carcinoma in situ (intraductal carcinoma) of the breast. N Engl J Med 1988;318:898–902.

71. Gleason DF. Histologic grade, clinical stage, and patient age in prostate cancer. Natl Cancer Inst Monogr 1988;7:15–19.

72. Elston CW. The assessment of histological differentiation in breast cancer. Aust N Z J Surg 1984;54:11–17.

73. Hill RP. Tumor progression: potential role of unstable genomic changes. Cancer Metastasis Rev 1990;9:137–142.

74. Nowell PC. Mechanisms of tumor progression. Cancer Res 1986;46:2203–2208.

2
Imaging Strategies and Perspectives in Oncology

E. Edmund Kim

In the past 30 years, there has been an enormous increase in the range of imaging techniques available to investigate patients with cancer. The value of ultrasonography, X-ray, computed tomography (CT), and nuclear imaging, including single photon emission computed tomgraphy (SPECT), positron emission tomography (PET), and magnetic resonance imaging (MRI), have often been assessed in cancer management. Some methods may have limited application in common diseases or only be useful in rare tumors, and confusion can arise about the role and value of these techniques.

Imaging plays a significant role in the diagnosis, staging, and follow-up of cancer patients. A large percentage of medical imaging is performed in cancer patients. In many patients, more than one imaging study is performed for a specific clinical indication that could have been addressed with one appropriate study. Oncologists must determine which tests are most accurate and economical for a specific clinical indication. A well-designed imaging strategy is an implicit component of the approach to a cancer patient. Patients are sometimes referred for oncological opinion without having simple imaging tests from which major therapeutic decisions can be made. In other situations, they may have been subjected to inappropriate or incomplete imaging studies that need to be repeated or multiple unnecessary tests. This situation creates extra work, wastes finite resources, and may delay treatment.

Cancer patients should undergo relevant investigations quickly and efficiently. The primary applications of imaging procedures in cancer patients are in tumor detection, staging, and follow-up. The challenge of oncological imaging is complex and varied with each organ site and, often, tumor type. Once the tumor is detected and a specific histological diagnosis has been established, the definition of the T (tumor) lesion is performed.

Imaging Strategies

Film-Screening Technique

Of all the common imaging procedures, the film-screen technique provides by far the greatest resolution, often more than can be used. The limiting problems with film radiography in tumor detection are tissue discrimination and resolution of low-contrast objects. Signal-to-noise problems often limit the ability of radionuclide imaging to resolve tumor masses. This is, in part, a deficiency corrected by the tomographic scanning. Radioimmunoimaging using a monoclonal antibody may allow the identification of many tumors at a smaller size than currently is possible. Signal-to-noise problems, suboptimal labeling, and lack of developing tumor-specific antibodies have been the major challenges.

Ultrasonography

Ultrasonography (US) uses high-frequency sound waves to image the body. When tissues change, if the change in speed of sound movement is great enough, part of the sound is reflected back from the tissue interface. When this interface is perpendicular to the path of the sound waves, the reflected sound will be reflected back at the crystal transducer, which can record its return. The time taken for the sound to return can be electronically converted into the distance traveled by the sound, permitting an image in depth to be made. Multiple images can be arrayed to create a two-dimensional image of the location of echo surfaces within the body. High-frequency sound waves propagate well through soft tissue and fluid spaces; they are stopped by air or bone. Fluid-filled structures, lymphomas masses, and some neurogenic tumors are usually anechoic. Air and calcium are markedly echogenic and stop the sound transmission. Large amounts of air or calcium prevent imaging.

Three different methods are used for recording the image: A-mode, B-mode, and M-mode. The A-mode image is like a line graph, and the height of the line represents the intensity of echogenicity. The length along the graph represents the depth of that echo source within the body. In the B-mode image, the intensity of echoes from a point in the body is related to the intensity of the light exposing the film and making the image. A two-dimensional image is constructed in which the top of the image represents the skin surface and the depth below the skin surface is proportional to the depth of the point imaged within the body. The horizontal axis reflects the movement of the transducer along the skin surface as the image is made. New B-mode real-time machines have special transducers and electrodes that permit the making of rapid sequential images. The M-mode image shows the motion of a structure such as a cardiac valve as it rapidly changes position over time.

The advantages of sonographic imaging are no radiation, relatively low cost, and high accuracy in pelvic and retroperitoneal as well as cardiac diseases. Among the disadvantages of sonographic imaging are included poor imaging of morbidly obese patients or interference by air, confusion of fluid-filled colon with masses, and poor screen due to sample error.

Computerized Tomography

In most body imaging, computerized tomography (CT) has been the standard against which other tumor imaging systems are measured. Image production for CT depends on the physical characteristics of the structure imaged (density, atomic number, and number of electrons per gram) and the energy of the X-ray beam. Advantages of CT are better contrast resolution than plain radiographs, the ability to obtain axial images, the ability to guide lesion biopsy and radiotherapy planning, and good depiction of bone detail. CT is superior to MRI in characterizing the margins, periosteal reaction, and matrix of a bone tumor [1]. Disadvantages of CT are the inability to obtain direct coronal or sagittal images of large body parts, inability to image the entire spine in one visit, insensitivity to bone marrow edema, and requirement for intravenous injection of the contrast agent.

Magnetic Resonance Imaging and Spectroscopy

In magnetic resonance imaging (MRI), a powerful unidirectional magnetic field is used to orient or polarize some of the body's hydrogen atoms in the direction of the magnetic field. Using a computer, the radiowave emissions from hydrogen atoms within the body can be used to synthesize a three-dimensional volume image.

Image production for MRI depends upon the inherent characteristics of the structure imaged (T_1 and T_2 relaxation times), the proton density of the structure, flow effects, and instrument parameters such as repetition time and echo time. The advantages found in the use of MRI include excellent tissue contrast resolution, direct multiplanar imaging, no ionizing radiation, ability to image blood flow, increased sensitivity to edema, and very low incidence of reactions to MRI contrast agents. The disadvantages of using MRI can be relatively high cost, poor cortical bone detail, and inherent contraindications with ferromagnetic foreign bodies or implants [2].

With the most commonly used MR imaging technique, known as spin-echo imaging, the T_1-weighted MR images require relatively short repetition and echo time (TR and TE) settings, but T_2-weighted images require long TR and TE sequences. Tumors appear relatively dark on T_1-weighted MR images when compared to surrounding normal tissues, and they appear relatively bright on T_2-weighted images. Anatomical detail is somewhat better on T_1-weighted images, whereas tumors and peritumoral edema as well as reactive tissues often stand out in better contrast to surrounding normal tissues on T_2-weighted images.

Nuclear Magnetic Resonance

The history of nuclear magnetic resonance (NMR) began with the discovery of the NMR phenomenon that led to the use of NMR as a spectroscopic technique to determine chemical composition and physical properties of a material and to probe the metabolism of a tissue [3]. Biochemical information relevant to energy status and metabolism can be used to characterize a tumor and indicate response to treatment and progress. It is now possible to do semiquantitative spectroscopic analyses of metabolites in tissues with magnetic resonance.

Positron Emission Tomography

Positron emission tomography (PET) is recognized as a powerful tool and its clinical applications are increasing, particularly since the basic considerations of whole-body scanning. The use of positron-emitting tracers is also likely to increase as gamma cameras are adapted with special collimators or coincidence electronics. Like the spectroscopic analyses, PET scanning provides unique information about the metabolic activities of tumors and includes metabolic changes that may occur with treatment. The short-lived positron-emitting radiopharmaceuticals are used to tag certain normal metabolites or drugs. The rate and intensity of accumulation of radiolabeled metabolites or drugs are analyzed with serial PET scans to evaluate tumor biology and therapeutic response or prediction.

Tumor Size

Tumor size or volume (the T component of the American Joint Committee staging system) has an obvious major impact on both the treatment decision process and patient outcome. Tumor size alone is only a part of the problem because similarly sized tumors show significantly different behaviors. However, the detection of a cancer at a smaller size or volume that can be effectively treated generally results in a more favorable outcome.

Threshold tumor size is difficult to define. From an imaging standpoint, the limits of resolution of the various imaging systems can be generally characterized. The limitations to detection variables relate to equipment (spatial and contrast resolution), patient and target organ considerations, and interobserver variations. Tumor growth has been shown to be exponential and proceeds along predictable lines until its volume reaches 3 to $4 \, mm^3$, receiving its nutrition from the extravascular space by diffusion. Subsequent to this growth volume, the cluster of cancer cells induces its own vascular supply, possibly through the elaboration of tumor angiogenesis factor [4]. From this time on, the tumor is able to stimulate new capillaries, to acquire nutrients by perfusion, and is capable of metastasizing.

With current imaging techniques, tumor nodules from 5 mm to 1 cm represent the smallest size of detection, and such lesions are biologically advanced. The improved and more sophisticated imaging techniques and procedures have advanced cancer staging by more accurate and specific characterization. The newer techniques also direct more aggressive treatment to both the primary tumor and, occasionally, its metastatic lesions.

Decision Theory Process

The value of cancer screening has been questioned, and random radiographic screening procedures have neither resulted in an improved survival for the cancer victim nor been justified from the standpoint of cost-effectiveness. The exception is the notable yield from mammographic screening. With lung cancers, as well as with most other primary tumor locations, the principal goal of imaging efforts should be tumor definition and staging, not random screening. The decision therapy process has largely been an intuitive one in clinical practice. A clear understanding of the decision theory process must accompany a knowledge of both the disease and imaging systems being applied to the clinical problem.

Most oncologists are familiar with the common terms of sensitivity, specificity, and positive and negative predictive tests. The more widespread use of computers in medical environments will require oncologists to become more familiar with these terms. The increasingly rigid demands of healthcare reimbursement policies will dictate term use in the prioritization of healthcare services. The sensitivity of a test is a function of the true-positive rate compared with the sum of the true positives and false negatives. The specificity is the relationship of the true-negative yield compared with the sum of true-negative plus false-positive rates. The predictive value is a more important variable of its potential usefulness. The positive predictive value is determined by the true-positive yield compared with the sum of the true- and false-positive rates.

Important components of the art of medicine are skills in repeatedly making decisions, formulating appropriate judgments, and being comfortable with risk and uncertainty. Logical medical reasoning is grounded in the development and evaluation of a hypothesis of disease and the comparison of the hypothesis with alternative hypotheses. Imaging specialists develop hypotheses on the basis of disease as it is revealed in observed signals or complexes of signals and differentiated from noise. Noise is a form of artifact, and signals are important because they affect the probability of a diagnostic hypothesis. Observation of a finding (signal) and true-positive assignment represent the determination of a personal probability with which the imaging specialist expresses certainty about the event, with the degree of certainty being conditioned by the existing knowledge of the signal. The Bayes theorem permits use of personal probabilities to combine observed evidence with existent prior information to reach a differential diagnosis [5]. The decision maker must keep in mind the inaccuracies of tests and the errors and bias that occur in the interpretation of test results.

Perspectives

Technological advances have already led to fundamental improvements used to visualize tumors and to assess their metabolic, as well as physical, effects on the body. They have not only improved cancer care and lessened patient suffering, but they also may have reduced overall medical expenditures by shortening and simplifying diagnostic procedures, lessening hospitalization requirements, and helping to tailor therapeutic approaches more appropriately to individual patient needs [6]. Even with these technological advances, it is necessary to emphasize that imaging studies cannot make a histological diagnosis or pathological grading, and that relevant clinical information is essential for a proper interpretation or consultation. Furthermore, modern ultrasonography, CT, and MRI have not replaced most of the standard radiological techniques, but they serve to complement the standard methods. Much research remains on the appropriate uses of diagnostic imaging in cancer management because the current applications of imaging techniques in clinical oncology are still less than optimal.

One area of continuing concern is the type and appropriate periodicity of imaging tests for following cancer patients after treatment. A number of new developments in diagnostic imaging have potential impact for the detection, diagnosis, staging, and follow-up of cancer patients. Some of the new diagnostic imaging developments include rapid CT and MR imaging, Doppler and endoluminal ultrasound techniques, new contrast and radiopharmaceutical agents, improved PET, single photon emission tomography (SPECT), and MR spectroscopy (MRS) or spectroscopic imaging. A plethora of imaging techniques is available without sufficient data to use them in the most efficient manner. Accelerating medical costs will force radiologists, nuclear physicians, and oncologists to take the difficult steps that are needed to evaluate our existing imaging methods systematically for their contributions to cancer management and to determine their appropriate uses or develop more concerted roles for them.

Imaging is entering its second century at the same time we are entering a new millennium. The development of molecular biology and genetics over the past 20 years has provided medical science with unprecedented chances to study the molecular basis of diseases. Imaging becomes involved in the age of molecular medicine by creating new contrast media and radiopharmaceuticals. New classes of contrast agents based on tissue-specific uptake will be developed. MRI agents will be designed to take advantage of new knowledge of receptor systems and metabolic pathways. Nuclear and MR imaging agents based on antisense technology will allow extraordinary specific tissue targeting. By designing the right nucleic acid sequences, artificial antisense molecules can selectively block DNA and RNA replication by binding to key areas along the molecule.

Imaging techniques will be used as probes of molecular and genetic phenomena to monitor the progress of gene therapy. The successful transfection of a cell with tyrosinase results in the expression of melanin, which sequesters metal ions intracellularly. Successfully transfected cells thus have altered magnetic susceptibility for MRI and also actively localized radioactive metals such as In-111 [7]. Genetic material causing the expression of cell-surface receptors can bind radioligands administered systematically, and the marker genes in gene therapy would then provide the opportunity to follow the expression of the treatment through imaging techniques.

Many drugs appear promising on the basis of biodistribution in experimental animals, but fail in clinical trials because of drastically different pharmacokinetics and pharmacodynamics of new therapeutic drugs. Higher field strengths of magnets to resolve spectra in small voxels will lead to increased use of spectroscopic imaging and true ability to characterize normal and abnormal tissues by their metabolic signatures for the definitive tissue diagnosis through imaging, eliminating the need for biopsy. Molecular imaging will move the capability for making diagnoses closer to the onset of disease and will increase diagnostic specificity [8].

References

1. Magid D. Two-dimensional and three-dimensional computed tomographic imaging in musculoskeletal tumors. Radiol Clin North Am 1993;31:425–447.
2. Shellock FG, Morisoli S, Lanal E. MR procedures and biomedical implants, material and devices: 1993 update. Radiology 1993;189:587–599.
3. Negendank WG, Brown TR, Evelhock JL. Proceedings of a National Cancer Institute Workshop: MR spectroscopy and tumor cell biology. Radiology 1992;185:875–883.
4. Folkman J, Merler E, Abernathy C, Williams G. Isolation of a tumor factor responsible for angiogenesis. J Exp Med 1971;133:275–288.
5. Steckel R, Kagan AR. Pitfalls in the diagnosis of metastatic disease or local tumor extension with modern imaging techniques. Invest Radiol 1990;25:818–824.
6. Wood BP. Decision making in radiology. Radiology 1999;211:601–603.
7. Weissleder R, Simonova M, Bogdanova A, et al. MRI and scintigraphy of gene expression through melanin induction. Radiology 1997;204:425–429.
8. Thrall JH. Directions in radiology for the next millennium. AJR 1998;171:1459–1462.

3
Principles of Single Photon Emission Computed Tomography and Positron Emission Tomography

Wai-Hoi "Gary" Wong and Jorge Uribe

Radionuclide-tracer targeted imaging is based on the detection of gamma rays emitted by the radionuclides embedded in biologically specific compounds after the injection of the compounds into human or experimental animals. The most common imaging radionuclides used for imaging emit gamma rays, which are uncorrelated, and these gamma rays are detected individually or singularly for imaging; this is called single photon imaging. The basic imaging devices used for single photon imaging are gamma cameras or the rotational version, single photon emission computed tomography (SPECT) cameras. Another radionuclide-tracer imaging technique uses positron emitting radionuclides that emit two 511-KeV gamma rays simultaneously, and this pair of gamma rays is detected simultaneously or coincidentally for imaging purposes; this is known as coincidence imaging or positron imaging. Positron emission tomography (PET) cameras or coincidence cameras are used for imaging such positron-labeled tracers. The imaging principles and design of single photon cameras and those of PET cameras are significantly different. This chapter describes the principles of these two imaging methods.

Basic Principle of Single Photon Imaging

The design of gamma cameras is most suitable for imaging radionuclides with gamma-ray energy between 80 and 300 KeV. The most common single photon radionuclides in this energy range are tabulated in Table 3.1.

Even though gamma-ray photons are electromagnetic waves similar to optical photons, their energies are sufficiently high that gamma photons cannot be bent, refracted, or reflected by optical lens systems. Hence, gamma rays cannot be imaged or focused by conventional optical systems or cameras. Because any form of imaging involves the detection of the direction of travel of the photons, the only way of determining the direction of an individual gamma photon is by collimation techniques. A gamma camera is basically a position-sensitive gamma-ray detector covered by a lead collimator (Figure 3.1). Hal Anger first described the present gamma camera design in 1953 using a pinhole collimator [1]. Hence, gamma cameras are also known as Anger cameras. The major refinement in modern cameras from the first design is in the area of electronics and the use of computers.

The Position-Sensitive Detector Head

The position-sensitive detector is made up of a large sodium iodide NaI(Tl) scintillation crystal with a typical size of 40 to 50 cm square and dozens of photomultiplier tubes (Figure 3.1). When a gamma ray interacts with the NaI(Tl) crystal, a burst of scintillation photons (optical wavelength) is emitted by the scintillation crystal at the location of interaction. The scintillation photons are detected by the photomultipliers behind the NaI(Tl) crystal.

TABLE 3.1. Common single photon radionuclides.

Radionuclide	Half-life ($T_{1/2}$)	Principal gamma energy (KeV)	Fractional emission
^{67}Ga	78 h	93	0.38
		185	0.24
		300	0.16
^{99m}Tc	6 h	140	0.88
^{111}In	2.81 d	172	0.9
		247	0.94
^{123}I	13 h	27	0.71
		159	0.84
^{131}I	8.06 d	284	0.06
		364	0.82
		637	0.06

Photomultiplier tubes (PMT) are light detectors that convert light into electrical signals and amplify the electrical signal by more than a million times so that the electrical signal from a single gamma ray is large enough to be received and processed by conventional electronic circuits. The PMT that is the nearest to the scintillation point receives the most scintillation light, and the PMT farther away receives less light. A position-decoding circuit connected to the outputs of all the PMTs analyzes the relative amount of scintillation light received by all PMTs. From the relative PMT signal outputs, the position-decoding circuit calculates the X–Y position or coordinates of the scintillation point. The signal sum of all the PMTs is a measure of the gamma-ray energy deposition. The energy deposition of the gamma ray is inspected by a "window/threshold" inspection circuit to determine if the gamma ray has deposited all its energy or just part of its energy on the crystal. Only the event that has deposited all its energy, equal to one of the main imaging gamma rays, are kept as an imaging event while the rest are discarded. This energy 'window' selection process is essential to maximize image quality because the process eliminates (a) imaging events that deposit only partial energy in the detector and (b) non-imaging scattered gamma rays which have been

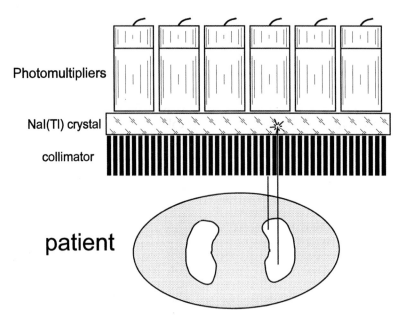

FIGURE 3.1. Basic components of a gamma camera detector head.

scattered once or twice in the body (scattering causes a change in gamma-ray direction). Scattered events, the major source of image degradation, create high background noise in the image to obscure the tracer uptake in the target organ.

The NaI(Tl) crystal used in a gamma camera is a large crystal, 8 to 12 mm thick, and encapsulated in a hermetically sealed canister with a glass window that allows the scintillation to be emitted. Because NaI(Tl) is hydroscopic, the crystal will be damaged if the hermetic seal is broken or becomes leaky after years of use. The glass window also serves as a light distribution device to spread the scintillation light optimally over more PMTs to improve the accuracy of position-decoding calculation. A thinner crystal, for example, 8 mm, provides higher intrinsic spatial resolution but lower detection efficiency, especially for imaging higher-energy gamma rays, for example, ^{131}I. Imaging efficiency is an important consideration because the lead collimator absorbs more than 99% of the gamma ray incident onto the camera. Gamma camera imaging is always count-limited. However, for imaging lower-energy gamma, such as the 140 KeV from ^{99m}Tc, an 8-mm-thick crystal is sufficient. The crystal, PMT array, and the front-end electronics are contained in a lighttight, lead-lined housing. This assembly or camera head is covered by a collimator system.

Collimators

Gamma-ray imaging involves the detection of (a) photons coming from each individual point in an object, and (b) the directions of travel of these photons. Because the gamma ray cannot be focused by optical lens systems because of its very short wavelengths, the only way to find the direction of travel of gamma photons is to use an absorptive collimator to selectively pass photons (from a fixed direction) onto the detector head. The collimator blocks and absorbs all other photons from reaching the detector (see Figure 3.1). The collimator is generally a lead structure with a honeycomb array of tunnels or holes. A collimator with longer septa length and smaller holes defines the photon direction better (higher resolution) but the "pass-through" efficiency is low; this is the inevitable compromise of a high-resolution collimator. On the other hand, a high-efficiency collimator has larger holes and shorter septa length, which degrade image resolution. Gamma cameras are designed to facilitate the changing of collimators depending on the imaging needs, and a set of different collimators are generally supplied with a gamma camera. Careful design and production of collimators are essential to imaging quality. For imaging higher-energy gamma rays, for example, ^{131}I, a "high-energy" collimator with thicker septa thickness is needed to lower septa penetration by the higher-energy gamma ray. Generally, a 5% septa penetration is an acceptable compromise.

Currently, the intrinsic resolution of the gamma camera is about 3 mm, which means that the NaI(Tl) and photomultiplier combination is capable of 3-mm resolution, but the practical resolution is poorer and is limited by the collimator used. There are four major types of collimators: pinhole, parallel hole, converging hole, and diverging hole collimators (Figure 3.2). The pinhole collimator is a cone made of lead or tungsten and has a small pinhole aperture at the end of the cone. The pinhole is typically a few millimeters in diameter; replacing inserts carrying the pinhole can alter the size of the pinhole. A larger pinhole has higher efficiency but lower resolution. With this collimator, a gamma camera functions like that of a basic optical pinhole camera. The imaged size (magnification) of an object changes with the distance between the object and the pinhole, which causes a distortion for three-dimensional objects. The magnification effect of a pinhole collimator is often used to magnify small objects (e.g., thyroid) by placing the object very close to the pinhole.

The parallel hole collimator is the most widely used, general purpose collimator. The parallel hole collimator has a magnification of one with neither minification nor magnification. The parallel holes are drilled in a piece of lead or formed by bending lead foils. The thickness of the lead wall (septa) is designed to prevent the gamma ray from entering one hole and exiting the next hole (septa penetration). For imaging higher-energy gamma rays, the septa thickness has to be greater. The converg-

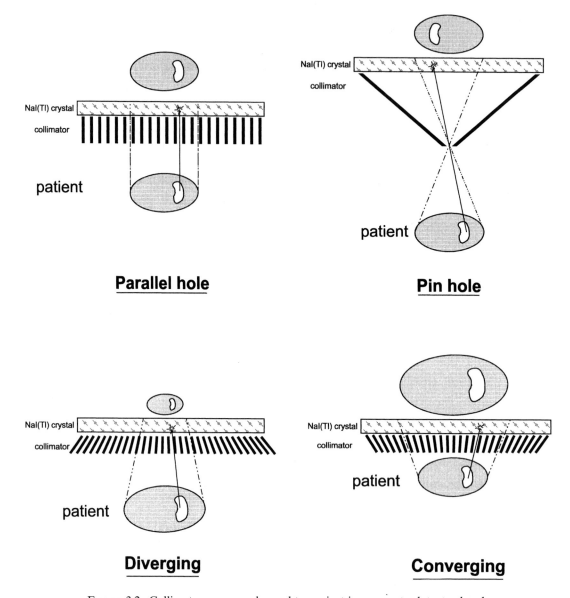

FIGURE 3.2. Collimators commonly used to project images onto detector heads.

ing collimator is similar to the parallel hole collimator except that the holes are not parallel but diverge from the detector head. This collimator produces a minified image of the object. The collimator is useful for imaging a large object with a smaller camera. The converging collimator is just the opposite of a diverging collimator. A converging collimator magnifies the object and allows the full utilization of a camera's detection surface for imaging a smaller object to improve the visualization of

small structures. For parallel, diverging, and converging collimators, the imaging resolution improves as the source is close to the collimators. Therefore, to obtain the best possible image resolution, the object should be brought as close to the collimator as physically allowed.

The intrinsic disadvantage of lead collimators is the low efficiency of gamma-ray utilization, as the collimator absorbs most of the gamma ray emitted by the subject. The typical efficiency of a low-energy, high-resolution collimator is 2×10^{-4} photons transmitted for each photon emitted by the subject. Even a high-sensitivity (low-resolution) collimator only transmits about 4×10^{-4} photons for each photon emitted. This intrinsic disadvantage of imaging tracers with single gamma photon emission is also carried from planar imaging (described above) to tomographic imaging.

Single Photon Emission Computed Tomography

The planar imaging technique just described maps a three-dimensional object into a two-dimensional image where the depth information of the tracer distribution is lost. Structures at one depth can be obscured by overlying structures at another depth. To render a three-dimensional image, tomographic imaging techniques are needed. Currently, single photon emission computed tomography (SPECT) is the most practical and commonly used tomographic imaging technique. The SPECT technique renders a three-dimensional object into cross-sectional slices. A SPECT camera is basically a regular gamma camera with the capability to rotate around the subject. The simplest SPECT camera has only one detector head while the more expensive SPECT cameras have two to three detector heads. To function in the SPECT mode, a camera acquires multiple projection (planar) images at different viewing angles in a step-and-shoot mode. Typically, 32 to 64 viewing projections are acquired, depending on the subject and image matrix sizes. For a single-detector-head SPECT, the number of angular views required should be $D/(2d)$ over a $180°$ rotation, where D is the diameter of the field of view (or object size) and d is the sampling distance or the pixel size of the data acquisition. For SPECT imaging, the projection images have typical matrix sizes of 64×64 or 128×128. The typical image slice thickness is 12 to 24 mm. Based on the multiple viewing projection data acquired, the image reconstruction computer reconstructs a three-dimensional image of the subject with the use of a mathematical technique (filtered backprojection) similar to that of a X-ray CT scan. The princi-

ple and mathematical detail of the computed tomographic technique used in SPECT can be found in publications by Budinger [2] and Croft [3].

Principle of Positron Imaging

A more sophisticated tracer imaging technique is positron imaging. These tracers are labeled with positron-emitting isotopes. Positron-emitting tracers are used because of their unique tomographic capability and the availability of metabolically important radionuclides. The tomographic capability comes from the simultaneous emission of two back-to-back, 511-KeV gamma rays from a positron-labeled molecule. With the detection of the gamma-ray pairs by detectors outside the object, the direction of gamma-ray emission can be found by drawing a line between the two locations of detection on two opposing detectors. Hence, no lead collimator is needed to define the gamma-ray directions, which leads to a detection efficiency 50- to 100 fold higher compared to SPECT or single photon imaging. A second important feature of positron imaging lies in the existence of its isotopes (^{11}C, ^{13}N, ^{15}O, ^{18}F), which are essential elements of all living organisms and their physiological processes. With the isotopes, more physiology-specific and chemistry-specific tracers can be synthesized to study the physiological functions of normal or pathological tissues in vivo. The distribution of these positron-labeled compounds, as depicted by the tomographic images, may be converted into images of functional parameters such as metabolic rates, blood perfusion rates, and receptor densities.

Basic Positron Properties

A positron ($\beta+$) is an antimatter of an electron ($\beta-$). It is basically an electron with a positive electrical charge that is emitted from the radionuclear decay of a nucleus which is deficient in neutrons. The neutrons provide an attractive, strong nuclear force for binding nuclear particles together to compensate for the repulsive electrostatic force experienced by

TABLE 3.2. Physical properties of common positron isotopes.

Positron isotopes	^{11}C	^{13}N	^{15}O	^{18}F	^{68}Ga[a]
Half-life (min)	20.4	9.96	2.07	109.7	68.3
Average β + energy (MeV)	0.3	0.4	0.6	0.2	0.7
Average positioning error (mm)	0.28	—	—	0.22	1.35

[a] ^{68}Ga is generated from a ^{68}Ga/^{68}Ge generator (the parent ^{68}Ge has a half-life of 275 days).

the protons. When a nucleus has a deficiency in neutrons, the nucleus is unstable, and a radiodecay will occur to transmute the nucleus into a more stable nucleus. Positrons can be produced by such a radiodecay. Because of nuclear instability and the physics of β-decay, positron-emitting nuclei have very short lives. Hence, the positron does not occur in nature but can be generated by nuclear reactions occurring in nuclear reactors or particle accelerators. Protons are accelerated in a small cyclotron to an energy of 10 to 17 MeV, which is sufficient to produce the nuclear reactions for biomedical positron imaging [4]. Small linear accelerators can also be used. The half-lives of the positron isotopes most often used in medical imaging are listed in Table 3.2.

The positrons are emitted from the nucleus with some kinetic energy (Table 3.2). The emitted positron slows down to nearly zero energy through electrostatic interactions in the tissue before it can annihilate with an electron to generate the two gamma rays used for tomographic imaging. Hence, the emitted positron traveled a short distance (0.2–2 mm) before generating the gamma-ray pair. This small distance, or positron range, causes a small imaging error, which generally is insignificant because it is usually smaller than the imaging resolution of a PET camera. However, tracers with higher positron energy, such as ^{82}Rb, may produce a larger imaging error that is observable. This positron-range error contributes to the fundamental resolution limit of PET imaging. The tomographic property of positron imaging is derived from the detection of the annihilation gamma-ray pair at the same time (coincidence detection) by detectors placed at opposite sides of the imaged subject. A true coincidental detection implies that a positron-tracer molecule existed along the line joining the two detectors (Figure 3.3). In a typical image acquisition, tens of millions of coincidence events (coincidence lines) are detected. These coincidence lines are used to reconstruct a three-dimensional tomographic image with the same mathematical technique (filtered backprojection) used in SPECT. The backprojection

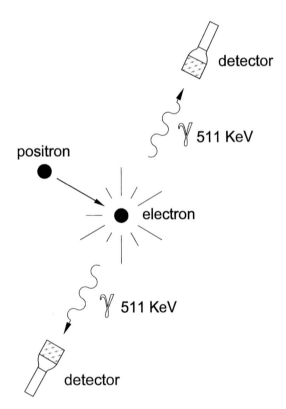

FIGURE 3.3. Principles of coincidence detection and imaging for positron tracers. The annihilation of a positron with an electron in tissue generates the two 180° gamma rays, which are detected in coincidence by two external scintillation detectors.

process is performed with a very fast computer [5–7].

A unique quantitative imaging property is also derived from the 180° emission of the gamma-ray pair. In conventional nuclear imaging or single photon imaging, the attenuation of gamma rays by the body cannot be exactly calculated or measured with an external radioactive source, which hinders the use of the image as a tool for in vivo quantitative measurement of the tracer distribution. However, with the 180° emission of two gamma rays, the positron tracer allows the attenuating effect of the body to be exactly measured with an external radioactive source. This attenuation correction process is mathematically exact and allows the PET camera to be used as an in vivo quantitative assay device. This quantitative property is very important for generating accurate tracer biodistribution and quantitative parametric images of physiological functions.

PET Cameras

There are three classes of positron emission tomography (PET) cameras (Figure 3.4): (a) a dual-head rotating NaI(Tl) camera (SPECT) with modified electronics for coincidence detection with the lead collimator removed; (b) a dedicated NaI(Tl) PET camera with the six large NaI(Tl) detectors forming a hexagonal ring; and (c) a dedicated PET camera using tens of thousands of small, high-density detector material (bismuth germanate or BGO). Class (c) can be further divided into two subclasses: one with a full detection ring and the other a partial detection ring.

Dual-Head Rotating NaI(Tl) PET Camera (Class a)

This camera is simply a dual-head SPECT camera with coincidence electronics added [8]. Elimination of the lead collimator increases the detection sensitivity by 20× or more over the regular gamma camera type. The thin NaI(Tl) detector used for SPECT still has low sensitivity for detecting 511-KeV gamma rays. The detection efficiency is just 9% for the coincidence gamma pairs incident onto the two opposing camera heads. When compared with a dedicated PET camera, which uses much thicker detectors made of BGO scintillation material, the sensitivity of this modified SPECT camera type is 9 to 10 fold lower if the detection areas are identical. However, the detection sensitivity of this class of camera is a substantial improvement over the lead collimator type. This camera type can detect structures or lesions as small as 1.5 to 2.0 cm in diameter.

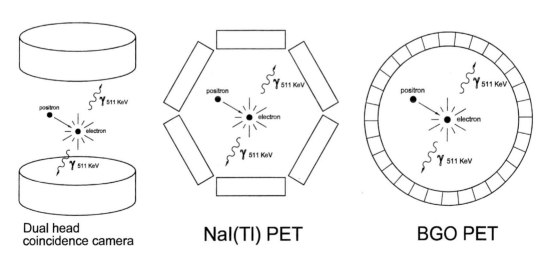

FIGURE 3.4. Three basic designs of PET cameras.

Dedicated PET Camera with a NaI(Tl) Detector Ring (Class b)

The dedicated PET camera with NaI(Tl) detector ring is an improvement over the SPECT camera type. This camera is similar to the dual-head NaI(Tl) gamma camera with coincidence detection electronics, but instead of having two heads, this PET type has six heads [9]. The six heads are configured to form a fixed ring around the patient. This six-head PET increases the detection sensitivity significantly. Furthermore, because the camera is designed to be a dedicated PET camera, the thickness of the NaI(Tl) detector has been increased from 1 to 2.5 cm to increase the camera's detection sensitivity. This increased detector thickness contributes to another fourfold increase in coincidence detection efficiency compared to a dual-head coincidence camera. Furthermore, with the detectors completely surrounding the patient, the detection efficiency is uniform in the transaxial field of view. However, because the detector design is basically that of a gamma camera, which has limited count-rate capabilities, the removal of the collimator forces the injected dose to be reduced. The injected dose is generally reduced by 60% to 80% from that of a dedicated PET that uses thousands of individual BGO scintillation detectors. The reduced dose decreases image quality.

Dedicated PET Camera with BGO Detector Rings (Class c)

The most sensitive camera with the highest image quality is the dedicated PET camera with BGO detector rings, but it is also the most expensive. Unlike the PET cameras discussed, which are based on the gamma camera technology using a single, large NaI(Tl) detector, the BGO camera uses tens of thousands of small, discrete BGO detectors [10,11]. The discrete BGO detectors are packed into many detector rings surrounding the patient. The multiplicity of detectors in this camera type allows the cameras to operate at much higher count-rates (3–6×), which translates to a higher injected dose to provide a higher quality image. Furthermore, BGO has a twofold higher density and

higher atomic number than NaI(Tl), and it has significantly higher detection sensitivity for the higher-energy gamma ray emitted by positron tracers. Hence, the detected counts per unit injected dose are also higher with the dedicated PET/BGO than with the other three camera types using NaI(Tl) detectors, which enables the camera to provide a further improvement in image quality. Practical resolution and image quality are highest with this camera type. Generally, the highest intrinsic spatial resolution of this camera type is 4.2 to 4.5 mm for human imaging, although an experimental PET has recently achieved 2.8 mm resolution [11,12]. The practical image resolution is lower depending on the number of counts collected. Under optimal conditions, the practical image resolution may achieve 6 mm. For human whole-body imaging, the image resolution will be lower because of severe gamma-ray attenuation by the body. With this camera type, smaller structures or lesions (6–10) mm are detectable.

Quantitation and Parametric Imaging

An advantage of PET imaging is that the tracer kinetics and uptake can be accurately quantified from the image data because of its accurate attenuation-correction capability, which is not possible in SPECT. With tracer-transport modeling and multiple scans over a time period (dynamic imaging), functional parameters can be quantified. Some current physiological parameters generated by PET include blood flow [13–15], metabolic rate [16], blood volume [17,18], and receptor densities. These quantified parameters are more useful than a tracer uptake image. A region with high tracer uptake may be either an area of high-blood volume/perfusion, especially if the images are taken right after injection, or an area of high metabolism; quantified parametric images of metabolic rate and blood space would differentiate this ambiguity. Quantitation can be carried out in two ways, depending on the complexity of the tracer transport model and the noise in the image data:

1. If the transport model is complex involving many parameters and if the image data is noisy, it is better to draw a region of interest in

the image data, and compute the average functional parameters within the region.

2. If the model is simple (1–2 parameters) and the image quality is high, it may be more useful to generate a parametric image set that is equivalent to perform a region-of-interest (ROI) parametric calculation on a pixel-by-pixel basis for the whole image set.

Quantitation is especially important for accurately monitoring the efficacy of therapy if a baseline quantitation is performed before the treatment.

Tracer modeling and parametric quantitation techniques for ^{18}F-deoxyglucose (FDG), ^{15}O-water, and ^{13}N-ammonia have been studied and used extensively. FDG is currently the most useful tracer for detecting and studying cancer. Most FDG methods are based on the three compartment models (Figure 3.5) [19]. The physiological parameters to be deduced are the rate constants k_1^*, k_2^*, k_3^*, and k_4^*. One way to find the rate constants of a lesion is by drawing an ROI in the image set and extracting the time-activity data within the ROI. The ROI time-activity data are then combined with the time-activity data of the blood plasma tracer activity levels as input to a curve-fitting computer program for the three-compartment model. The curve-fitting program would output the rate constants [20]. This procedure generates the average rate constants in the ROI instead of a set of parametric images of the rate constants. Conceptually, the same method can be applied pixel by pixel to generate a set of parametric images of the rate constants. However, such an image processing procedure requires the image quality of the original uptake data to be very high so that the statistical errors for all the pixels are small. Furthermore, the curve-fitting time for all the image

pixels may be impracticably lengthy with the present computing technology.

A practical method of generating FDG metabolic images uses the unidirectional flow model [17,18], sometimes called the Patlak-plot method. This method is a three-compartment model with k_4 equal to zero. A negligible k_4 implies that that there is no leakage of the tracer from the trapped cell space. This simplifies the model from having four parameters (k_1^*, k_2^*, k_3^*, and k_4^*) to two parameters (K_i, V_d), where K_i is the macrometabolic rate constant and V_d is the blood distribution volume and vascular space. This method is computationally fast and less demanding on the quality of the raw image data. This simplified method still requires the measurement of the tracer input function or the blood time–activity curve. Generally, all parametric imaging methods require the measurement of the tracer input function.

A widely used semiquantitative parameter is the standard uptake value (SUV) or differential uptake ratio (DUR) [21,22], defined as

$$\text{SUV (DUR)} = [\text{tissue activity in } \mu\text{Ci/g}]/$$
$$[\text{injected dose in mCi/kg body weight}]$$

For FDG, the tissue activity used is generally the tracer uptake between 30 and 60 min. There is much variability in this measurement depending on the exact implementation in each clinical site. To minimize variability for comparison purposes, all the studies in this same site should follow the same quality control parameters such as the waiting time after injection, the duration of imaging, and fasting protocols. To further minimize variability, plasma glucose level correction [23,24] should also be applied:

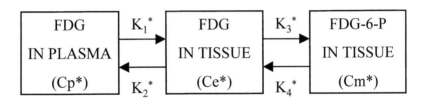

FIGURE 3.5. The three-compartment kinetic model of ^{18}F-deoxyglucose (FDG).

SUV (corrected)=SUV×[plasma glucose/100]

In addition, there should be a body fat correction term [22,25] to account for the reduced uptake of FDG in body fat. The SUV can be extracted either as the peak value in an ROI or displaying the SUV pixel by pixel as a pseudo-color-quantitation SUV image. The SUV quantitation is not as accurate as the three-compartment model or the unidirectional model, but it is very simple to implement and requires no blood sampling, which is more practical.

References

1. Anger HO. Radioisotope cameras. In: Hine GJ, ed. Instrumentation in Nuclear Medicine, Vol. 1. New York: Academic Press, 1967:485–552.
2. Budinger TF. Physical attributes of single-photon tomography. J Nucl Med 1980;21:579–592.
3. Croft BY. Single Photon Emission Computed Tomography. Chicago: Year Book, 1986.
4. Fowler JS, Wolf AP. Positron emitter-labeled compounds: priorities and problems. In: Phelps M, Mazziotta J, Schelbert H, eds. Positron Emission Tomography and Autoradiography: Principles and Applications for the Brain and Heart. New York: Raven Press, 1986:391–450.
5. Phelps ME, Mazziotta JC, Schelbert HR, eds. Positron Emission Tomography and Autoradiography: Principles and Applications for the Brain and Heart. New York: Raven Press, 1986.
6. Bracewell RN, Riddle AC. Inversion of fan-beam scans in radioastronomy. Astrophys J 1967;150:427–434.
7. Brooks RA, DiChiro G. Theory of image reconstruction in computed tomography. Radiology 1975;117:561–572.
8. Muehllehner M, Geagan P, Countryman P, et al. SPECT scanner with PET coincidence capability. J Nucl Med 1995;36(5):70.
9. Muehllehner G, Karp JS. A positron camera using position sensitive detectors: PENN-PET. J Nucl Med 1986;27:90–98.
10. Adam LE, Zaers J, Ostertag H, et al. Performance evaluation of the whole-body PET scanner ECAT EXACT HR+ following the IEC standard. IEEE Trans Nucl Sci 1997;44(3):1172–1179.
11. Wong W-H, Uribe J, Lu W, et al. Design of a Variable Field of View PET Camera. IEEE Transactions on Nuclear Science 1996;43(3):1915–1920.
12. Uribe J, Baghaei H, Li H, et al. Basic imaging performance characteristics of a variable field of view PET camera using quadrant sharing detector design. IEEE Trans Nucl Sci 1999;46(3):491–449.
13. Frackowiak RSJ, Lenzi G-L, Jones T, et al. Quantitative measurement of emission tomography: theory, procedure and normal values. J Comput Assist Tomogr 1980;4:727–736.
14. Huang S-C, Carson RE, Hoffman EJ, et al. Quantitative measurement of local cerebral blood flow in humans by positron computed tomography and ^{15}O-water. J Cereb Blood Flow Metab 1983;3:141–153.
15. Ruotsalainen U, Raitakari M, Nuutila P, et al. Quantitative blood flow measurement of skeletal muscle using oxygen-15-water and PET. J Nucl Med 1997;38(2):314–319.
16. Phelps ME, Huang SC, Hoffman EJ, et al. Tomographic measurements of local cerebral glucose metabolic rate in humans with [^{18}F]2-fluoro-2-deoxy-D-glucose: validation of method. Ann Neurol 1979;6:371–388.
17. Patlak C, Blasberg R, Fenstermacher J. Graphical evaluation of blood-to-brain transfer constants from multiple-time uptake data. J Cereb Blood Flow Metab 1983;3:1–7.
18. Gjedde A. Calculation of cerebral glucose phosphorylation from brain uptake of glucose analogs in vivo: a re-examination. Brain Res Rev 1982;4:237–274.
19. Sokoloff L, Reivich M, Kennedy C, et al. The (^{14}C)-deoxyglucose method for the measurement of local cerebral glucose utilization: theory, procedure and normal values in the conscious and anesthetized albino rat. J Neurochem 1977;28:897–916.
20. Carson RE. Parameter estimation in positron emission tomography. In: Phelps M, Mazziotta J, Schelbert H, eds. Positron Emission Tomography and Autoradiography: Principles and Applications for the Brain and Heart. New York: Raven Press, 1986:347–390.
21. Hanburg LM, Hunter GT, Alpert NM, et al. The dose uptake ratio as an index of glucose metabolism: useful parameter or over simplification? J Nucl Med 1994;35:1308–1312.
22. Zasadny KR, Wahl RL. Standardized uptake values of normal tissues at PET with 2-[fluorine-18-]-fluoro-2-deoxy-D-glucose: variations with body weight and a method for correction. Radiology 1993;189:847–850.

23. Lindholm P, Minn H, Leskinen-Kallio S, et al. Influence of the blood glucose concentration on FDG uptake in cancer—a PET study. J Nucl Med 1993;34:1–6.

24. Langen K-J, Braun U, Kops ER, et al. The influence of plasma glucose levels on fluorine-18-fluorodeoxyglucose uptake in bronchial carcinomas. J Nucl Med 1993;34:355–359.

25. Kim CK, Gupta NC, Chandramouli B, Alavi A. Standardized uptake values of FDG: body surface area correction is preferable to body weight correction. J Nucl Med 1994;35:164–167.

4
Principles of Magnetic Resonance Imaging and Magnetic Resonance Spectroscopy

Edward F. Jackson

The wide range of contrast that can be obtained using magnetic resonance imaging (MRI) has made it the modality of choice for the imaging of soft tissues. The mechanisms underlying the wide range of contrast depend on numerous intrinsic and extrinsic parameters. The inherent intrinsic parameters include, but are not limited to, proton density, spin-lattice (T_1) relaxation times, spin-spin (T_2) relaxation times, chemical environment, velocity, temperature, and the rate at which the protons diffuse. Extrinsic parameters, on the other hand, are those parameters that can be utilized to select which of the intrinsic parameters will be the primary contributor to image contrast. Such parameters include the choice of pulse sequence, the timing parameters for a given sequence, that is, the echo time (TE) and the repetition time (TR), various types of preparation pulses, and, for gradient-echo sequences, the flip angle. Other acquisition parameters, such as the slice thickness, acquisition matrix, field of view, and the type of radiofrequency coil used to acquire the signal, primarily affect the image resolution and signal-to-noise ratio. By appropriately choosing values for the extensive number of available extrinsic parameters, an incredibly wide range of image contrasts can be obtained and tailored to the need of assessing anatomy, pathophysiology, and, more recently, function. In addition, localized biochemical information can be obtained in a totally noninvasive manner using magnetic resonance spectroscopy (MRS) techniques. In this chapter, the underlying physical principles of MRI and MRS are briefly

reviewed, with particular interest paid to techniques that may be useful in targeted imaging studies in oncology. Given the short length of the chapter, the level of detail of the discussions is relatively superficial. For more detailed discussion of the basic principles and applications, the reader is referred to existing texts and review literature for MRI [1–7] and MRS [8–12].

Basic Principles and Applications of MRI

Signal Creation and Detection

To form a MR image, three basic requirements must be satisfied. First, the nuclei of interest must possess a nonzero nuclear magnetic moment. Such nuclei have an odd number of protons and/or neutrons and behave classically as if they were very small dipole magnets. In the absence of an applied magnetic field, the individual "magnetic dipoles" are randomly distributed and there is no net magnetization. When placed in a static magnetic field, spin-1/2 nuclei, such as protons, have two allowed energy levels: a lower energy level that occurs when the magnetic moment is parallel to the applied field, and a higher energy level that occurs when the magnetic moment is antiparallel to the applied field. The lower energy of the parallel state energy level results in a slight preferential alignment of the dipoles with the applied magnetic field, which gives rise to a net magnetization vector parallel to the applied field. It should be noted that the percentage of nuclear magnetic moments that are preferentially aligned with the applied field is quite small; for ^{1}H-MRI at an applied field of 1.5 tesla (T) and room temperature, the net excess of preferentially aligned dipoles accounts for only 10 of 1 million magnetic dipoles. Therefore, the inherent sensitivity of MRI is rather low, and it is not surprising that the proton, with the greatest in vivo natural abundance and MR sensitivity, is the primary nucleus of interest for MRI. It is the sole nucleus considered in the MRI sections of this chapter.

Thus far, the application of an external static magnetic field to a collection of nuclear spins with nonzero magnetic moments has resulted in a net magnetization that is parallel to the applied field. This *longitudinal* magnetization, however, is not what is detected. Instead, the longitudinal magnetization must be converted into *transverse* magnetization, perpendicular to the applied static field, before it can be detected. This conversion can be accomplished by the application of a time-varying magnetic field applied perpendicular to the applied static field and at a specific frequency known as the Larmor frequency, given by the expression $v_0 = \gamma B_0$, where γ is the gyromagnetic ratio, a constant for a given nucleus, and B_0 is the applied magnetic field strength. For protons at 1.5 T, this frequency is approximately 64 MHz and corresponds to the frequency necessary to induce transitions between the two allowed energy levels of the proton when placed in the applied static field. The time-varying radiofrequency field that induces the transitions is commonly noted as the B_1 field. By varying the amplitude or duration of the B_1 radiofrequency pulse, the longitudinal magnetization can be nutated to an arbitrary angle with respect to the applied static field. This angle is known as the *flip angle* and most commonly ranges between 20° and 180°. A 90° flip angle converts all available longitudinal magnetization into transverse magnetization, which is what ultimately gives rise to the detected signal. Immediately following such a 90° pulse, the transverse component of the magnetization begins to precess around the longitudinal

axis at the Larmor frequency. The resulting time-varying magnetic field gives rise to a time-varying voltage signal, known as the free induction decay (FID), in a properly tuned and oriented radiofrequency coil.

The transverse magnetization created by the B_1 field does not, of course, remain in the transverse plane indefinitely. After the B_1 pulse is terminated, two independent relaxation processes occur. The first, known as spin-lattice relaxation, describes the manner by which the transverse magnetization components recover to the equilibrium longitudinal magnetization established by the applied static field, B_0. The rate at which the recovery occurs is determined by the spin-lattice relaxation time, T_1. Fortunately, the T_1 relaxation times vary among tissue types, providing a highly useful means of generating image contrast. Simultaneous with the T_1 relaxation, spin-spin relaxation occurs. In addition to converting the longitudinal magnetization into transverse magnetization, the B_1 pulse causes the individual magnetic moments to precess coherently. When the pulse is terminated, however, spin-spin interactions cause the magnetic moments to dephase at a rate characterized by the spin-spin relaxation time, T_2. The T_2 relaxation times also vary with tissue type, providing another useful means of generating image contrast. It should be noted that the T_1 relaxation times are field strength dependent whereas the T_2 relaxation times are nearly independent of the applied field strength. The increasing T_1 relaxation time with field strength dependence is important when designing imaging protocols at different field strengths if similar image contrasts are required. (The signal-to-noise ratio of the MR signal and the chemical shift also increase with increasing field strength.) Although tables of the relaxation times exist [13], some general trends can be summarized as follows. In general, at 1.5 T the T_1 relaxation times vary from approximately 250 to 3000 ms, with lipid protons having the shortest relaxation times and pure fluids such as cerebrospinal fluid and vitreous humor having the longest relaxation times. The T_2 relaxation times range from approximately 30 ms (muscle) to 2000 ms (cerebrospinal fluid and vitreous humor). The T_2 relaxation time for any tissue is always less than the corresponding T_1 relaxation time.

Spin-spin relaxation ultimately yields dephasing of the measured signal, but does give rise to a clinically useful image contrast mechanism. Unfortunately, other processes can also cause dephasing of the transverse magnetization and, uncorrected, yield a loss of signal to noise in the resulting images. With the exception of applications to perfusion imaging and other susceptibility mapping techniques (discussed later), such dephasing phenomena are detrimental in MRI. The most common source of such increased dephasing is local magnetic field inhomogeneities caused by poor static magnetic field homogeneity or, much more commonly, by magnetic susceptibility variations at the interfaces between tissues. Such susceptibility variations, most evident at tissue–air or tissue–bone interfaces, give rise to apparent inhomogeneity of the applied static field and cause a decrease in the "apparent T_2", or T_2^*, relaxation time. The larger the apparent inhomogeneity, the smaller the value of T_2^* and the more rapidly the transverse magnetization dephases. In routine clinical imaging, such effects are clearly detrimental. Fortunately, these effects can be minimized by using *spin-echo* imaging techniques. The spin-echo signal, which occurs at the echo time, TE, is created by the combination of 90° and 180° pulses, separated by a period given by TE/2. During the first TE/2 period between the 90° and 180° pulses, the FID created by the 90° pulse decays at a rate determined by T_2^*. The 180° pulse inverts the phase at TE/2, resulting in a rephasing of the transverse magnetization at TE. The spin-echo signal thus obtained compensates for the effects of local field inhomogeneities, but maintains the useful contrast resulting from the non-reversible, that is, true, T_2 spin-spin dephasing.

Spatial Localization

Thus far, the application of the static magnetic field, B_0, and time-varying field, B_1, has resulted in a measurable MR signal. However, as yet the signal is not localized in space. To encode spatial information, three additional spatially varying, or gradient, magnetic fields are utilized. The three gradient fields are mutually perpendicular such that the z-component of the magnetic field increases in either the x-, y-, or z-direction, depending on which coil is producing the field. In classical two-dimensional spin-echo imaging experiments, one gradient is used to select a slice. This slice selection is accomplished with the simultaneous application of a radiofrequency pulse of bandwidth Δv_{rf} and a magnetic field gradient pulse of amplitude G_r, where r can represent the x-, y-, or z-direction. The thickness of the selected slice is then given by $\Delta v_{rf}/(\gamma G_r)$. In practice, it is the amplitude of the gradient pulse, not the bandwidth of the B_1 pulse, that is commonly used to select the slice thickness.

To spatially encode the measured MR signals in the remaining two dimensions, two additional gradient fields are utilized. The first is a frequency-encoding gradient that is applied at the same time the echo is detected. If this encoding is performed using the x-gradient, for example, then the effect is to modify the Larmor equation such that $v_{freq} = \gamma(B_0 + x\ G_x)$. Therefore, the frequency-encoding gradient creates a one-to-one correspondence between the frequency and spatial position, that is, positional information is encoded as frequency information. Therefore, if we can determine the precessional frequencies of the nuclear spins, we can determine their position. Taking the Fourier transform of the detected signal accomplishes this task.

The spatial information in the third direction is encoded using a phase-encoding gradient pulse that is typically placed immediately following the slice selective B_1 pulse. The phase-encoding gradient creates a one-to-one correspondence between the phase of the detected signal and the position in the phase-encoding direction. Typically, the phase-encoding gradient is applied 128 to 256 times, once per TR interval in conventional spin-echo imaging. At each repetition of the phase-encoding gradient, its amplitude is changed by a fixed amount. Therefore, each detected echo will have slightly different phase information that is directly related to the spatial location of the nuclear spins contributing to the MR signal. If the phase information can be extracted from the

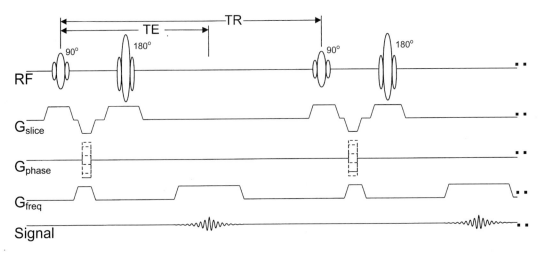

FIGURE 4.1. Generic spin-echo pulse sequence timing diagram. RF, applied B_1 radiofrequency pulses; G_{slice}, slice-selection gradient; G_{phase}, phase-encoding gradient; G_{freq}, frequency-encoding gradient; Signal, detected spin echo; TE, echo time; TR, repetition time.

measured echoes, then the spatial distribution of the spins can be completely defined in the second in-plane direction. This phase information is extracted using a second Fourier transform. A generic pulse sequence for a spin-echo image acquisition (Figure 4.1) shows the slice selective, frequency-encoding, and phase-encoding gradients, as well as the TE and TR intervals.

Basic MR Image Contrast Mechanisms

As mentioned, a large number of intrinsic parameters can be made to affect the image contrast by the appropriate choices of extrinsic parameters, such as the values of TE and TR. Historically, the most widely utilized types of image contrast have been provided by intertissue differences in proton density, T_1-relaxation times, and/or T_2-relaxation times. When using a conventional spin-echo acquisition technique, the values of TE and TR are the primary determinants. If TE is short, minimal dephasing of the signal from spin-spin (T_2) interactions will occur, and T_2 effects will not play a dominant role in the image contrast. If TR is long, the transverse magnetization from all tissues will significantly recover to the equilibrium values, and the image contrast will not be significantly affected by T_1 effects. Therefore, if an image is acquired with long values of TR and short values of TE, T_1 and T_2 effects are both minimized and the image will be proton density-weighted. If TE is long and TR is long, T_1 effects are minimized while T_2 effects are emphasized; the resulting image is T_2-weighted. Finally, if TE is short (minimizing T_2 effects) and TR is short (emphasizing T_1 effects), the resulting image contrast is T_1-weighted. In general, nonproteinaceous fluids are dark on T_1-weighted images (long T_1 relaxation times), but bright on T_2-weighted images (long T_2 relaxation times). Lipids, on the other hand, are bright on T_1-weighted images (short T_1 relaxation times) and intermediate on T_2-weighted images (intermediate T_2 relaxation times). Expected signal intensities of other common tissues relative to normal brain cortex on T_1-, T_2-, and proton density-weighted images in neuroimaging are given in Table 4.1, and illustrate the wide range of contrast available in MRI even using these relative simple types of image weightings.

Paramagnetic Contrast Agents

The initial, and still most widely utilized, MR contrast agents are all based on the paramagnetic gadolinium (Gd) atom. As gadolinium is

TABLE 4.1. Appearance of various substances relative to brain cortex on T_1-weighted (T1W), T_2-weighted (T2W), and proton density-weighted (PDW) spin-echo images.

Substance	T1W	T2W	PDW
Fat and yellow marrow	+++	+	++
Proteinaceous material	++ (Variable)	Variable	Variable
Intracellular methemoglobin	+++	–	–
Extracellular methemoglobin	+++	++	++
Deoxyhemoglobin	–	—	–
Hemosiderin	—	—	—
Melanin	++	–	Isointense
Calcium (some states)	+/–	–	–
Paramagnetic contrast agent	+++	Minimal effect	Minimal effect
Cyst	–	+++	++
Edema	–	+++	++
Vitreous humor	—	++	Isointense
Cerebrospinal fluid	—	+++	Isointense
Multiple sclerosis plaques	–	++	++
Tumors (most)	–	+ (Complex)	+ (Complex)
Abscess	–	+ (Complex)	+ (Complex)
Infarct	–	++	++
Iron (e.g., in globus pallidus)	—	—	—
Air	No signal	No signal	No signal
Cortical bone	No signal	No signal	No signal

toxic, it is tightly chelated to a readily eliminated agent, such as DTPA (diethylenetriaminepentaacetic acid), to prevent dissociation of the Gd. The three most commonly used Gd-based contrast agents differ only in the chelating agents; two are nonionic and one is ionic. The mean molecular weight of each of the three common contrast agents is about 550 Da, and the osmolality of each agent is fairly similar and much less than that of common radiopaque X-ray imaging contrast agents. Given the molecular weight of the agents, none of them cross an intact blood–brain barrier, but all can cross the endothelial cells of tissues outside the central nervous system. Paramagnetic substances, in close proximity to the free water protons that contribute signal to the MR image, cause a shortening of both the T_1 and T_2 relaxation times. The magnitude of the decrease in relaxation times depends upon the Gd concentration and the spin-lattice and spin-spin relaxivities, R_1 and R_2, respectively:

$$\frac{1}{T_1}=\frac{1}{T_{1,0}}+R_1[Gd] \quad \text{and} \quad \frac{1}{T_2}=\frac{1}{T_{2,0}}+R_2[Gd]$$

where $T_{1,0}$ and $T_{2,0}$ are the spin-lattice and spin-spin relaxation times in the absence of gadolinium, and [Gd] is the gadolinium concentration. The relaxivities vary with the chemical structure, and hence spatial density of Gd atoms, of the particular contrast agent. For the three commonly used Gd-based contrast agents, R_1 is about $4.5\,mM^{-1}s^{-1}$ and R_2 is about $5.5\,mM^{-1}s^{-1}$. The effects of increasing Gd concentration on the T_1 and T_2 relaxation times for gray matter (where the $T_{1,0}$ and $T_{2,0}$ are assumed to be 1055 ms and 68 ms, respectively) are shown in Figure 4.2, where it is readily appreciated that the primary effect is a decrease in the T_1 relaxation time. Therefore, at the recommended clinical dose level of 0.1 mmol/kg, the Gd-based contrast agents cause a preferential decrease in T_1 and hence an increase in signal intensity on T_1-weighted images in regions where the contrast agent accumulates. The increase in T_1-based tissue contrast with the administration of Gd contrast agents can be quite dramatic (Figure 4.3), and has proved extremely useful in oncological imaging. The minor contrast agent-induced decrease in T_2 relaxation times is

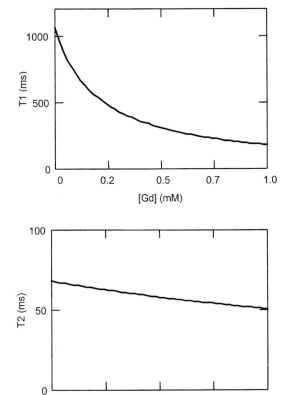

usually of minimal consequence for routine MR imaging. (It is useful, however, in bolus contrast agent dynamic susceptibility techniques for blood volume mapping, as discussed later.)

Not all MR contrast agents are Gd based. Some are based on other paramagnetic, superparamagnetic, or ferromagnetic materials. Several of the various agents approved for clinical use, or in clinical trials, are reviewed in the recent literature [see, for example, issues 7(1) and 10(3) of the *Journal of Magnetic Resonance Imaging*]. Undoubtedly, the development of more highly specific contrast agents using, for example, Gd bound to monoclonal antibodies or other targeted delivery systems, will have a tremendous impact in oncological imaging using MRI. Some of these agents are discussed in detail in Chapter 12.

For many years, pre- and postcontrast agent enhanced T_1-, T_2-, and proton density-weighted images formed the standard MR imaging protocol for oncological imaging, and examples of some of these types of images are the case of a patient with an anaplastic astrocytoma (Figure 4.4) and the case of a patient with invasive rectal carcinoma (Figure 4.5).

FIGURE 4.2. Effect on Gd-DTPA concentration on T_1 (*top*) and T_2 (*bottom*) relaxation times for gray matter tissue, with relaxation times in the absence of Gd-DTPA assumed to be $T_{1,0} = 1065$ ms and $T_{2,0} = 68$ ms.

Preparation Pulses

In addition to the extrinsic parameters TE and TR, a variety of "magnetization preparation"

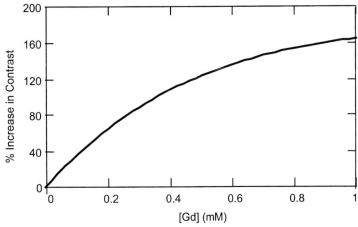

FIGURE 4.3. Percent increase in contrast of gray matter in the absence of Gd-DTPA versus gray matter in the presence of Gd-DTPA as a function of Gd-DTPA concentration for a spin-echo sequence with TR = 400 ms and TE = 18 ms.

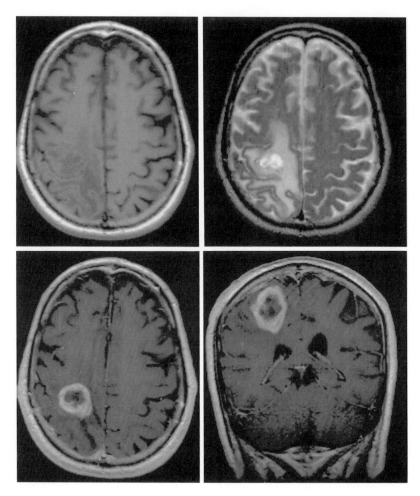

FIGURE 4.4. Spin-echo images from a patient with an anaplastic astrocytoma. *Top left*: T₁-weighted axial image before administration of Gd-DTPA. *Top right*: T₂-weighted image. *Bottom left*: T₁-weighted axial image following administration of Gd-DTPA. *Bottom right*: T₁-weighted coronal image following administration of Gd-DTPA.

pulses can be used to strongly influence image contrast [1,2,4]. There are four very common preparation pulse techniques. In the first, a bandwidth-limited RF pulse and gradient pulse combination is utilized to selectively saturate, that is, apply a 90° pulse to, a given spatial range of protons. If the protons that have experienced such a 90° pulse are then subjected to a spin-echo (SE) imaging sequence, the magnetization from the selectively saturated protons will be in the longitudinal direction at TE (90° saturation plus 90° slice selection plus 180° spin-echo pulse) and, as a result, will not be detected. Such "spatial saturation" pulses are commonly used

to null the signal from certain regions of the patient. For example, spatial saturation techniques are commonly used to suppress the signal from blood flowing through a given imaging plane to eliminate flow-related artifacts. The second common type of preparation pulse technique involves the use of frequency-selective RF pulses. These pulses apply a 90° pulse to a given range of resonant frequencies. Because water and fat protons resonate at different frequencies (~215 Hz separation at 1.5 T), such pulses can be used to selectively saturate either the water or, much more commonly, fat protons. If this selective 90° pulse is applied

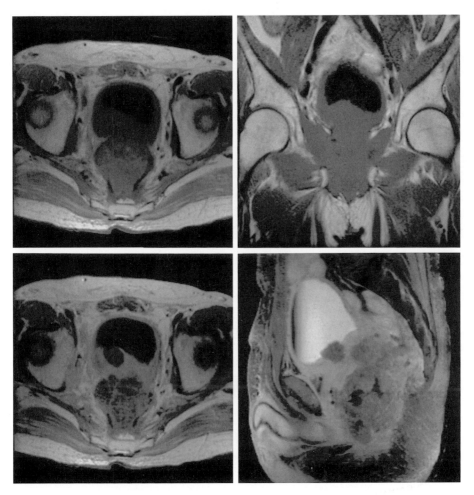

FIGURE 4.5. Spin-echo images from a patient with invasive rectal carcinoma. *Top left*: T_1-weighted axial image before administration of Gd-DTPA. *Top right*: T_1-weighted coronal image before administration of Gd-DTPA. *Bottom left*: T_1-weighted axial image following administration of Gd-DTPA. *Bottom right*: T_2-weighted fast spin-echo sagittal image.

to the fat protons before a SE sequence is applied, the magnetization from the fat protons will be in the longitudinal direction at the echo time and, therefore, will not be detected. Such pulses are based on the chemically selective suppression, or CHESS, pulses proposed by Haase et al. [14], and are commonly known as chem-sat or fat-sat pulses. An example of fat suppression using such frequency selective saturation techniques is given in Figure 4.6. The fourth commonly utilized class of magnetization preparation pulses, known as inversion pulses, are 180° pulses applied at a given time interval, the inversion time (TI), before a SE sequence. These pulses are neither frequency nor spatially selective but invert all protons within a given slice. The protons recover to the equilibrium longitudinal direction at a rate determined by their T_1 relaxation times. If the magnetization from a particular species of protons has recovered to the transverse plane at the end of the inversion time, the 90° and 180° SE sequence pulses leave this magnetization in the longitudinal direction and it will not be detected. Therefore, one of the common uses of inversion pulses is to selectively null the signal from certain tissues based on their T_1 relaxation times. Two commonly used inversion sequences

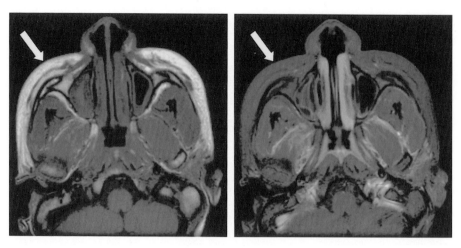

FIGURE 4.6. T_1-weighted axial spin-echo images without (*left*) and with (*right*) fat suppression (*arrows*).

are the short tau inversioΩn recovery (STIR) sequence, used to suppress the signal from fat protons, and the fluid attenuated inversion recovery (FLAIR) sequence, used to suppress the signal from "free fluids" such as cerebrospinal fluid and many cysts (Figure 4.7).

Faster Imaging Techniques

Although the spin-echo imaging sequence is still widely utilized in MRI, other sequences have been introduced with the primary goal of decreasing the image acquisition time. The first of these techniques is commonly known as the "gradient recalled echo" (GRE) sequence. In this sequence, the 180° spin-echo refocusing pulse is removed, allowing for decreasing the TE and TR times, thereby decreasing the scan time (with all other parameters constant). Furthermore, the longitudinal magnetization is partially maintained in the GRE sequence because of the use of a "partial flip angle" exci-

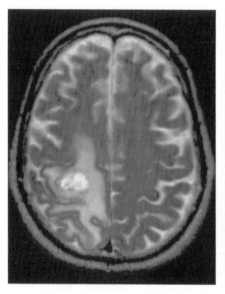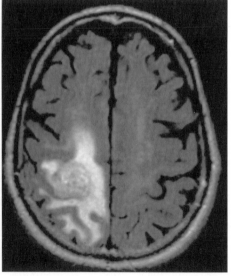

FIGURE 4.7. T_2-weighted fast spin-echo image (*left*) and fluid attenuated inversion recovery (FLAIR) image (*right*) of a patient with anaplastic astrocytoma.

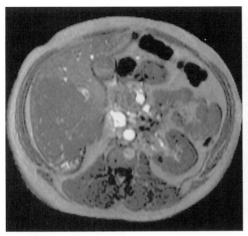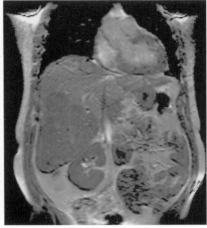

FIGURE 4.8. T_1-weighted breath-hold gradient-echo axial (*left*) and coronal (*right*) images from a patient with liver cancer.

tation pulse rather than the 90° pulse used in the SE sequence. With these modifications of the SE sequence, GRE sequences with very short TE and TR values (down to ~1.5 ms and ~8 ms, respectively, on state-of-the-art scanners) are possible. As the goal of such sequences is to decrease the acquisition times, the TR values are always made as low as practically possible given signal-to-noise and anatomical coverage requirements. Therefore, TR is not typically used as an extrinsic parameter to control the degree of T_1-weighted image contrast as it is in SE imaging. Instead the flip angle is the parameter used to control the amount of T_1-weighting obtained in a given GRE acquisition. Typical values range from 20° to 90°, with smaller flip angles providing minimal T_1-weighting and large flip angles providing increased T_1-weighting. As the 180° pulse is no longer used, images with increasing TE values have increasing amounts of T_2*-weighting as opposed to T_2-weighting obtained in SE imaging. Therefore, with TR fixed to a small value to decrease acquisition time, the combination of a small flip angle (10°–20°) and small value of TE (~2–8 ms) yields a proton density-weighted GRE image, the combination of a small flip angle (~10°–20°) and moderately large TE (~15–20 ms) yields a T_2*-weighted image, and the combination of a large flip angle (~60°–90°) and a small value of TE (~2–8 ms) yields a T_1-weighted image.

Gradient recalled echo sequences are widely used for obtaining (1) very rapid breath-hold T_1-weighted images (Figure 4.8), where motion artifacts limit the image quality of SE imaging; (2) high-resolution T_1-weighted "volume" scans (Figure 4.9), where comparable quality SE imaging times are prohibitive; and (3) magnetic resonance angiography images [15,16] (Figure 4.10), where the rapid imaging time and enhanced flow related enhancement

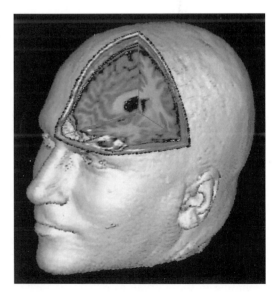

FIGURE 4.9. Three-dimensional shaded surface view of T_1-weighted fast gradient-echo volume scan data.

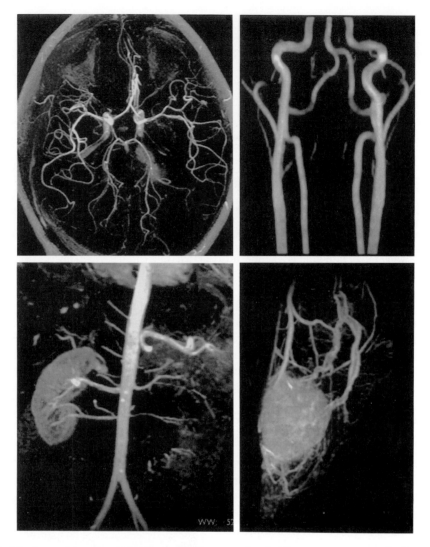

FIGURE 4.10. Maximum intensity projections of MR angiography. *Top left*: Three-dimensional (3-D) time-of-flight angiogram of the circle of Willis (without contrast agent). *Top right*: Two-dimensional (2-D) time-of-flight angiogram of the carotid and vertebral arteries (without contrast agent). *Bottom left*: 3-D contrast agent-enhanced renal angiogram. *Bottom right*: 3-D contrast agent-enhanced angiogram of the foot (giant cell tumor).

relative to the SE imaging sequences make the GRE sequence the technique of choice. A problem with obtaining T_2^*-weighted images with GRE sequences, however, is the often dramatic image signal loss in areas of magnetic field inhomogeneity (due to the rapid T_2^* signal dephasing in these areas, as discussed earlier). Often such areas of "signal void" are unwanted and have limited the use of GRE sequences for

acquiring rapid "T_2-like" images. However, there are certain cases in which such signal loss is advantageous. One example is in the detection of blood. If the blood products are paramagnetic, such as deoxyhemoglobin, or superparamagnetic, like hemosiderin, they give rise to dramatic decreases in T_2^* and result in areas of conspicuous signal loss on T_2^*-weighted images. Transient T_2^* signal losses also occur as a bolus of paramagnetic contrast agent passes through the microcirculation, and this is the basis of bolus contrast agent enhancement of dynamic susceptibility blood volume mapping, as discussed later.

Because the GRE sequences provided inadequate T_2-weighted image quality, other imaging sequences were developed to provide the necessary T_2-weighting without the relatively long acquisition times required when using the SE sequence. In the early 1990s, the fast spin-echo (FSE) technique, based on the rapid acquisition with relaxation enhancement (RARE) imaging sequence introduced by Hennig et al. [17], became a clinically viable means of obtaining high-quality T_2-weighted images in a fraction of the time required by comparable SE sequences. In this technique, numerous 180° pulses are applied each TR; the number of 180° pulses applied per TR is commonly known as the echo train length, or ETL. Each 180° pulse generates an echo, and each echo is uniquely phase encoded by applying separate phase-encoding gradient pulses for each echo. In this way, the image acquisition time can be decreased by up to a factor of ETL. Currently, FSE sequences are the technique most commonly used to acquire T_2-weighted images. However, there are some issues that must be considered when comparing the image quality of FSE with conventional SE imaging. First, fat is significantly brighter on FSE images relative to SE images with comparable TE and TR values, most probably because of the decreased diffusion effects and decreased J-coupling effects [18,19]. However, fat suppression techniques, such as chemical shift selective suppression pulses and short tau inversion recovery sequences (discussed earlier), can be used to suppress the fat signal as necessary. Second, when using FSE sequences to obtain short TE proton density- or T_1-weighted images, the resulting images may exhibit "T_2 blurring" in the phase-encoding direction, particularly for large values of ETL [20]. This phenomenon arises because each of the echoes in the echo train has a unique T_2 weighting, which has a detrimental effect on the point spread function, and hence resolution, as the ETL increases or TE decreases. Finally, for comparable values of TE and TR, FSE images have more T_2-weighting than SE images, again because the multiple echoes per TR have a range of T_2-weightings, not a single unique value.

In recent years, dramatic improvements in the gradient field subsystems of the MR system have allowed the commercial implementation of echo planar imaging (EPI) and spiral imaging sequences (see reviews [1,21]). Both these techniques provide the ability to obtain images extremely rapidly, for example, as fast as 30 to 300 ms per image. Such "snapshot" imaging techniques have allowed MR imaging to move from a means of providing exquisite anatomical images to a means of assessing tissue function and physiology.

Snapshot EPI imaging is similar to FSE imaging, but to the extreme. In a snapshot EPI scan, all the required phase-encoded echoes are acquired in a single TR. To obtain high-quality EPI scans, therefore, requires extremely fast gradient subsystems and the ability to acquire the necessary data in very rapid fashion, that is, high bandwidth receiver electronics. Although the spatial resolution and image quality of such scans are not nearly as good as those obtained using SE, GRE, or FSE sequences, the temporal resolution of the EPI scans is far superior. Today all major manufacturers of MR scanners offer EPI capabilities on their state-of-the-art scanners, providing a means for translating what have to date been basic research imaging capabilities to clinical applications.

Advanced MRI Techniques Based on High-Speed MR Imaging

As previously noted, the greatly improved gradient subsystems have allowed for the very rapid acquisition of MR images. This increase in temporal resolution has provided a means for pushing the state of the art in MR imaging from a modality capable of providing exquisite images of anatomy and pathology to a modality capable of providing a way to assess tissue function and physiology. Some of these more recent advances that may have a significant impact on oncological imaging are very briefly outlined next.

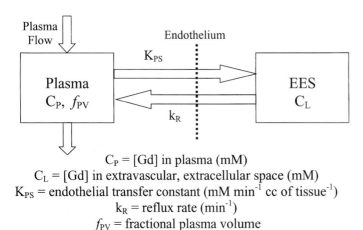

FIGURE 4.11. A two-compartment model used in the pharmacokinetic modeling of dynamic contrast agent-enhanced image data to obtain measures of fractional plasma volume and permeability-surface area product.

C_P = [Gd] in plasma (mM)
C_L = [Gd] in extravascular, extracellular space (mM)
K_{PS} = endothelial transfer constant (mM min^{-1} cc of tissue^{-1})
k_R = reflux rate (min^{-1})
f_{PV} = fractional plasma volume

Dynamic Contrast Agent-Enhanced MRI

Although the use of paramagnetic contrast agents has been common, particularly in oncological imaging, only static images have commonly been obtained and then qualitatively evaluated; that is, T_1-weighted images are acquired before and after the administration of the contrast agent and then visually compared. With improved temporal resolution, however, scans can be acquired before, during, and following the contrast agent infusion. Monitoring the kinetics of the contrast agent uptake by various lesions may then provide information that is useful in the differentiation of benign versus malignant lesions or treatment-related changes versus tumor progression. Several studies have suggested the advantages of such quantitative or semiquantitative dynamic studies in a variety of lesions, including, but not limited to, those in brain, breast, cervical, bladder, prostate, and musculoskeletal tissues [22–51]. If analyzed using pharmacokinetic models, such as the two-compartment model depicted in Figure 4.11, data from dynamic contrast agent-enhanced MRI study can provide noninvasive measures of blood volume fraction and permeability-surface area product. Each of these parameters may prove quite useful as surrogate markers for assessing the efficacy of antiangiogenesis drugs, in addition to providing information that may be useful in differential diagnosis of treatment related changes *vs* tumor progression. Examples of parametric maps of blood volume fraction and perme-

ability-surface area product are given in Figure 4.12.

Bolus Contrast Agent Dynamic Susceptibility Studies

As mentioned, a bolus of paramagnetic contrast agent passing through the microvasculature producing intravoxel susceptibility effects (decreased T_2^* relaxation times; more rapid dephasing of transverse magnetization) causes a transient decrease in signal intensity in nearby tissues. In Figure 4.13, the area under the signal intensity–time curve is proportional to the local blood volume. Therefore, this dynamic susceptibility technique provides a means of mapping regional blood volume (rBV) [52–55]. Furthermore, if the mean transit time (MTT) of the blood can be computed from the first pass data, the regional blood flow (rBF) can be computed from the central volume theorem, rBF=rBV/MTT. Note that this approach assumes that the contrast agent remains intravascular, and if relatively rapid leakage of the agent occurs, two effects detrimental to rBV mapping accuracy result. First, the dynamic susceptibility effects are weakened (less intravoxel dephasing), and second, the signal intensity may partially increase as a result of the shortened T_1 relaxation times secondary to the contrast agent leakage into the extravascular space. Both these effects cause an underestimation of the blood volume. Therefore, most dynamic susceptibility blood volume mapping studies have been performed in the

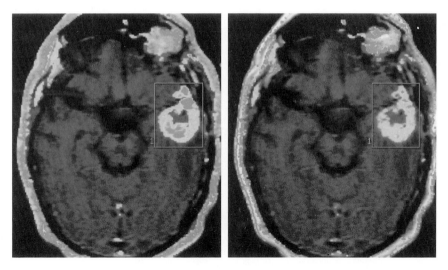

FIGURE 4.12. Pharmacokinetic model results in a patient with recurrent astrocytoma. *Left*: Fractional plasma volume map. *Right*: Permeability-surface area product map.

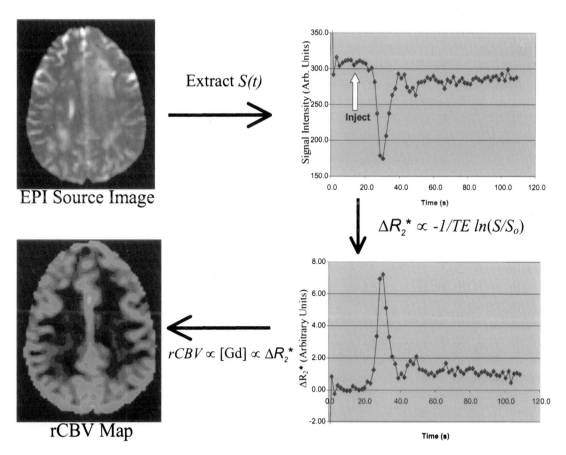

FIGURE 4.13. Process used in the generation of regional cerebral blood volume maps from T_2^*-weighed dynamic susceptibility EPI source data. $S(t)$, signal intensity as a function of time from a chosen region of interest; S_0, signal intensity from the region of interest before infusion of contrast agent; $rCBV$, regional cerebral blood volume; R_2^*, apparent T_2 relaxation rate; [Gd], gadolinium concentration.

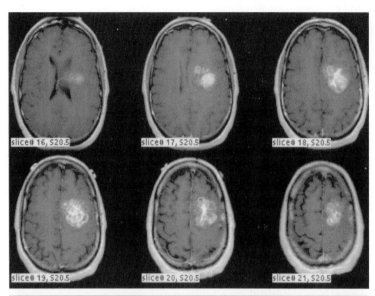

FIGURE 4.14. Spin-echo T_1-weighted axial images following contrast agent infusion (*top*) and regional cerebral blood volume maps (*bottom*) from a patient with glioblastoma multiforme.

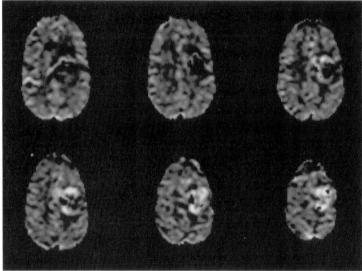

brain where the presence of the blood–brain barrier typically results in no to minimal leakage of the contrast agent, except in lesions associated with highly fenestrated blood–brain barriers. In the future, higher molecular weight contrast agents, which remain in the vascular system for a longer duration, should play an important role in the expansion of these techniques.

Several studies have demonstrated the utility of this technique in the assessment of brain tumors [54,56–60], and an example of a rBV map in a patient with glioblastoma multiforme is given in Figure 4.14.

Diffusion Imaging

Ultrafast imaging techniques have also provided a means of generating images in which the pixel intensity is proportional to the rate of random, Brownian motion of the water protons [54,61–63]. Thus far, the primary application of diffusion imaging has been in the central nervous system where diffusion is anisotropic;

that is, water protons diffuse along the myeli-
nated white matter tracts much more easily
than across them [64]. This anisotropy is both
disadvantageous and advantageous. If one is
solely interested in obtaining an image of the
"apparent" diffusion coefficient without regard
to direction, then the anisotropy is somewhat of
a hindrance because diffusion-weighted images
must be obtained with diffusion-sensitizing
gradient pulses applied in all three directions
and then combined appropriately to remove
the directional dependence. Otherwise, image
intensity variations from normal white matter
tract diffusion anisotropy may be indistinguishable from variations caused by pathology. Such

"averaged" images (more technically, diffusion
tensor trace images) are often used in the evaluation of patients with symptoms of acute
stroke as diffusion imaging has been shown
to detect ischemic injury much earlier than
T_1-, T_2-, or proton density-weighted imaging
[54,65,66]. On the other hand, the anisotropic
nature of diffusion in the white matter allows
for exquisite visualization of the white matter
tracts in the brain [54,67–70] and how the tracts
are displaced or destroyed by lesions (Figure
4.15). Finally, quantitative diffusion imaging, by
providing a means of noninvasively measuring
the degree of cellularity [71], may prove useful
in the characterization of lesions.

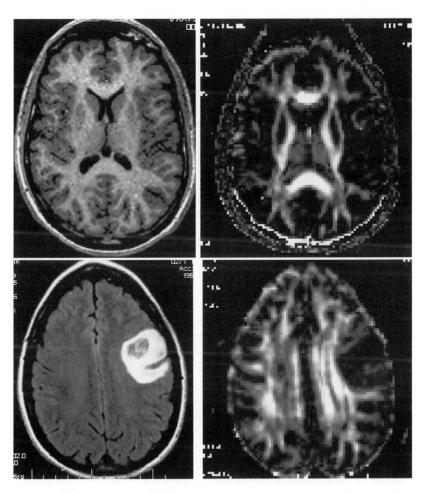

FIGURE 4.15. *Top*: T_1-weighted axial (*left*) and diffusion MR tractogram (*right*) in normal brain. *Bottom*:
Fluid attenuated inversion recovery (FLAIR) image
(*left*) and diffusion MR tractogram (*right*) in a
glioma patient. The distortion of the normal white
matter tracts is clear in the tractogram.

Basic Principles of Magnetic Resonance Spectroscopy

While recent advances in MRI have allowed for new methods of probing tissue function and physiology, magnetic resonance spectroscopy (MRS) offers a means of obtaining noninvasive biochemical information from normal and diseased tissues. Because one of the primary applications of the nuclear magnetic resonance phenomenon has been the determination of chemical structure based on MR spectra, it is not surprising that investigators began developing and implementing in vivo spectroscopy techniques in parallel with imaging techniques in the mid-1980s. However, clinical MRS applications have lagged significantly behind MRI applications. Nevertheless, the tantalizing ability to obtain information akin to a "noninvasive biopsy" has continued to drive MRS research and the goal of transitioning MRS from the research laboratories to the clinic.

Many of the important physical principles discussed in regard to MRI are also important in regard to MRS. For example, any nucleus with nonzero spin can theoretically be utilized for MRS studies, just as any nonzero spin nucleus can theoretically be used for MRI studies. For in vivo applications, however, only a few nuclei are readily studied, with the most common two being proton and phosphorus nuclei. Although each of these nuclei has its own advantages and disadvantages for in vivo studies, the basic physical principles forming the foundation of the MRS examination is the same.

Recall that following the application of a 90° pulse the excited protons precess in the transverse plane at the Larmor frequency given by $\nu = \gamma\, B_{nucleus}$, where γ is the gyromagnetic ratio and $B_{nucleus}$ is the magnetic field at the nucleus, which is the applied magnetic field B_0 modified by the local chemical environment. Therefore, nuclei in differing chemical environments have slightly different resonant frequencies depending on the amount of local nuclear shielding [72]. If the nuclear shielding constant is given by σ, then the modified resonant frequency is $\nu = \gamma\, B_0\, (1 - \sigma)$. Therefore, the local shielding effect, which arises from the electron configuration at the nucleus of interest, results in spectra with multiple peaks for a given nuclear species where the peak positions depend upon the local chemical environment. The position of a given spectral peak is usually given in terms of its *chemical shift*, δ, with respect to a reference peak. For in vivo applications, the reference peak is commonly chosen to be the water resonance in ^1H spectroscopic studies and the phosphocreatine resonance in ^{31}P studies of those tissues that have a detectable amount of this high-energy substrate, for example, muscle. As the separation between the peaks in a given spectrum increases linearly with the strength of the static magnetic field, the chemical shifts of the spectral peaks in direct frequency units normally require specifying the static field strength at which the spectrum was acquired, making comparison of spectra acquired at different field strengths difficult. To remove the field strength dependence of the chemical shifts of the spectral peaks, the shifts are most often reported in terms of a field strength independent parts-per-million (ppm) scale, as defined by

$$\delta = \frac{\nu_{peak} - \nu_{reference}}{\nu_{reference}}$$

where ν_{peak} and $\nu_{reference}$ are the resonance frequencies of the peak of interest and the reference peak, respectively.

Localization

A simple chemical spectrum from a sample, or patient, can be obtained by a one-dimensional Fourier transformation of the free-induction decay that follows a single 90° pulse. However, for in vivo spectral data to have any significance, the region from which the spectrum is obtained must be accurately known. Therefore, a localization technique must be utilized, and this should satisfy several basic criteria. First, it should be image based such that the volume of interest (VOI) from which the spectra are acquired can be selected on a standard MR image. Second, it should be possible to locate the VOI anywhere within the field of view of the image while retaining high-quality localization. Third, it should be possible to obtain a spectrum from the VOI in a single acquisition to facilitate optimization of the magnetic field homogeneity within the VOI by automated or interactive adjustment of the currents in the magnetic field correction coils or linear gradient coils. Finally, for patient safety and comfort the localization technique should deposit as little radiofrequency (RF) power as possible and should require minimal setup and acquisition times. The goal of maintaining short acquisition times is also critical to minimize the deleterious effects of voluntary or involuntary patient motion on the spectral quality. In addition to these general requirements, there are also some nucleus-specific requirements. For example, in ^{1}H-MRS studies it is necessary to have an efficient water suppression scheme to detect signals from metabolites of interest that typically have concentrations approximately 10,000 times less than the concentration of water. Several localization techniques have been used for in vivo MRS [10,73]. However,

given the length and nature of this chapter, only the techniques most commonly used for in vivo MRS studies are reviewed. Other techniques are reviewed in the general MRS references given earlier.

The most common localization techniques can be divided into two basic categories: single voxel (SV) and spectroscopic imaging (SI) techniques. In SV techniques, the spectral data are acquired from a single VOI at a time, typically by applying three orthogonal slice selective gradient/RF pulse combinations to define three slabs, with the intersection of the slabs defining the VOI (Figure 4.16a). On the other hand, SI techniques (Figure 4.16b) acquire spectra from a number of VOIs simultaneously [74,75]. A clear advantage of SV techniques is the ability to highly optimize the magnetic field homogeneity within the selected VOI. As the magnetic field homogeneity is improved, so is the spectral resolution and, in the case of ^{1}H-MRS, the degree of water suppression.

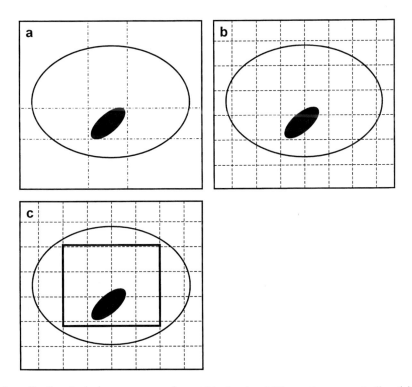

FIGURE 4.16. Localization techniques commonly used in in vivo MR spectroscopy studies. (**a**) Single voxel (SV) localization. (**b**) Two-dimensional spectroscopy imaging (SI) localization. (**c**) Hybrid SV–SI localization.

Single Voxel Localization Techniques

For ¹H-MRS studies, the most commonly used SV techniques are variants of the stimulated-echo acquisition mode (STEAM) sequence [76–78] and the point-resolved spectroscopy (PRESS) sequence [79]. Both these sequences have all the characteristics of ideal localization techniques outlined. For ³¹P-MRS studies, which require minimal T_2-weighting because of the short apparent T_2 relaxation times of the ATP resonances, the image-selected in vivo spectroscopy (ISIS) technique [80] has been commonly used, but this is not discussed further in this chapter.

STEAM Sequences

In the STEAM-based localization sequences, there are three orthogonal slice-selecting gradient/RF pulse combinations, each acting identically to the slice-selection pulses in a MR imaging sequence. The localized VOI is the intersection of the three orthogonal slices (see Figure 4.16a). The volume of the selected VOI can be set by adjustment of the individual slice thicknesses, and the position of the VOI can be set by appropriate selection of the offset frequencies of the three RF pulses.

Although the slice selective pulses do generate the desired signal from the VOI, it can be shown that the three RF pulses actually give rise to a maximum of five echoes [81]. However, in STEAM MRS, only one of the echoes is localized to the VOI, while the others arise from columns of spins rather than a well-defined three-dimensional VOI. To ensure that the unwanted echoes containing information from spins outside the VOI are not detected, "spoiler gradient" pulses are applied following each slice selective radiofrequency–gradient pulse. The spoilers destroy unwanted coherences that would otherwise arise from spins outside the VOI and degrade the localization and spectral quality [76,78,82]. In addition, eight or more signal averages are typically required to obtain adequate signal-to-noise ratio in the resulting spectra, and appropriate phase cycling of the radiofrequency pulses and receiver during data acquisition will further suppress the signal from outside the VOI [81].

The high quality of localization obtained with STEAM has made it one of the most frequently utilized SV techniques, despite the fact that only half the available signal from the VOI is obtained in the stimulated echo. (The remaining available signal is distributed among the other two-pulse and three-pulse echoes that are not localized completely in the VOI.) An example of a STEAM localized ¹H spectrum from normal human brain is given in Figure 4.17.

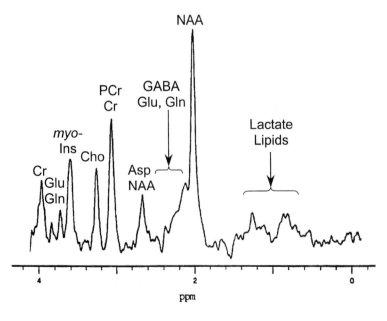

FIGURE 4.17. In vivo ¹H-MR spectrum from normal human white matter (TE=20 ms, TR=3000 ms). NAA, *N*-acetyl-aspartate; Cr, creatine; PCr, phosphocreatine; Cho, choline compounds; Glu, glutamate; Gln, glutamine; Ins, *myo*-inositol; *Asp*, aspartate; GABA, γ-aminobutyric acid.

PRESS Sequences

The PRESS-based localization sequences differ from the STEAM sequences primarily in that PRESS acquires a localized *spin* echo whereas STEAM acquires a localized *stimulated* echo. The primary advantage of PRESS compared to STEAM is the fact that all available signal from the localized VOI is detected in the form of the spin echo using PRESS, whereas only 50% of the available signal is detected in the form of the stimulated echo using STEAM. The primary disadvantage of PRESS relative to STEAM is the lengthened minimum echo time when using PRESS, which can be an important limitation if the metabolites of interest have short T_2 relaxation times. Also, due to the non-linearity of the spin system response to the radiofrequency pulses, it is more difficult to achieve well-defined slice profiles using 180° slice selective pulses compared to the 90° slice selective pulses used in the STEAM sequence. Recent "designer radiofrequency pulses" [83], however, have significantly improved 180° slice selective pulse profiles in PRESS sequences.

Spectroscopic Imaging Techniques

2D SI Localization

The 2D (two-dimensional) SI localization sequence first uses a slice-selection radiofrequency pulse–gradient combination to define the plane of interest. Localization within the plane is then accomplished using phase encoding, in a manner that is totally analogous to phase encoding in 2D MRI. With this technique, spectra from a number of contiguous VOIs are acquired simultaneously, allowing for the assessment of lesion heterogeneity and, where possible, comparing spectral findings in a lesion with those obtained from contralateral normal-appearing regions. Another advantage is in the acquisition of spectral data from small VOIs, which results from the phase-encoding localization of the VOIs as compared to the slice-selection localization of the VOI in STEAM or PRESS. Small voxels are obtained using SV techniques by increasing the amplitude of the slice-selection gradient pulse or by increasing the duration of the gradient–RF pulse combination. As increasing the length of the pulses comes at the cost of increased minimum echo time, the gradient pulse amplitude is usually increased instead. Large-amplitude, rapidly switched gradient fields, however, frequently yield significant eddy currents, and the time-varying magnetic fields induced by these eddy currents result in distortions of the ideal gradient fields. The eddy current fields can also be of long enough duration that they result in distortions in the FID or echo signals, and these distortions cannot be easily corrected. On the other hand, obtaining small voxel dimensions using phase-encoding techniques, like those utilized in SI, does not require such large gradient pulse amplitudes. Therefore, while the typical voxel volumes in SV localization are of the order of 1 to $10\,cm^3$, volumes of $0.125\,cm^3$ or less can be achieved using SI localization and $1\text{-}cm^3$ voxel volumes are fairly common.

Another primary advantage of SI techniques over SV techniques is the ability to reconstruct low-resolution images from the spectral data in which the pixel intensity is proportional to the relative concentrations of the metabolites of interest. Typically, the relative concentration in each voxel is determined by integrating the area under the peak of interest. Such metabolic maps, or "met-maps," are quite useful in visually assessing the spatial variation in the concentrations of the metabolites. However, their quality depends strongly on the accuracy of the integration of the peak areas, so care should be taken in selection of the limits of integration. In general, although the met-maps provide a quick means of assessing the spatial variations in concentration, the individual spectra should also be inspected.

Disadvantages of SI techniques relative to SV techniques include difficulty in optimizing the magnetic field over a large volume of tissue when using SI localization as opposed to a relatively small volume when using SV localization, typically long acquisition times, and the possibility of significant spectral bleed from one voxel to its neighbors [84–86]. The first of these disadvantages is typically the most significant because inadequate field homogeneity results in poor resolution of the spectral peaks and unacceptable water suppression. However, the long acquisition times, commonly 15 to 30 min for ^{1}H 2D SI studies, are also a significant problem because patient motion during the MRS acquisition will have a deleterious, and uncorrectable, effect on the quality of the spectra. With the recent advances in echo-planar imaging-compatible MR scanners, however, EPI-based SI [87] could dramatically decrease the imaging acquisition times and potentially eliminate this disadvantage relative to SV localization.

The spectral bleed artifacts are also important to consider when acquiring SI MRS data. The result of intervoxel spectral bleed is the contamination of the spectrum from a given voxel by the spectral components in neighboring voxels. This can be quite serious, for example, in ^{1}H-MRS studies of human brain, where large-amplitude lipid signals from the skull can contaminate voxels located within the brain parenchyma by spectral bleed. The false lipid peaks from the spectral bleed appear in the same chemical shift range as lactate and "true" lipid peaks and can give rise to misleading results. The origin of the spectral bleed phenomenon is the same as the truncation artifact in MRI; there is insufficient sampling of the k-space data in the phase-encoding directions. The effects are decreased as the number of phase-encoding steps increases, but at the cost of increased scan time and decreased voxel sizes. Fortunately, the effects can also be decreased during processing of the spectral data.

Hybrid SI–SV Methods

In an effort to maintain the advantages of both SI and SV localization methods, while decreasing the impact of the disadvantages of either method, a common approach to acquiring in vivo MRS data is to combine a SV sequence with a SI sequence (see Figure 4.16c). The SV technique is used to localize a relatively large, but well-localized VOI, and phase-encoding gradients are used to subdivide the large VOI into smaller voxels. The advantage of SI localization in obtaining spectra from multiple voxels is retained, while the use of the SV technique to preselect the large VOI greatly minimizes spectral bleed contamination from lipid

signals outside of the VOI. It also allows for improved magnetic field optimization, with the concomitant improvement in spectral resolution and water suppression. As an alternative to the use of an SV technique to preselect a VOI to minimize spectral bleed, multiple spatial saturation bands (discussed in the MRI section) can be used to saturate the lipid signals outside the true region of interest immediately before the application of the SI sequence. This method of "outer volume suppression" [88–91] allows tailoring the definition of the VOI that will subsequently be subdivided into SI-encoded voxels; that is, by using multiple spatial saturation bands applied at various angles, the lipid protons in the skull can be suppressed while allowing spectra to be acquired from nearly all the brain parenchyma.

Water Suppression Techniques

There are numerous techniques for accomplishing the water suppression required for ^{1}H-MRS [92]; however, the technique most commonly utilized for in vivo MRS is the application of multiple saturation pulses. These pulses are most commonly known as chemical shift selective (CHESS) pulses [14,93]. They are narrow bandwidth pulses (typically ~50 Hz) that selectively saturate the water resonance in ^{1}H-MRS studies, and the basic idea behind their mechanism of action is no different than discussed in regard to frequency-selective fat suppression techniques in MRI. If the water protons are saturated by these pulses, and the subsequent localization sequence results in the application of an odd number of multiples of 90° pulses to the water protons, the water proton magnetization is in the longitudinal direction during data acquisition and is not detected. However, the frequency-selective nature of the saturation pulses means that the magnetization due to protons with resonant frequencies that differ from the resonant frequency of water is minimally affected. The use of multiple (typically three) saturation pulses is necessary in the case of in vivo MRS to increase the degree of suppression of the water signal. With the appropriate flip angles of the CHESS pulses and associated spoiler gradient pulses to prevent unwanted stimulated echoes from forming after the suppression pulses are applied, water suppression factors of 1000 or greater can be obtained in vivo and are sufficient to allow spectral peaks from several metabolites of interest to be observed.

Spectral Quantification

Having acquired the localized time domain data and transformed it into spectral information, the decision now to be made is how to interpret the results. The most common approaches to spectral quantification are, in order of increasing complexity, (1) simple visual assessment of the spectral peaks, (2) computing the relative spectral peak heights, (3) computing the relative spectral peak areas, or (4) computing the absolute concentration of the metabolites based on the peak areas. Option 1 provides little information other than allowing for the assessment of the presence or absence of a particular metabolite, or a substantial decrease or increase in metabolite concentrations. Option 2 is more quantitative, but peak height measurements can be very misleading when comparing multiple spectra unless extreme care is taken. The difficulty lies in the fact that the peak height depends upon, among other things, the spin-spin relaxation time, which varies from metabolite to metabolite, and the field homogeneity, which typically varies from scan to scan (in SV and SI studies) and from voxel to voxel (even in a given SI study). This problem is minimized if the spectra are analyzed using option 3 because the peak areas for a given concentration (and acquisition parameters, TE and TR) are independent of the field homogeneity (so long as the resulting spectral resolution is adequate to allow the peaks to be resolved).

A problem with both peak height and peak area calculations, however, is that both these measures depends on many acquisition parameters, including the TE, TR, number of signal averages, and voxel size. Therefore, of all the options for spectral analysis, option 4 appears to be preferred because it results in actual concentration measurements for the metabolites of interest that are independent of the data acquisition parameters. It is, however, the most difficult option as some reference standard must be used to allow the calculation of the absolute concentrations. Investigators seeking to obtain absolute concentrations have typically used either an external standard [82,94–98], such as a vial of known concentration of a standard reagent in the field of view, or an internal standard [99–102], such as the assumed concentration of water in the tissue occupying the VOI. Both means of obtaining the "standard reference" are fraught with difficulties, and the relative strengths and weaknesses of both techniques have been recently reviewed [103].

A very common approach to quantification, which seeks to minimize the dependence of the peak areas or heights on data acquisition parameters, is to report ratios of peak areas or ratios of peak heights with respect to a chosen standard reference peak. However, care must be taken in interpreting the results as changes in peak area or height of either spectral peak used in the calculation will change the resulting ratio. Furthermore, there are regional variations in the concentrations of some metabolites whereas concentrations of other metabolites are relatively constant. This finding reinforces the need for interpreting peak area (or height) ratio values with care. Finally, it is important to remember that T_1 and T_2 relaxation times vary among the metabolites of interest. Therefore, when comparing peak areas, heights, or even ratios to values in the literature or from previously acquired spectra, it is imperative to remember that individual peak areas and heights change with the TE and TR values used during data acquisition. As a result, comparisons between spectra acquired with differing TE or TR times should be performed with caution, and the peak areas, heights, or ratios must be corrected using known T_1 and T_2 relaxation times of the various metabolites if the TE or TR times differed between acquisitions.

Regardless of the technique used to acquire the MRS data or the spectral processing and quantification methodologies used, the reproducibility of MRS results should be carefully validated. Such validation is particularly important if the studies involve longitudinal follow-up scans in a given disease state, or, for example, if the studies require the acquisition of spectra from "MRS-difficult" regions near sources of local magnetic field inhomogeneities, such as areas near the skull base. Because both acquisition and processing variations can strongly affect the quantitative results, reproducibility studies are important for a given site [86,104] or for multicenter trials [105].

Finally, in vivo MRS voxel sizes are typically rather large and contain a mixture of tissue types. For example, in an MRS exam of intracranial lesions a voxel may contain a mixture of lesion, white matter, gray matter, edema, and cerebrospinal fluid; this makes comparisons difficult if the relative concentrations of the metabolites are not corrected for the heterogeneous distribution of tissues within the voxel. Several investigators have sought to address this issue by utilizing automated or manual image segmentation techniques to determine the percentage of each tissue in a given voxel and then to correct the relative peak area ratios or heights based on these determinations [106–108].

Clinical Applications of In Vivo MRS

In vivo MRS has a rather long history, and several review articles and texts have discussed applications of MRS to a variety of normal and pathological conditions [8,10–12,109–118]. Restrictions on the length of this introductory chapter prevent a discussion of the variety of multinuclear MRS studies previously reported. Therefore, the applications presented are restricted to those that address ^{1}H-MRS studies, particularly more recent studies specific to oncology. Currently, ^{1}H-MRS in vivo studies are much more common than those involving other nuclei, and readers interested in studies involving nuclei other than ^{1}H are encouraged to utilize the references just given.

Central Nervous System Applications

The water-suppressed ^{1}H spectrum acquired from a normal human brain shown earlier in Figure 4.17 demonstrates several spectral peaks, or resonances. In general, resonances from *myo*-inositol, total creatine (creatine and phosphocreatine), choline, and N-acetylaspartate are clearly resolved in normal brain spectra acquired at 1.5 T, and other weaker resonances can also be observed.

The dominant peak at approximately 2.0 ppm in [1]H-MR spectra from normal brain results from N-acetylaspartate (NAA). Although the exact biochemical role of NAA has not been fully elucidated [119], it is present in abundance only in viable mature neurons, and has been widely used as an indicator of neuronal integrity. The concentration of NAA increases during the development of the normal neonate [120,121] and reaches approximately 8 to 12 mM in adults [82,98]. In general, most disease processes, including neoplasms [100,106,117,122–138], result in decreased levels of NAA. The spatial distributions of NAA and other metabolites have been investigated using both SV and SI techniques [96,98,107,108,131,139–142]. NAA, in particular, has been shown to vary depending on tissue type (white matter versus gray matter) and location within the cranium. Finally, it should be noted that the NAA peak also has contributions from N-acetylaspartylglutamate (NAAG) at about 2.05 ppm [11,116].

The next most prominent spectral peaks in the normal brain spectrum are from total creatine and choline-containing compounds. The total creatine peak at 3.0 ppm has components from creatine (Cr) and phosphocreatine (PCr). The choline (Cho) peak at 3.2 ppm has components from compounds associated with membrane synthesis and breakdown, such as phosphorylcholine and glycerophosphorylcholine. Elevated Cho levels have been reported in many neoplasms [106,122,124,127,129,131,133,134, 138,143–146]. The most probable explanation for the increase in Cho levels in focal and inflammatory processes is the production of Cho-containing breakdown products of myelin, but other possible mechanisms have not been fully investigated. Levels of Cr, typically present at about 10 mM in normal brain, have been shown to decrease in some neoplasms [106,122,127, 129,131,133,134,138,144,146] and in stroke [147–152].

Even though myelin is rich in lipids, the rigid structure makes the lipid "MRS invisible" in normal brain parenchyma. However, measurable lipid levels have been reported in certain disease states, such as some but not all neoplasms [90,106,122,127,144,153]. It is believed that the lipids and other macromolecules observed in these cases result from the release of MR-visible lipids and other membrane breakdown products when the normal rigid myelin structure is disrupted. The signals from the lipids and other membrane breakdown products are seen only at short echo times because of their relatively short spin-spin relaxation times and significant *J*-modulation. As extracranial lipid signals can contaminate the localized VOI because of poor localization quality or, in the case of SI techniques, spectral bleed, one must interpret such signals with care, particularly if the voxel showing significant lipid signals is near the skull.

Lactate is typically maintained at very low levels in normal brain (<0.5 mM) and is not detected using ^{1}H-MRS. However, in certain pathological conditions, such as some but not all neoplasms [106,124–126,129,131–135,144, 154–156] a doublet resonance from the methyl protons can be observed at 1.35 ppm. A potential difficulty with lactate detection, however, lies in the fact that the lactate methyl protons and the methylene lipid protons resonate at very similar frequencies and the peaks can overlap. Therefore, it can be difficult, if not impossible, to determine whether an elevation of lactate or an elevation of lipids is responsible for peaks around 1.3 ppm. One common technique used to distinguish lactate from lipids is to acquire spectra at appropriately chosen short and long echo times. The short echo time spectrum will provide information regarding the lipid *and* lactate levels, while a judicious choice of longer echo time (~135 ms for 1.5 T systems) will selectively invert the lactate doublet and greatly decrease the contribution of the lipid signals, which have short spin-spin relaxation times. A spectrum from a patient with a glioblastoma multiforme, demonstrating elevated lactate and choline levels, is given in Figure 4.18.

Other resonances from *myo*-inositol (3.58 ppm, with additional contributions from inositol monophosphates and glycine), glucose (3.43 and 3.80 ppm), γ-aminobutyric acid (GABA) and glutamate/glutamine (2.1–2.5 ppm), and alanine (doublet at 1.47 ppm) and other amino acids have also been reported [11,116]. Quantitation of peaks closer to the residual water peak than Cho have, until more recently, been exceedingly difficult because of insufficient water suppression. However, improvements in automated field homogeneity corrections and water-suppression optimization have made quantitative analysis of several

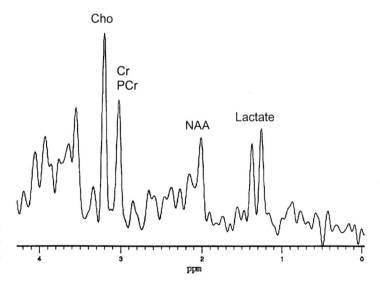

FIGURE 4.18. In vivo [1]H-MR spectrum from a patient with glioblastoma multiforme (abbreviations as defined in Figure 4.17).

peaks in this region possible. Biochemicals with spectral peaks in this region include *myo*-inositol, glucose, and additional signals from Cr and glutamate/glutamine [11]. Decreased *myo*-inositol levels have been reported in some neoplasms [11]. However, because of the large number of overlapping peaks in the glutamate/glutamine region of the spectrum, absolute quantitation is exceedingly difficult without sophisticated spectral editing techniques [157]. Similarly, spectral editing techniques are required for the detection of GABA [158–160].

In general, the most consistent findings of ¹H-MRS studies of intracranial neoplasms are that Cho levels are elevated, NAA levels are decreased, and Cr levels are decreased. Lactate and lipids and other membrane breakdown products may or may not be present.

Applications Outside the CNS

The ¹H spectra acquired from extracranial tissues exhibit relatively few quantifiable spectral peaks, and this has severely limited in vivo MRS applications outside the CNS. For example, the water-suppressed localized spectrum from human muscle tissue consists primarily of peaks from residual water (~4.7 ppm), Cho+carnosine (3.2 ppm), Cr+PCr (3.0 ppm), carnosine (~8 ppm), and lipids. The lipid spectrum itself is rather complex, with resonances due to the following protons: —CH_3 (~1.0 ppm), —CH_2—CH_2— (~1.4 ppm), —CH_2—CH=CH— (~2.1 ppm), and —CH=CH— (~5.5 ppm). Because the concentrations of water and lipids (~3.5 M in muscle and up to 60 M in adipose tissue and marrow) are quite large relative to the concentrations of other metabolites of interest, either the residual water peak or one or more of the lipid peaks typically masks resonances from other metabolites. Suppression of the lipid resonances using either frequency-selective saturation techniques or inversion recovery techniques usually results in suppression of the signal from many of the metabolites of interest as well. In oncological applications, some groups have attempted to use ¹H-MRS as a tool to monitor leukemia therapy by observing the lipid level variations

in the marrow and have reported that successful chemotherapy results in a reduction of the water-to-fat ratio in the marrow [161–163]. Lipid signals in bone tumors have also been characterized [164]. Another report summarized the effects of radiation therapy on normal muscle tissue of a single subject as being a dramatic decrease in Cho+carnitine and PCr+Cr levels [165]. Furthermore, in prostate cancer patients several groups have reported that the level of citrate, which is present in sufficient concentration in the prostate to be detected via in vivo ¹H-MRS (~70 mM concentration with a multiplet resonance at 2.6 ppm), allows the differentiation between neoplasm and benign prostate hyperplasia (BPH), with neoplasms demonstrating consistently lower citrate levels than BPH or normal peripheral zone tissue [166–170]. In general, however, applications of in vivo ¹H-MRS to oncology in anatomical sites outside the CNS have been quite limited.

Conclusion

This chapter has provided a brief introduction to the physical principles of magnetic resonance imaging and magnetic resonance spectroscopy and outlined some of the more recent developments that are poised to greatly advance the use of magnetic resonance in oncology. The use of these techniques, along with the development of more targeted contrast agents, should greatly advance our ability to noninvasively characterize lesions and evaluate the efficacy of current and novel oncological therapies.

References

1. Haacke EM, Brown RW, Thompson MR, Venkatesan R. Magnetic resonance imaging. Physical Principles and Sequence Design. New York: Wiley-Liss, 1999:914.
2. Jackson EF. Magnetic resonance imaging: physical principles to advanced applications. In: Kim EE, Jackson EF, eds. Molecular Imaging in Oncology. Berlin: Springer, 1999:17–45.
3. Sanders JA. Magnetic resonance imaging. In: Orrison WWJ, Lewine JD, Sanders JA,

Hartshorne MF, eds. Functional Brain Imaging. St. Louis: Mosby, 1995:145–186.

4. Elster AD. Questions and Answers in Magnetic Resonance Imaging. St Louis: Mosby, 1994.

5. Wehrli FW, Haacke EM. Principles of MR imaging. In: Potchen EJ, Haacke EM, Siebert JE, Gottschalk A, eds. Magnetic Resonance Angiography. St. Louis: Mosby, 1993:9–34.

6. Wehrli FW. Principles of magnetic resonance. In: Stark DD, Bradley WG, eds. Magnetic Resonance Imaging, Vol. 1. St. Louis: Mosby Year-Book, 1992:3–20.

7. Edelman RR, Kleefield J, Wentz KU, Atkinson DJ. Basic principles of magnetic resonance imaging. In: Edelman RR, Hesselink JR, eds. Clinical Magnetic Resonance Imaging. Philadelphia: Saunders, 1990:3–38.

8. Danielsen ER, Ross BD. Magnetic Resonance Spectroscopy Diagnosis of Neurological Diseases. New York: Dekker, 1999.

9. De Graaf RA. In Vivo NMR Spectroscopy: Principles and Techniques. New York: Wiley, 1999.

10. Jackson EF. Magnetic resonance spectroscopy: physical principles and applications. In: Kim EE, Jackson EF, eds. Molecular Imaging in Oncology. Berlin: Springer, 1999:47–70.

11. Ross B, Michaelis T. Clinical applications of magnetic resonance spectroscopy. Magn Reson Q 1994;10:191–247.

12. Cady EB. Clinical Magnetic Resonance Spectroscopy. New York: Plenum Press, 1990: 250–254.

13. Wood ML, Bronskill MJ, Mulkern RV, Santyr GE. Physical MR desktop data. J Magn Reson Imaging 1994;3S:19–26.

14. Haase A, Frahm J, Hänicke W, Matthei D. ^{1}H-NMR chemical shift selective (CHESS) imaging. Phys Med Biol 1985;30:341–344.

15. Potchen EJ, Haacke EM, Siebert JE, Gottschalk A. Magnetic Resonance Angiography. St. Louis: Mosby, 1993.

16. Prince MR, Grist TM, Debatin JF. 3D Contrast MR Angiography. New York: Springer-Verlag, 1997.

17. Hennig J, Nauerth A, Friedburg H. RARE imaging: a fast imaging method for clinical MR. Magn Reson Med 1986;3:823–833.

18. Constable RT, Anderson AW, Zhong J, Gore JC. Factors influencing contrast in fast spin-echo MR imaging. Magn Reson Imaging 1992; 10:497–511.

19. Henkelman RM, Hardy PA, Bishop JE, Poon CS, Plewes DB. Why fat is bright in RARE and fast spin-echo imaging. J Magn Reson Imaging 1992;2:533–540.

20. Constable RT, Gore JC. The loss of small objects in variable TE imaging: implications for FSE, RARE, and EPI. Magn Reson Med 1992; 28:9–24.

21. Cho ZH, Jones JP, Singh M. Foundations of Medical Imaging. New York: Wiley, 1993.

22. Barentsz JO, Engelbrecht M, Jager GJ, et al. Fast dynamic gadolinium-enhanced MR imaging of urinary bladder and prostate cancer. J Magn Reson Imaging 1999;10:295–304.

23. Hawighorst H, Libicher M, Knopp MV, Moehler T, Kauffmann GW, van Kaick G. Evaluation of angiogenesis and perfusion of bone marrow lesions: role of semiquantitative and quantitative dynamic MRI. J Magn Reson Imaging 1999;10:286–294.

24. Mayr NA, Hawighorst H, Yuh WTC, Essig M, Magnotta VA, Knopp MV. MR microcirculation assessment in cervical cancer: correlations with histomorphological tumor markers and clinical outcome. J Magn Reson Imaging 1999; 10:267–276.

25. Knopp MV, Weiss E, Sinn HP, et al. Pathophysiologic basis of contrast enhancement in breast tumors. J Magn Reson Imaging 1999;10:260–266.

26. Reddick WE, Taylor JS, Fletcher BD. Dynamic MR imaging (DEMRI) of microcirculation in bone sarcoma. J Magn Reson Imaging 1999; 10:277–285.

27. Wong ET, Jackson EF, Hess K, et al. Correlations between dynamic MRI and outcome in patients with malignant glioma. Neurology 1998;50:777–781.

28. Buckley DL, Drew PJ, Mussurakis S, Monson JRT, Horsman A. Microvessel density in invasive breast cancer assessed by dynamic Gd-DTPA enhanced MRI. J Magn Reson Imaging 1997;7:461–464.

29. Hazle JD, Jackson EF, Schomer DF, Leeds NE. Dynamic imaging of intracranial lesions using fast spin-echo imaging: differentiation of brain tumors and treatment effects. J Magn Reson Imaging 1997;7:1084–1093.

30. den Boer J, Hoenderop R, Smink J, et al. Pharmacokinetic analysis of Gd-DTPA enhancement in dynamic three-dimensional MRI of breast lesions. J Magn Reson Imaging 1997;7:702–715.

31. Griebel J, Mayr N, de Vries A, et al. Assessment of tumor microcirculation: a new role of

dynamic contrast MR imaging. J Magn Reson Imaging 1997;7:111–119.

32. Hawighorst H, Knapstein P, Weikel W, et al. Cervical carcinoma: comparison of standard and pharmacokinetic MR imaging. Radiology 1996;201:531–539.

33. Hawighorst H, Knapstein P, Schaeffer U, et al. Pelvic lesions in patients with treated cervical carcinoma: efficacy of pharmacokinetic analysis of dynamic MR images in distinguishing recurrent tumors from benign conditions. AJR 1996;166:401–408.

34. Buadu LD, Maurakami J, Murayama S, et al. Breast lesions: correlation of contrast medium enhancement patterns on MR images with histopathologic findings and tumor angiogenesis. Radiology 1996;200:639–649.

35. Mussurakis S, Buckley D, Bowsley S, et al. Dynamic contrast-enhanced magnetic resonance imaging of the breast combined with pharmacokinetic analysis of gadolinium-DTPA uptake in the diagnosis of local recurrence of early stage breast carcinoma. Invest Radiol 1995;30:650–662.

36. Hoffmann U, Brix G, Knopp M, Hess T, Lorenz WJ. Pharmacokinetic mapping of the breast: a new method for dynamic MR mammography. Magn Reson Med 1995;33:506–514.

37. Tofts PS, Berkowitz B, Schnall MD. Quantitative analysis of dynamic Gd-DTPA enhancement in breast tumors using a permeability model. Magn Reson Med 1995;33:564–568.

38. Reddick WE, Bhargava R, Taylor JS, Meyer WH, Fletcher BD. Dynamic contrast-enhanced MR imaging evaluation of osteosarcoma response to neoadjuvant chemotherapy. J Magn Reson Imaging 1995;5:689–694.

39. Verstraete KL, De Deene Y, Roels H, Dierick A, Uyttendaele D, Kunnen M. Benign and malignant musculoskeletal lesions: dynamic contrast-enhanced MR imaging—parametric "first-pass" images depict tissue vascularization and perfusion. Radiology 1994;192:835–843.

40. Knopp M, Brix G, Junkermann H, Sinn H. MR mammography with pharmacokinetic mapping for monitoring of breast cancer treatment during neoadjuvant therapy. Magn Reson Imaging 1994;2:633–658.

41. Turkat TJ, Klein BD, Polan RL, Richman R. Dynamic MR mammography: a technique for potentially reducing the biopsy rate for benign breast disease. J Magn Reson Imaging 1994; 4:563–568.

42. Kucharczyk W, Bishop JE, Plewes DB, Keller MA, George S. Detection of pituitary micro-adenomas: comparison of dynamic keyhole fast spin-echo, unenhanced, and conventional contrast-enhanced MR imaging. AJR 1994;163: 671–679.

43. Müller-Schimpfle M, Brix G, Layer G, et al. Recurrent rectal cancer: diagnosis with dynamic MR imaging. Radiology 1993;189:881–889.

44. Hanna SL, Reddick WE, Parham DM, Gronemeyer SA, Taylor JS, Fletcher BD. Automated pixel-by-pixel mapping of dynamic contrast-enhanced MR images for evaluation of osteosarcoma response to chemotherapy: preliminary results. J Magn Reson Imaging 1993;3:849–853.

45. Nägele T, Petersen D, Klose U, et al. Dynamic contrast enhancement of intracranial tumors with snapshot-FLASH MR imaging. AJNR 1993;14:89–98.

46. Tofts PS, Kermode AG. Measurement of the blood-brain barrier permeability and leakage space using dynamic MR imaging. 1. Fundamental concepts. Magn Reson Med 1991;17: 357–367.

47. Mirowitz SA, Totty WG, Lee JKT. Characterization of musculoskeletal masses using dynamic Gd-DTPA enhanced spin-echo MRI. J Comput Assist Tomogr 1992;16:120–125.

48. Fletcher BD, Hanna SL, Fairclough D, Gronemeyer SA. Pediatric musculoskeletal tumors: use of dynamic, contrast-enhanced MR imaging to monitor response to chemotherapy. Radiology 1992;184:243–248.

49. Hanna SL, Parham DM, Fairclough DL, Meyer WH, Le AH, Fletcher BD. Assessment of osteosarcoma response to preoperative chemotherapy using dynamic FLASH gadolinium-DTPA-enhanced magnetic resonance mapping. Invest Radiol 1992;27:367–373.

50. Bullock PR, Mansfield P, Gowland P, Worthington BS, Firth JL. Dynamic imaging of contrast enhancement in brain tumors. Magn Reson Med 1991;19:293–298.

51. Larsson HBW, Stubgaard M, Frederiksen JL, Jensen M, Henriksen O, Paulson OB. Quantitation of blood-brain barrier defect by magnetic resonance imaging and gadolinium-DTPA in patients with multiple sclerosis and brain tumors. Magn Reson Med 1990;16:117–131.

52. Ostergaard L, Weisskoff RM, Chesler DA, Gyldensted C, Rosen BR. High resolution measurement of cerebral blood flow using intravascular tracer bolus passages. Part I: Mathematical approach and statistical analysis. Magn Reson Med 1996;36:715–725.

53. Ostergaard L, Sorensen AG, Kwong KK, Weisskoff RM, Gyldensted C, Rosen BR. High resolution measurement of cerebral blood flow using intravascular tracer bolus passages. Part II: Experimental comparison and preliminary results. Magn Reson Med 1996;36:726–736.

54. Sorenson AG, Rosen BR. Functional MRI of the brain. In: Atlas SW, ed. Magnetic Resonance Imaging of the Brain and Spine. Philadelphia: Lippincott-Raven, 1996:1501–1545.

55. Rosen BR, Belliveau JW, Vevea JM, Brady TJ. Perfusion imaging with NMR contrast agents. Magn Reson Med 1990;14:249–265.

56. Aronen HJ, Cohen MS, Belliveau JW, Fordham JA, Rosen BR. Ultrafast imaging of brain tumors. Top Magn Reson Imaging 1993;5:14–24.

57. Aronen HJ, Gazit IE, Louis DN, et al. Cerebral blood volume maps of gliomas: comparison with tumor grade and histologic findings. Radiology 1994;191:41–51.

58. Aronen HJ, Glass J, Pardo FS, et al. Echo-planar MR cerebral blood volume mapping of gliomas. Clinical utility. Acta Radiol 1995;36:520–528.

59. Rosen BR, Belliveau JW, Aronen HJ, et al. Susceptibility contrast imaging of cerebral blood volume: human experience. Magn Reson Med 1991;22:293–299.

60. Sorenson AG, Tievsky AL, Ostergaard L, Weisskoff RM, Rosen BR. Contrast agents in functional MR imaging. J Magn Reson Imaging 1997;7:47–55.

61. Le Bihan D, Turner R, Moonen CTW, Pekar J. Imaging of diffusion and microcirculation with gradient sensitization: design, strategy, and significance. J Magn Reson Imaging 1991;1:7–28.

62. Le Bihan D, Turner R, Douek P, Patronas N. Diffusion MR imaging: clinical applications. AJR 1992;159:591–599.

63. Le Bihan D, Turner R. Diffusion and perfusion nuclear magnetic resonance imaging. In: Potchen EJ, Haacke EM, Siebert JE, Gottschalk A, eds. Magnetic Resonance Angiography. Concepts & Applications. St. Louis: Mosby Year-Book, 1993:323–342.

64. Moseley ME, Cohen Y, Kucharczyk J, et al. Diffusion-weighted MR imaging of anisotropic water diffusion in cat central nervous system. Radiology 1990;176:439–445.

65. Beauchamp NJJ, Ulug AM, Passe TJ, van Zijl PCM. MR diffusion imaging in stroke: review and controversies. RadioGraphics 1998;18:1269–1283.

66. van Gelderen P, de Vleeschouwer MHM, DesPres D, Pekar J, van Zijl PCM, Moonen CTW. Water diffusion and acute stroke. Magn Reson Med 1994;31:154–163.

67. Pajevic S, Pierpaoli C. Color schemes to represent the orientation of anisotropic tissues from diffusion tensor data: application to white matter fiber tract mapping in the human brain. Magn Reson Med 1999;42:526–540.

68. Virta A, Barnett A, Pierpaoli C. Visualizing and characterizing white matter fiber structure and architecture in the human pyramidal tract using diffusion tensor MRI. Magn Reson Imaging 1999;17:1121–1133.

69. Pierpaoli C, Jezzard P, Basser PJ, Barnett A, Di Chiro G. Diffusion tensor MR imaging of the human brain. Radiology 1996;201:637–648.

70. Basser PJ, Mattiello J, LeBihan D. MR imaging of fiber-tract direction and diffusion in anisotropic tissues. In: Twelfth Annual Meeting of the Society of Magnetic Resonance in Medicine, New York, 1993, Vol. 1. Society of Magnetic Resonance in Medicine, New York.

71. Chenevert TL, McKeever PE, Ross BD. Monitoring early response of experimental brain tumors to therapy using diffusion magnetic resonance imaging. Clin Cancer Res 1997;3:1457–1466.

72. Becker ED. High Resolution NMR. Theory and Chemical Applications. New York: Academic Press, 1980.

73. Aue WP. Localization methods for in vivo NMR spectroscopy. Rev Magn Reson Med 1986;1:21–72.

74. Brown TR, Kincaid BM, Ugurbil K. NMR chemical shift imaging in three dimensions. Proc Natl Acad Sci USA 1982;79:3523–3526.

75. Maudsley AA, Hilal SK, Perman WH, Simon HE. Spatially resolved high resolution spectroscopy by "four-dimensional" NMR. J Magn Reson 1983;51:147–152.

76. Granot J. Selected volume excitation using stimulated echoes (VEST): application to spatially localized spectroscopy and imaging. J Magn Reson 1986;70:488–492.

77. Frahm J, Merboldt K-D, Hänicke W. Localized proton spectroscopy using stimulated echoes. J Magn Reson 1987;72:502–508.

78. Kimmich R, Hoepfel D. Volume-selective multipulse spin-echo spectroscopy. J Magn Reson 1987;72:379–384.

79. Bottomley PA. Selective volume method for performing localized NMR spectroscopy. U.S. Patent 4,480,228, 1984.

80. Ordidge RJ, Connelly A, Lohman JAB. Image-selected in vivo spectroscopy (ISIS). A new technique for spatially selective NMR spectroscopy. J Magn Reson 1986;66:283–294.

81. Fauth J-M, Schweiger A, Braunschweiler L, Forrer J, Ernst RR. Elimination of unwanted echoes and reduction of dead time in three-pulse electron spin-echo spectroscopy. J Magn Reson 1986;66:74–85.

82. Frahm J, Bruhn H, Gyngell ML, Merboldt KD, Hänicke W, Sauter R. Localized proton NMR spectroscopy in different regions of the human brain in vivo. Relaxation times and concentrations of cerebral metabolites. Magn Reson Med 1989;11:47–63.

83. Pauly J, Le Roux P, Nishimura D, Macovski A. Parameter relations for the Shinnar-Le Roux selective excitation pulse design algorithm. IEEE Trans Med Imaging 1991;10:53–65.

84. Jackson EF, Narayana PA, Flamig DP. One-dimensional spectroscopic imaging with stimulated echoes. Phantom and human leg studies. Magn Reson Imaging 1990;8:153–159.

85. Moonen CTW, Sobering G, van Zijl PCM, Gillen J, von Kienlin M, Bizzi A. Proton spectroscopic imaging of human brain. J Magn Reson 1992;98:556–575.

86. Jackson EF, Doyle TJ, Wolinsky JS, Narayana PA. Short TE hydrogen-1 spectroscopic MR imaging of normal human brain: reproducibility studies. J Magn Reson Imaging 1994;4:5445–5551.

87. Posse S, Tedeschi G, Risinger R, Ogg R, Le Bihan D. High speed ^{1}H spectroscopic imaging in human brain by echo planar spatial-spectral encoding. Magn Reson Med 1995;33:34–40.

88. de Crespigny AJS, Carpenter TA, Hall LD. Region-of-interest selection by outer-volume saturation. J Magn Reson 1989;85:595–603.

89. Dunn JH, Matson GB, Maudsley AA, Weiner MW. 3D phase encoding ^{1}H spectroscopic imaging of human brain. Magn Reson Imaging 1992;10:315–319.

90. Posse S, Schuknecht B, Smith ME, van Zijl PCM, Herschkowitz N, Moonen CTW. Short echo time proton MR spectroscopic imaging. J Comput Assist Tomogr 1993;17:1–14.

91. Shungu DC, Glickson JD. Sensitivity and localization enhancement in multinuclear in vivo NMR spectroscopy by outer volume presaturation. Magn Reson Med 1993;30:661–671.

92. Hore PJ. Solvent suppression. In: Oppenheimer NJ, James TL, eds. Nuclear Magnetic Resonance, Part A: Spectral Techniques and Dynam-ics, Vol. 176. New York: Academic Press, 1989: 64–77.

93. Doddrell DM, Galloway GJ, Brooks WM, et al. Water signal elimination in vivo using "suppression by mistimed echo and repetive gradient episodes." J Magn Reson 1986;70: 176–180.

94. Soher BJ, van Zijl PCM, Duyn JH, Barker PB. Quantitative proton MR spectroscopic imaging of the human brain. Magn Reson Med 1996;35: 356–363.

95. Husted CA, Duijn JH, Matson GB, Maudsley AA, Weiner MW. Molar quantitation of in vivo proton metabolites in human brain with 3D magnetic resonance spectroscopy imaging. Magn Reson Imaging 1994;12:661–667.

96. Michaelis T, Merboldt K-D, Bruhn H, Hänicke W, Frahm J. Absolute concentration of metabolites in the adult human brain in vivo: quantification of localized proton MR spectra. Radiology 1993;187:219–227.

97. Kreis R, Ernst T, Ross BD. Development of the human brain: in vivo quantification of metabolite and water content with proton magnetic resonance spectroscopy. Magn Reson Med 1993;30:424–437.

98. Narayana PA, Fotedar LK, Jackson EF, Bohan TP, Butler IJ, Wolinsky JS. Regional in vivo proton magnetic resonance spectroscopy of brain. J Magn Reson 1989;83:44–52.

99. Davie CA, Barker GJ, Webb S, et al. Persistent functional deficit in multiple sclerosis and autosomal dominant cerebellar ataxia is associated with axon loss. Brain 1995;118:1583–1592.

100. Usenius J-PR, Kauppinen RA, Vainio PA, et al. Quantitative metabolite patterns of human brain tumors: detection by ^{1}H NMR spectroscopy in vivo and in vitro. J Comput Assist Tomogr 1994;18:705–713.

101. Christiansen P, Henriksen O, Stubgaard M, Gideon P, Larsson HBW. In vivo quantification of brain metabolites by ^{1}H-MRS using water as an internal standard. Magn Reson Imaging 1993;11:107–118.

102. Pan JW, Hetherington HP, Hamm JR, Shulman RG. Quantitation of metabolites by ^{1}H NMR. Magn Reson Med 1991;20:48–56.

103. Danielsen ER, Michaelis T, Ross BD. Three methods of calibration in quantitative proton MR spectroscopy. J Magn Reson Ser B 1995; 106:287–291.

104. Charles HC, Lazeyras F, Tupler LA, Krishnan RR. Reproducibility of high spatial resolution

proton magnetic resonance spectroscopic imaging of the human brain. Magn Reson Med 1996;35:606–610.

105. Webb PG, Sailasuta N, Kohler SJ, Raidy T, Moats RA, Hurd RE. Automated single-voxel proton MRS: technical development and multisite verification. Magn Reson Med 1994;31:365–373.

106. Negendank WG, Sauter R, Brown TR, et al. Proton magnetic resonance spectroscopy in patients with glial tumors: a multicenter study. J Neurosurg 1996;84:449–458.

107. Doyle TJ, Bedell BJ, Narayana PA. Relative concentrations of proton MR visible neurochemicals in gray and white matter in human brain. Magn Reson Med 1995;33:755–759.

108. Hetherington HP, Pan JW, Mason GF, et al. Quantitative ^{1}H spectroscopic imaging of human brain at 4.1 T using imaging segmentation. Magn Reson Med 1996;36:21–29.

109. Jackson EF, Meyers CA. Introduction to hippocampal spectroscopy. In: Tien RD, ed. Neuroimaging Clinics of North America, Vol. 7. Philadelphia: Saunders, 1997:143–154.

110. Ross B, Michaelis T. MR spectroscopy of the brain: neurospectroscopy. In: Edelman RR, Hesselink JR, Zlatkin MB, eds. Clinical Magnetic Resonance Imaging, Vol. 1. Philadelphia: Saunders, 1996:928–981.

111. Cox IJ. Development and applications of in vivo clinical magnetic resonance spectroscopy. Prog Biophys Mol Biol 1996;65:45–81.

112. Falini A, Calabrese G, Origgi D, et al. Proton magnetic resonance spectroscopy and intracranial tumors: clinical perspectives. J Neurol 1996;243:706–714.

113. Vion-Dury J, Meyerhoff DJ, Cozzone PJ, Weiner MW. What might be the impact on neurology of the analysis of brain metabolism by in vivo magnetic resonance spectroscopy? J Neurol 1994;241:354–371.

114. Leach MO. Magnetic resonance spectroscopy applied to clinical oncology. Tech Health Care 1994;2:235–246.

115. Barker PB, Glickson JD, Bryan RN. In vivo magnetic resonance spectroscopy of human brain tumors. Top Magn Reson Imaging 1993;5:32–45.

116. Howe FA, Maxwell RJ, Saunders DE, Brown MM, Griffiths JR. Proton spectroscopy in vivo. Magn Reson Q 1993;9:31–59.

117. Negendank W. Studies of human tumors by MRS: a review. NMR Biomed 1992;5:303–324.

118. Bottomley PA. Human in vivo NMR spectroscopy in diagnostic medicine: clinical tool or research probe? Radiology 1989;170:1–15.

119. Birken DL, Oldendorf WH. N-Acetyl-L-aspartic acid: a literature review of a compound prominent in ^{1}H-NMR spectroscopic studies of brain. Neurosci Biobehav Rev 1989;13:23–31.

120. Kreis R, Ernst T, Ross BD. Development of the human brain: in vivo quantification of metabolite and water content with ^{1}H-MRS. In: Twelfth Annual Meeting of the Society of Magnetic Resonance in Medicine, New York, 1993, Vol. 1. Society of Magnetic Resonance in Medicine, New York.

121. van der Knaap MS, van der Grond J, van Rijen PC, Faber JA, Valk J, Willemse K. Age-dependent changes in localized proton and phosphorus MR spectroscopy of the brain. Radiology 1990;176:509–515.

122. Bizzi A, Movsas B, Tedeschi G, et al. Response of non-Hodgkin lymphoma to radiation therapy: early and long-term assessment with H-1 MR spectroscopic imaging. Radiology 1995;194:271–276.

123. Sijens PE, Knopp MV, Brunett A, et al. ^{1}H MR spectroscopy in patients with metastatic brain tumors: a multicenter study. Magn Reson Med 1995;33:818–826.

124. McBride DQ, Miller BL, Nikas DL, et al. Analysis of brain tumors using ^{1}H magnetic resonance spectroscopy. Surg Neurol 1995;44:137–144.

125. Kugel H, Heindel W, Bunke J, Du Mesnil R, Friedmann G. Human brain tumors: spectral patterns detected with localized H-1 MR spectroscopy. Radiology 1994;183:701–709.

126. Yamagata NT, Miller BL, McBride D, et al. In vivo proton spectroscopy of intracranial infections and neoplasms. J Neuroimaging 1994;4:23–28.

127. Ott D, Hennig J, Ernst T. Human brain tumors: Assessment with in vivo proton MR spectroscopy. Radiology 1993;186:745–752.

128. Sutton LN, Wang Z, Gusnard D, et al. Proton magnetic resonance spectroscopy of pediatric brain tumors. Neurosurgery (Baltim) 1992;31:195–202.

129. Fulham MJ, Bizzi A, Dietz MJ, et al. Mapping of brain tumor metabolites with proton MR spectroscopic imaging: clinical relevance. Radiology 1992;185:675–686.

130. Demaeral P, Johannik K, van Hecke P, et al. Localized ^{1}H NMR spectroscopy in fifty cases

of newly diagnosed intracranial tumors. J Comput Assist Tomogr 1991;15:67–76.

131. Frahm J, Bruhn H, Hänicke W, Merboldt K-D, Mursch K, Markakis E. Localized proton NMR spectroscopy of brain tumors using short-echo time STEAM sequences. J Comput Assist Tomogr 1991;15:915–922.

132. Henriksen O, Wieslander S, Gjerris F, Jensen KM. In vivo ^{1}H spectroscopy of human intracranial tumors at 1.5 T. Acta Radiol 1991;32:95–99.

133. Alger JR, Frank JA, Bizzi A, et al. Metabolism of human gliomas: assessment with H-1 MR spectroscopy and F-18 fluorodeoxyglucose PET. Radiology 1990;177:633–641.

134. Gill SS, Thomas DG, van Bruggen N, et al. Proton MR spectroscopy of intracranial tumors: in vivo and in vitro studies. J Comput Assist Tomogr 1990;14:497–504.

135. Luyten PR, Marien AJH, Heindel W, et al. Metabolic imaging of patients with intracranial tumors: H-1 MR spectroscopic imaging and PET. Radiology 1990;176:791–799.

136. Segebarth CM, Baleriaux DF, Luyten PR, den-Hollander JA. Detection of metabolic heterogeneity of human intracranial tumors in vivo by ^{1}H NMR spectroscopic imaging. Magn Reson Med 1990;13:62–76.

137. Arnold DL, Shoubridge EA, Emrich J, Feindel W, Villemure JG. Early metabolic changes following chemotherapy of human gliomas in vivo demonstrated by phosphorus magnetic resonance spectroscopy. Invest Radiol 1989;24:958–961.

138. Bruhn H, Frahm J, Gyngell ML, et al. Noninvasive differentiation of tumors with use of localized H-1 MR spectroscopy in vivo: initial experience in patients with cerebral tumors. Radiology 1989;172:541–548.

139. Tedeschi G, Bertolino A, Campbell G, et al. Brain regional distribution pattern of metabolite signal intensities in young adults by proton magnetic resonance spectroscopic imaging. Neurology 1995;45:1384–1391.

140. Tedeschi G, Righini A, Bizzi A, Barnett AS, Alger J. Cerebral white matter in the centrum semiovale exhibits a larger N-acetyl signal than does gray matter in long echo time ^{1}H-magnetic resonance spectroscopic imaging. Magn Reson Med 1995;33:127–133.

141. Hetherington HP, Mason GF, Pan JW, et al. Evaluation of cerebral gray and white matter metabolite differences by spectroscopic imaging at 4.1 T. Magn Reson Med 1994;32:565–571.

142. Narayana PA, Johnston D, Flamig DP. In vivo proton magnetic resonance spectroscopy studies of human brain. Magn Reson Imaging 1991;9:303–308.

143. Tedeschi G, Lundbom N, Raman R, et al. Increased choline signal coinciding with malignant degeneration of cerebral gliomas: a serial proton magnetic resonance spectroscopy imaging study. J Neurosurg 1997;87:516–524.

144. Tien RD, Lai PH, Smith JS, Lazeyras F. Single-voxel proton brain spectroscopy exam (PROBE/SV) in patients with primary brain tumors. AJR 1996;167:201–209.

145. Miller BL, Chang L, Booth R, et al. In vivo ^{1}H MRS choline: correlation with in vitro chemistry/histology. Life Sci 1996;58:1929–1935.

146. Tzika AA, Ball WS, Vigneron DB, Dunn RS, Kirks DR. Clinical proton MR spectroscopy of neurodegenerative disease in childhood. AJNR 1993;14:1267–1281.

147. Gideon P, Henriksen O. In vivo relaxation of N-acetyl-aspartate, creatine plus phosphocreatine, and choline containing compounds during the course of brain infarction: a proton MRS study. Magn Reson Imaging 1992;10:983–988.

148. Henriksen O, Gideon P, Sperling B, Olsen TS, Jørgensen HS, Arlien-Søborg P. Cerebral lactate production and blood flow in acute stroke. J Magn Reson Imaging 1992;2:511–517.

149. Mathews VP, Barker PB, Bryan RN. Magnetic resonance evaluation of stroke. Magn Reson Q 1992;8:245–263.

150. Sappey-Marinier D, Calabrese G, Hetherington H, et al. Proton magnetic resonance spectroscopy of human brain: applications to normal white matter, chronic infarction, and MRI white matter signal hyperintensities. Magn Reson Med 1992;26:313–327.

151. Fenstermacher MJ, Narayana PA. Serial proton magnetic resonance spectroscopy of ischemic brain injury in humans. Invest Radiol 1990;25:1034–1039.

152. Bruhn H, Frahm J, Gyngell ML, Merboldt KD, Hänicke W, Sauter R. Cerebral metabolism in man after acute stroke: new observations using localized proton NMR spectroscopy. Magn Reson Med 1989;9:126–131.

153. Tzika AA, Vigneron DB, Ball WSJ, Dunn RS, Kirks DR. Localized proton MR spectroscopy of the brain in children. J Magn Reson Imaging 1993;3:719–729.

154. Poptani H, Gupta RK, Jain VK, Roy R, Pandey R. Cystic intracranial mass lesions: possible role of in vivo MR spectroscopy in its differential

diagnosis. Magn Reson Imaging 1995;13:1019–1029.

155. Chang L, McBride D, Miller BL, et al. Localized in vivo ^{1}H magnetic-resonance spectroscopy and in vitro analysis of heterogeneous brain tumors. J Neuroimaging 1995;5:157–163.

156. Arnold DL, Shoubridge EA, Villemure JG, Feindel W. Proton and phosphorus magnetic resonance spectroscopy of human astrocytomas in vivo. Preliminary observations on tumor grading. NMR Biomed 1990;3:184–189.

157. Pan JW, Mason GF, Pohost GM, Hetherington HP. Spectroscopic imaging of human brain glutamate by water-suppressed *J*-refocused coherence transfer at 4.1 T. Magn Reson Med 1996;36:7–12.

158. Keltner JR, Wald LL, Frederick BdB, Renshaw PF. In vivo detection of GABA in human brain using a localized double-quantum filter technique. Magn Reson Med 1997;37:366–371.

159. Keltner JR, Wald LL, Christensen JD, et al. A technique for detecting GABA in the human brain with PRESS localization and optimized refocusing spectral editing radiofrequency pulses. Magn Reson Med 1996;36:458–461.

160. Rothman DL, Petroff OA, Behar KL, Mattson RH. Localized ^{1}H NMR measurements of gamma-aminobutyric acid in human brain in vivo. Proc Natl Acad Sci USA 1993;90:5662–5666.

161. Schick F, Einsele H, Kost R, et al. Hematopoietic reconstitution after bone marrow transplantation: assessment with MR imaging and H-1 localized spectroscopy. J Magn Reson Imaging 1994;4:71–78.

162. Schick F, Bongers H, Jung W-I, Skalej M, Lutz O, Claussen CD. Volume-selective proton MRS in vertebral bodies. Magn Reson Med 1992;26:207–217.

163. Jensen KE, Jensen M, Grundtvig P, Thomsen C, Karle H, Henriksen O. Localized in vivo proton spectroscopy of the bone marrow in patients with leukemia. Magn Reson Imaging 1990;8:779–789.

164. Schick F, Duda SH, Lutz O, Claussen CD. Lipids in bone tumors assessed by magnetic resonance: chemical shift imaging and proton spectroscopy in vivo. Anticancer Res 1996;16:1569–1574.

165. Bongers H, Schick F, Skalej M, Jung W-I, Stevens A. Localized in vivo ^{1}H spectroscopy of human skeletal muscle: normal and pathologic findings. Magn Reson Imaging 1992;10:957–964.

166. Garcia-Segura JM, Sanvhez-Chapado M, Ibarburen C, et al. In vivo proton magnetic resonance spectroscopy of diseased prostate: spectroscopic features of malignant versus benign pathology. Magn Reson Imaging 1999;17:755–765.

167. Liney GP, Turnbull LW, Knowles AJ. In vivo magnetic resonance spectroscopy and dynamic contrast enhanced imaging of the prostate gland. NMR Biomed 1999;12:39–44.

168. Hahn P, Smith IC, Leboldus L, Somorjai RL, Bezabeh T. The classification of benign and malignant human prostate tissue by multivariate analysis of ^{1}H magnetic resonance spectra. Cancer Res 1997;57:3398–3401.

169. Heerschap A, Jager GJ, van der Graaf M, et al. In vivo proton MR spectroscopy reveals altered metabolite content in malignant prostate tissue. Anticancer Res 1997;17:1455–1460.

170. Kurhanewicz J, Vigneron DB, Nelson SJ, et al. In vivo citrate levels in the normal and pathologic human prostate. In: Twelfth Annual Meeting of the Society of Magnetic Resonance in Medicine, New York, 1993, Vol. 1. Society of Magnetic Resonance in Medicine, New York.

5
Radiopharmaceuticals for Tumor-Targeted Imaging: Overview

David J. Yang, Tomio Inoue, and E. Edmund Kim

Improvement of scintigraphic tumor diagnosis, prognosis, planning, and monitoring of cancer treatment is clearly determined by development of more tumor-specific radiopharmaceuticals. Application of molecular targets for cancer imaging, therapy, and prevention are the major focus of research projects. Radionuclide imaging modalities (positron emission tomography, PET; single photon emission computed tomography, SPECT) are diagnostic cross-sectional imaging techniques that map the location and concentration of radionuclide-labeled radiotracers. Although computed tomography (CT) and magnetic resonance imaging (MRI) provide considerable anatomical information about the location and the extent of tumors, these imaging modalities cannot adequately differentiate invasive lesions from edema, radiation necrosis, or gliosis. PET and SPECT can be used to localize and characterize tumors by measuring metabolic activity [1].

Recent findings in the field of molecular and cellular biology have led to the development of molecular markers in the following research areas:

- Apoptosis/hypoxia: annexin/tirapazamine, misonidazole
- Anti/angiogenesis: integrins, paclitaxel, colchicine, vincristine, endostatin
- Invasion/metastasis: TNP470, marimastat
- Cell-cycle progression: thymidine, adenosine
- Immunological:

Tumor antigen: CD4$^+$ and CD8$^+$ T cells
Tumor vaccines: designer vectors

To characterize tumor tissue, radiolabeled ligands, radiolabeled antibodies [2], and signal transduction agents have opened a new era in scintigraphic detection of tumors and undergone extensive preclinical development and evaluation. Development of molecular nuclear medicine has been focused on the prediction of therapeutic response, differential diagnosis, and monitoring tumor response to treatment. Because of favorable physical characteristics and low price ($0.21/mCi versus $50/mCi of ^{18}F), ^{99m}Tc has been preferred to label radiopharmaceuticals. Although it has been reported that DTPA–drug conjugate could be labeled with ^{99m}Tc effectively, the DTPA (diethylene triaminepentaacetic acid) moiety does not chelate with ^{99m}Tc as stably as with ^{111}In [3].

bis-Aminoethanethiol tetradentate ligands, also called diaminodithiol compounds, are known to form very stable Tc(V)O complexes on the basis of efficient binding of the oxotechnetium group to two thiolsulfur and two amine nitrogen atoms [4]. ^{99m}Tc-ethylenedicysteine (^{99m}Tc-EC) is a successful example of N_2S_2 chelates [5–9]. ^{99m}Tc-EC-drug conjugates were then developed to characterize tumor tissues. In this chapter, we evaluate the potential of these tracers, which may be used to redirect early cancer diagnosis and therapeutics.

TABLE 5.1. Rf values determined by radio-TLC (ITLC-SG).

	System A[a]	System B[b]
^{99m}Tc-EC-folate	0	1 (>95%)
^{99m}Tc-EC	0	1 (>95%)
Free ^{99m}Tc	1	1
Reduced ^{99m}Tc	0	0

[a] Acetone (1 M in water):methanol (4:1).
[b] Ammonium acetate (1 M in water):methanol (4:1).

Tumor Folate Receptor Targeting

EC-folate was prepared according to the previously described methods [10]. Radiosynthesis of ^{99m}Tc-EC-folate was achieved by adding ^{99m}Tc-pertechnetate into a homemade kit containing EC-NIM (ethylenedicysteine-nitroimidazole) or EC (3 mg), SnCl$_2$ (100 µg), Na$_2$HPO$_4$ (13.5 mg), ascorbic acid (0.5 mg), and Na-EDTA (0.5 mg). Radiochemical purity was determined by TLC (ITLC SG; Gelman Sciences, Ann Arbor, MI) and eluted with acetone (system A) and ammonium acetate (1 M in water):methanol (4:1) (system B). Radio-TLC data are summarized in Table 5.1. The synthesis of ^{99m}Tc-EC-folate is shown in Figure 5.1.

Stability Assay of ^{99m}Tc-EC-Folate

Stability of ^{99m}Tc-EC-folate was tested in serum samples. Briefly, 740 kBq of 1 mg ^{99m}Tc-EC-folate was incubated in dog serum (200 µl) at 37°C for 4 h. The serum samples were diluted with 50% methanol in water, and radio-TLC was repeated at 0.5 to 4 h as described (see Table 5.1).

Tissue Distribution Studies

Female Fischer-344 rats (150±25 g) (Harlan Sprague-Dawley, Indianapolis, IN) were inoculated subcutaneously with 0.1 ml of mammary tumor cells from the 13762 tumor cell line suspension (10^6 cells/rat, a tumor cell line specific to Fischer rats) into the hind legs. Studies were performed 14 to 17 days after implantation when tumors reached approximately 1 cm diameter.

In tissue distribution studies, each animal was injected intravenously (i.v.) with ^{99m}Tc-EC-folate or ^{99m}Tc-EC (10 µCi/rat; $n=3$/time point). The injected mass of each ligand was 10 µg per rat. At 20 min, and 1, 2, and 4 h following administration of the radiopharmaceuticals, the animals were killed and the tumor and selected tissues were excised, weighed, and counted for radioactivity by a gamma counter (Packard, Downers Grove, IL). The biodistribution of tracer in each sample was calculated as percentage of the injected dose per gram of tissue wet weight (%ID/g). Student's t-test was used to assess the significance of differences between two groups. In a separate experiment, blocking studies were performed to determine the receptor-mediated process. In blocking studies, ^{99m}Tc-EC-folate was coadministrated intravenously with 50 and 150 µmol/kg folic acid to tumor-bearing rats ($n=3$/group). Animals were killed 1 h post injection and data were collected.

Scintigraphic and Autoradiography Studies

Scintigraphic images, using a gamma camera (Siemens Medical Systems, Hoffman Estates, IL) equipped with a low-energy, parallel hole collimator, were obtained 0.5 to 4 h after i.v. injection of 100 µCi of ^{99m}Tc-labeled radiotracer. Whole-body autoradiograms were obtained by a quantitative image analyzer (Cyclone Storage Phosphor System; Packard, Meridian, CT). Following i.v. injection of ^{99m}Tc-EC-folate, the animal was killed at 1 h and the body was fixed in carboxymethyl cellulose (4%). The frozen body was mounted onto a cryostat (LKB 2250 cryomicrotome) and cut into 100-µm coronal sections. Each section was thawed and mounted on a slide. The slide was then placed in contact with a multipurpose phosphor storage screen (MP, 7001480) and exposed for 15 h.

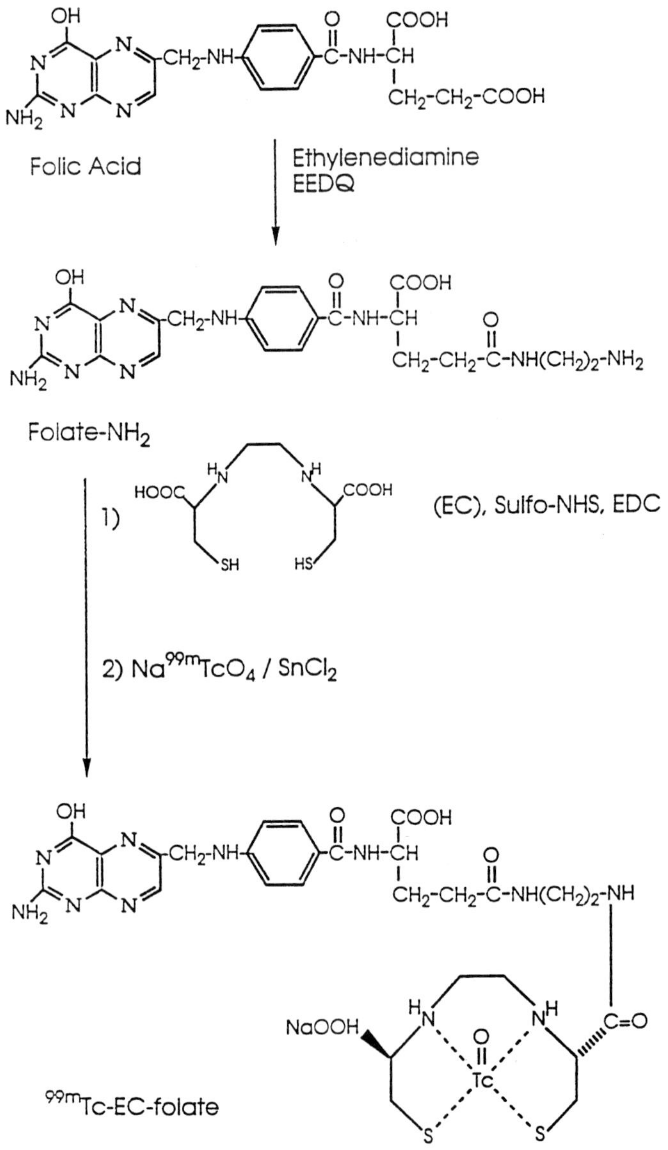

FIGURE 5.1. Synthesis of ^{99m}Tc-ethyl-enedicysteine-folate (^{99m}Tc-EC-folate).

Targeting Tumor Hypoxia

To a stirred mixture containing 2-nitroimida-zole (1 g) and Cs_2CO_3 (2.9 g) in dimethylfor-mamide (DMF) (50 ml), 1,3-ditosylpropane (3.84 g) was added. The reaction was heated at 80°C for 3 h. The solvent was evaporated and the residue was suspended in ethylacetate, loaded on a silica gel-packed column, and eluted with hexane:ethylacetate (1:1); yield was 1.67 g (57.5%) with m.p. 108°–111°C. ^{1}H-NMR (CDCl$_3$) was at δ 2.23 (m, 2 H), 2.48 (S, 3 H), 4.06 (t, 2 H, J=5.7 Hz), 4.52 (t, 2 H, J= 6.8 Hz), 7.09 (S, 1 H), 7.24 (S, 1 H), 7.40 (d, 2 H, J=8.2 Hz), 7.77 (d, 2 H, J=8.2 Hz).

Tosylated 2-nitroimidazole (1.33 g) was reacted with sodium azide (0.29 g) in DMF (10 ml) at 100°C for 3 h. After cooling, water (20 ml) was added and the product was extracted from ethylacetate. The solvent was evaporated to dryness to afford the azido ana-logue (0.6 g, 75%). ^{1}H-NMR (CDCl$_3$): δ 2.14 (m, 2 H), 3.41 (t, 2 H, J=6.2 Hz), 4.54 (t, 2 H, J=6.9 Hz), 7.17 (S, 2 H).

The azido analogue (0.57 g) was reduced by triphenyl phosphine (1.14 g) in tetrahydrofuran (THF) for 4 h. Concentrate HCl (12 ml) was added and heated for an additional 5 h. The product was extracted from ethylacetate to afford the amine hydrochloride analogue (360 mg, 60%). ^{1}H-NMR (D$_2$O): δ 2.29 (m, 2 H), 3.13 (t, 2 H, J = 7.8 Hz), 3.60 (br, 2 H), 4.35 (t, 2 H, J = 7.4 Hz), 7.50 (d, 1 H, J = 2.1 Hz), 7.63 (d, 1 H, J = 2.1 Hz).

Synthesis of Ethylenedicysteine-nitroimidazole (EC-NIM)

Sodium hydroxide (2 N, 0.6 ml) was added to a stirred solution of EC (134 mg) in water (2 ml). To this colorless solution, sulfo-NHS (260.6 mg), EDC (230 mg), and sodium hydroxide (2 N, 1 ml) were added. NIM-NH$_2$ hydrochloride salt (206.6 mg) was then added. The mixture was stirred for 24 h and dialyzed for 48 h (MW cutoff at 500). After dialysis, the product was frozen, dried, and weighed (594.8 mg; yield, 98%).

Radiolabeling of EC-NIM with ^{99m}Tc

Radiosynthesis of ^{99m}Tc-EC-NIM was achieved by using the same method described for ^{99m}Tc-EC-folate except EC-NIM (3 mg) was used instead of EC-folate. Radiochemical purity was determined by ITLC and eluted with ammonium acetate (1 M in water):methanol (4:1). The synthetic scheme is shown in Figure 5.2.

Scintigraphic Studies

Using the same procedure described for ^{99m}Tc-EC-folate, scintigraphic images were obtained. To ascertain whether ^{99m}Tc-EC-NIM could monitor tumor response to chemotherapy, a group of rats with tumor volume 1.5 cm and ovarian tumor-bearing mice were treated with paclitaxel (40 mg/kg, i.v.) at one single dose. The image was taken on day 4 after paclitaxel treatment. Following administration of the radiotracers, computer-outlined region of interest (ROI) was used to determine tumor and background changes.

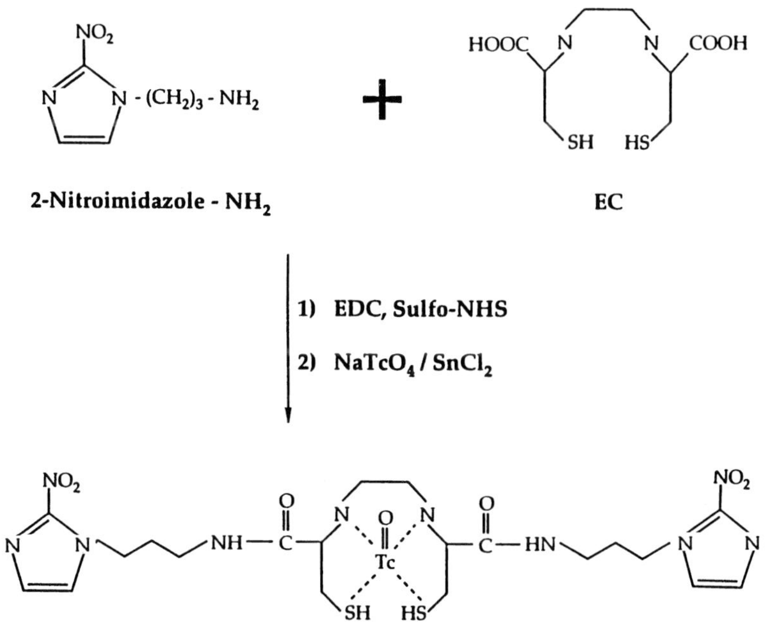

FIGURE 5.2. Synthesis of ^{99m}Tc-ethylenedicysteine-nitroimidazole (^{99m}Tc-EC-NIM).

Polarographic Oxygen Microelectrode pO₂ Measurements

To confirm tumor hypoxia, intratumoral pO_2 measurements were performed using the Eppendorf computerized histographic system; 20 to 25 pO_2 measurements along each of two to three linear tracks were made at 0.4-mm intervals on each tumor (40–75 measurements total). Tumor pO_2 measurements were made on three tumor-bearing rats. Using an online computer system, the pO_2 measurements of each track were expressed as absolute values relative to the location of the measuring point along the track, and as the relative frequencies within a pO_2 histogram between 0 and 100 mmHg with a class width of 2.5 mm.

Peptide Imaging of Cancer

Sodium hydroxide (1 N, 1 ml) was added to a stirred solution of EC (200 mg, 0.75 mmol) in water (10 ml). To this colorless solution, sulfo-NHS (162 mg, 0.75 mmol) and EDC (143 mg, 0.75 mmol) were added. Pentaglutamate sodium salt (GAP M.W. 750–1500; Sigma) (500 mg, 0.67 mmol) was then added. The mixture was stirred at room temperature for 24 h. The mixture was dialyzed for 48 h using Spectra/POR molecular porous membrane with cutoff at 500 (Spectrum, Houston, TX). After dialysis, the product was frozen dried using lyophilizer (Labconco, Kansas City, MO). The product in the salt form weighed 0.95 g. The synthetic scheme of ^{99m}Tc-EC-GAP is shown in Figure 5.3.

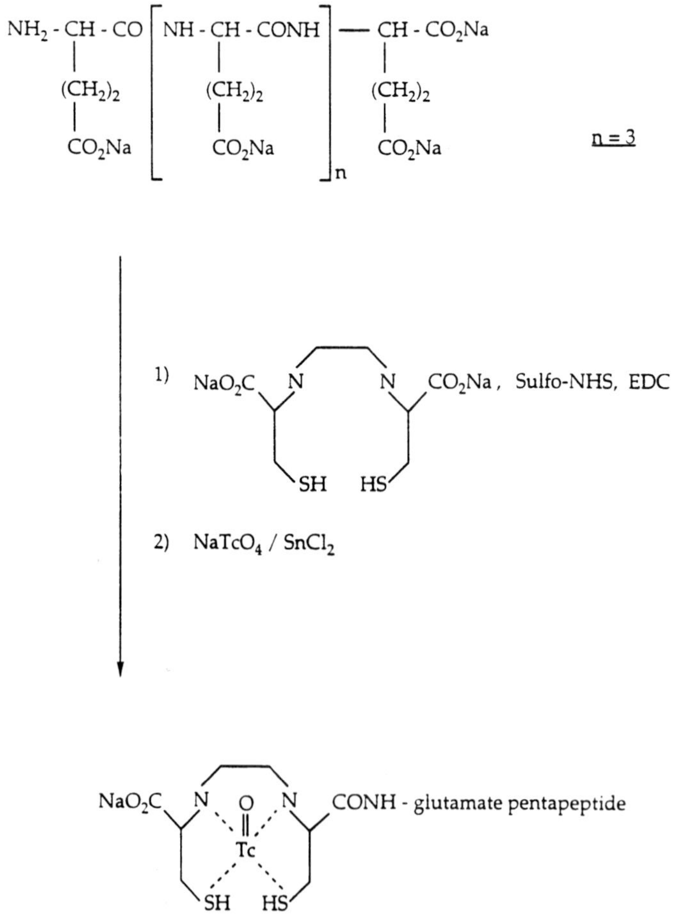

FIGURE 5.3. Radiosynthesis of ^{99m}Tc-EC-pentaglutamate.

Tissue Distribution Studies

In tissue distribution studies, the same procedure was used as described for ^{99m}Tc-EC-folate. Briefly, each animal was injected intravenously (i.v.) with ^{99m}Tc-EC-GAP or ^{99m}Tc-EC ($10\,\mu$Ci/rat, $n=3$/time point). Following administration of the radiopharmaceuticals, the animals were killed and the tumor and selected tissues were excised, weighed, and counted for radioactivity by a gamma counter.

Scintigraphic Studies

Scintigraphic images were obtained 0.5 to 4h after i.v. injection of $100\,\mu$Ci of each radiotracer.

Imaging Tumor Apoptotic Cells

Sodium bicarbonate (1 N, 1 ml) was added to a stirred solution of EC (5 mg, 0.019 mmol). To this colorless solution, sulfo-NHS (4 mg, 0.019 mmol) and EDC (4 mg, 0.019 mmol) were added. Annexin V (M.W. 33 kDa, human, Sigma) (0.3 mg) was then added. The mixture was stirred at room temperature for 24 h. The mixture was dialyzed for 48 h with cutoff at M.W. 10,000. After dialysis, the product (salt form) weighed 12 mg. Radiosynthesis of ^{99m}Tc-EC-annexin V was achieved using the same procedure as described for ^{99m}Tc-EC-folate.

Scintigraphic Studies

After i.v. injection of $100\,\mu$Ci of the radiotracer, scintigraphic images were obtained at 0.5 to 4 h. The animal models used were breast, ovarian, and sarcoma. Both breast and ovarian-tumor bearing rats are known to overexpress high apoptotic cells. The imaging studies were conducted on day 14 after tumor cell inoculation.

Imaging Tumor Angiogenesis

EC-COL (ethylenedicysteine-eolchicine) was prepared according to the previously described methods [11]. Radiosynthesis of ^{99m}Tc-EC-COL was achieved using the same procedure as described in Example 1.

Scintigraphic Studies

Scintigraphic images were obtained after i.v. injection of ^{99m}Tc-EC-COL and ^{99m}Tc-EC. Computer-outlined ROI was used to quantitate (counts per pixel) the tumor uptake versus normal muscle uptake.

Examples

Example 1: Targeting Tumor Folate Receptor

Chemistry and Biodistribution of ^{99m}Tc-EC-Folate

A simple, fast and high yield of ^{99m}Tc-EC-folate was developed. Radiochemical purity of ^{99m}Tc-EC-folate was greater than 95%. ^{99m}Tc-EC-folate was found to be stable at 20 min to 4 h in dog serum samples.

Biodistribution studies showed that tumor/blood count density ratios at 20 min to 4 h gradually increased for ^{99m}Tc-EC-folate, whereas these values decreased for ^{99m}Tc-EC in the same time period (Figure 5.4). In blocking studies, tumor/muscle and tumor/blood count density ratios were significantly decreased ($p<0.01$) with folic acid coadministrations (Figure 5.5).

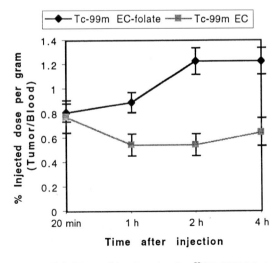

FIGURE 5.4. Tumor/blood ratios for ^{99m}Tc-EC-folate and ^{99m}Tc-EC.

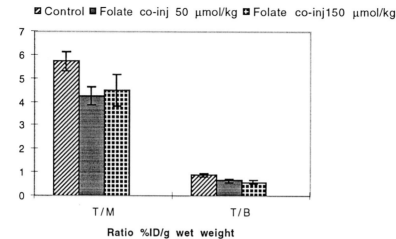

FIGURE 5.5. Tumor/blood and tumor/muscle ratios for ^{99m}Tc-EC-folate significantly de-creased (*$p < 0.01$) with different doses of folate coinjections.

Scintigraphic and Autoradiography Studies

Scintigraphic images obtained at different time points showed visualization of tumor in the ^{99m}Tc-EC-folate-injected group. Contrary, there was no apparent tumor uptake in the ^{99m}Tc-EC-injected group (Figure 5.6). Both radiotracers showed evident kidney uptake in all images. Autoradiograms performed at 1 h after injection of ^{99m}Tc-EC-folate clearly demonstrated tumor activity.

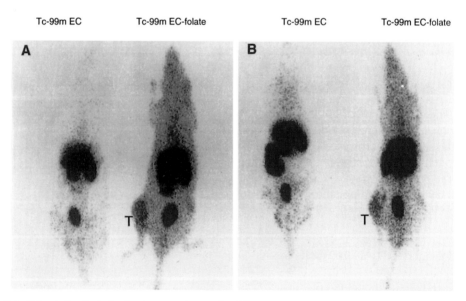

FIGURE 5.6. Selected whole-body images (ventral view) of rats with a subcutaneous breast tumor in the right hind leg 1 h (**A**) and 4 h (**B**) following i.v. administration of ^{99m}Tc-EC and ^{99m}Tc-EC-folate. ^{99m}Tc-EC-folate uptake was evident in the tumor (*T*) up to 4 h. There was no apparent radiotracer uptake in the tumor area with ^{99m}Tc-EC. Kidney and bladder activity were noted with both radiotracers. Tumor sizes were same (1 cm) in both animals.

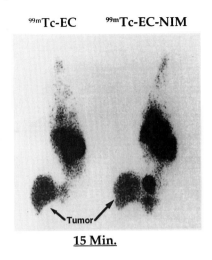
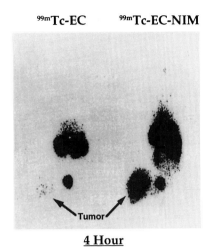

FIGURE 5.7. Whole-body images of breast tumor-bearing rats following administration of ^{99m}Tc-EC and ^{99m}Tc-EC-NIM (300μCi/rat, i.v., on day 14). Tumor uptake was higher in ^{99m}Tc-EC-NIM when compared to ^{99m}Tc-EC at 4h (*right*).

Example 2: Targeting Tumor Hypoxia

Scintigraphic Studies

Proton NMR confirmed the structure of EC-NIM. The radiochemical purity of ^{99m}Tc-EC-NIM was greater than 90%. In planar imaging of tumor-bearing rats following administration of ^{99m}Tc-EC and ^{99m}Tc-EC-NIM, the tumor uptake was higher in the ^{99m}Tc-EC-NIM group (Figure 5.7); however, the tumor uptake decreased after paclitaxel treatment (Figure 5.8). Similar findings were observed in ovarian tumor-bearing mice and sarcoma tumor-bearing mice (Figures 5.9, 5.10). ROI indicated that there was a marked difference of tumor/background ratios at pre- and postpacli-

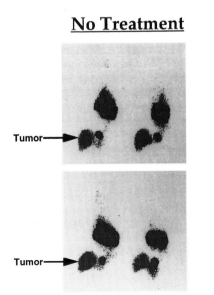
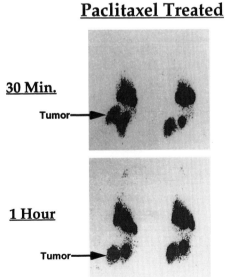

FIGURE 5.8. Whole-body images of breast tumor-bearing rats without (*left*) and with (*right*) paclitaxel treatment (40mg/kg, i.v., single injection on day 14) following the administration of ^{99m}Tc-EC-NIM (300 μCi/rat, i.v.) on day 18 showed decreased tumor volume and tumor uptake after paclitaxel treatment.

⁹⁹ᵐTc-EC-Nitroimidazole (NIM)

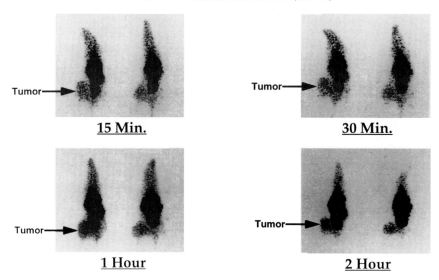

FIGURE 5.9. Whole-body images of sarcoma-bearing mice (low apoptosis) after administration of ⁹⁹ᵐTc-EC-NIM (100μCi/mouse, i.v.) showed the tumor well visualized from 15min to 2h post injection.

⁹⁹ᵐTc-EC-Nitroimidazole (NIM)
(100μCi/mouse, iv.)

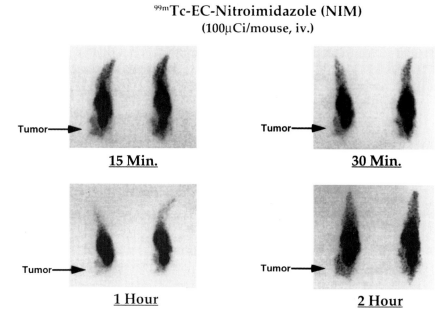

FIGURE 5.10. Whole-body images of sarcoma-bearing mice (low apoptosis) on day 18, after paclitaxel treatment (80mg/kg, i.v., single injection on day 14) showed a minimal uptake of ⁹⁹ᵐTc-EC-NIM.

FIGURE 5.11. Histological staining of tumor cells without treatment (control) showed viable
tumor cells.

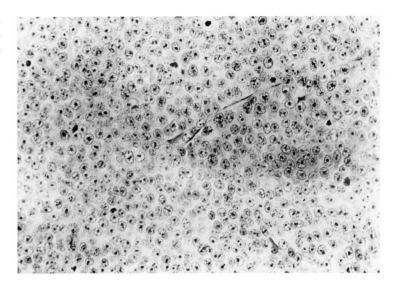

taxel treatment of ovarian tumors with [99m]Tc-
EC-NIM uptake (4.4±0.27 versus 2.8±0.03).
Histopathology findings revealed that extensive necrosis was observed after paclitaxel
treatment (Figures 5.11, 5.12).

Polarographic Oxygen Microelectrode pO₂ Measurements

Intratumoral pO_2 measurements of tumors
indicated the tumor oxygen tension range was
4.6±1.4 mmHg, as compared to normal muscle,
35±10 mmHg. The data indicate that the
tumors are hypoxic.

Example 3: Peptide Imaging of Cancer

Biodistribution and Scintigraphic Studies

^{99m}Tc-EC-glutamic acid pentapeptide (GAP)
was found to be stable at 0.5 to 4 h in dog serum
samples. No degradation products were observed. %ID/g uptake values, tumor/blood,
and tumor/muscle ratios for ^{99m}Tc-EC-GAP
and ^{99m}Tc-EC are given in Tables 5.2 and
5.3. Scintigraphic images obtained at different
time points showed visualization of tumor
in the ^{99m}Tc-EC-GAP group. The optimum
uptake is at 1 to 2 h post administration (Figure
5.13).

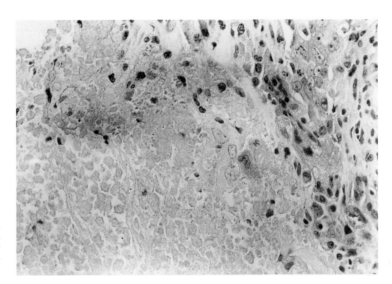

FIGURE 5.12. Histological staining of tumor cells after paclitaxel
treatment showed extensive necrotic tumor cells.

TABLE 5.2. Biodistribution of ^{99m}Tc-EC-GAP (glutamic acid pentapeptide) in tumor-bearing rats.

	Percent of injected ^{99m}Tc-EC-GAP dose per organ or tissue		
	20 min	2 h	4 h
Blood	0.607±0.068	0.220±0.014	0.161±0.012
Lung	0.390±0.045	0.134±0.011	0.105±0.005
Liver	0.787±0.163	0.368±0.025	0.337±0.052
Stomach	0.251±0.033	0.079±0.012	0.068±0.008
Kidney	10.477±0.464	10.644±1.032	9.048±0.506
Thyroid	0.365±0.054	0.121±0.010	0.111±0.007
Muscle	0.090±0.016	0.025±0.004	0.019±0.001
Intestine	0.245±0.083	0.111±0.051	0.237±0.151
Urine	19.235±5.471	13.234±1.311	4.297±0.256
Tumor	0.425±0.046	0.169±0.024	0.144±0.017
Tumor/blood	0.700±0.010	0.758±0.056	0.890±0.042
Tumor/lung	1.091±0.012	1.251±0.087	1.364±0.097
Tumor/muscle	4.873±0.564	6.867±0.821	7.583±0.406

Values represent the mean±standard deviation of data from three animals.

Example 4: Imaging Tumor Apoptotic Cells

Stability Assay of ^{99m}Tc-EC-Annexin

^{99m}Tc-EC-annexin was found to be stable at 0.5, 2, and 4h in dog serum samples. No degradation products were observed.

Scintigraphic Studies

Scintigraphic images obtained at different time points showed visualization of tumor in the ^{99m}Tc-EC-annexin group (Figures 5.14, 5.15). The images indicated that highly apoptotic cells have more uptake of ^{99m}Tc-EC-annexin.

TABLE 5.3. Biodistribution of ^{99m}Tc-EC in breast tumor-bearing rats.

	Percent of injected ^{99m}Tc-EC dose per organ or tissue			
	20 min	1 h	2 h	4 h
Blood	0.435±0.029	0.273±0.039	0.211±0.001	0.149±0.008
Lung	0.272±0.019	0.187±0.029	0.144±0.002	0.120±0.012
Liver	0.508±0.062	0.367±0.006	0.286±0.073	0.234±0.016
Stomach	0.136±0.060	0.127±0.106	0.037±0.027	0.043±0.014
Kidney	7.914±0.896	8.991±0.268	9.116±0.053	7.834±1.018
Thyroid	0.219±0.036	0.229±0.118	0.106±0.003	0.083±0.005
Muscle	0.060±0.006	0.043±0.002	0.028±0.009	0.019±0.001
Intestine	0.173±0.029	0.787±0.106	0.401±0.093	0.103±0.009
Urine	9.124±0.808	11.045±6.158	13.192±4.505	8.693±2.981
Tumor	0.342±0.163	0.149±0.020	0.115±0.002	0.096±0.005
Tumor/blood	0.776±0.322	0.544±0.004	0.546±0.010	0.649±0.005
Tumor/lung	1.256±0.430	0.797±0.022	0.797±0.002	0.798±0.007
Tumor/muscle	5.841±3.253	3.414±0.325	4.425±1.397	5.093±0.223

Values represent the mean±standard deviation of data from three animals.

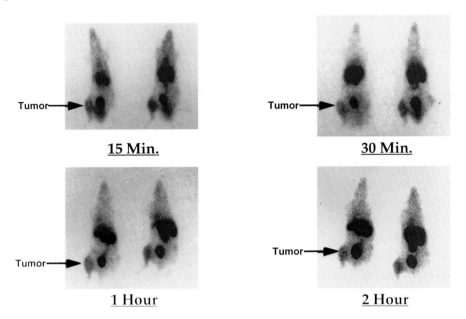

FIGURE 5.13. Whole-body images of breast tumor-bearing rats following intravenous administration of ^{99m}Tc-EC-pentaglutamate (300 μCi/rat) showed the tumors visualized from 15 min to 2h post injection.

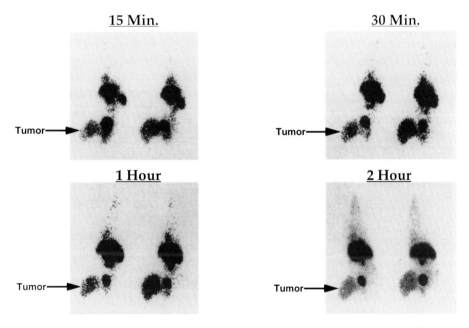

FIGURE 5.14. Whole-body images of breast tumor-bearing rats following administration of ^{99m}Tc-EC-annexin V (300 μCi/rat, i.v.) showed the tumors visualized from 15 min to 2h.

15 Min.   **30 Min.**

1 Hour   **2 Hour**

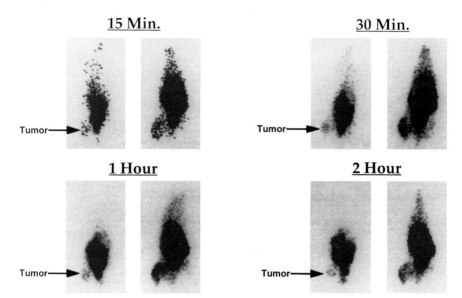

FIGURE 5.15. Whole-body images of ovarian (OCA-1) tumor-bearing mice after administration of ^{99m}Tc-EC (*left*) and ^{99m}Tc-EC-annexin V (*right*) (100 μCi/ mouse, i.v.) demonstrated the tumors clearly visualized from 15 min to 2 h post injection with ^{99m}Tc-EC-annexin V.

Example 5: Imaging Tumor Angiogenesis

Scintigraphic Study of ^{99m}Tc-EC-Colchicine (COL) in Breast Tumor-Bearing Rats

In vivo imaging studies in three breast tumor-bearing rats at 1 h post administration indicated that the tumor could be visualized well with ^{99m}Tc-EC-COL group (Figure 5.16), whereas less tumor uptake in the ^{99m}Tc-EC group was observed. Computer-outlined ROI showed that tumor/background ratios in the ^{99m}Tc-EC-COL group were significantly higher than in the ^{99m}Tc-EC group (Figure 5.17).

Approaches of Tumor-Targeted Imaging

To evaluate the biochemical process and pharmacological response using radiopharmaceuticals, the trends in molecular nuclear medicine have been assessed in the following several fields.

Cell-Cycle Control Imaging

Research on the relationship between intracellular signal transduction, cell cycles, and cell growth is likely to detect specific mechanisms to induce normal cell cycling and apoptosis in tumor cells without damaging normal cells. One approach for nuclear oncology focuses on tyrosine kinase-specific and Ras farnesyltransferase inhibitors for signal transduction in cancer cells. In conjunction, tyrosine kinase inhibitor with chemotherapy should have great potential to be effective in cancer therapeutics.

Natural tyrosine kinase inhibitors such as quercetin, genistein, and erbastatin have low affinity; however, there are several good candidates of tyrosine kinase inhibitors. For instance, the chloro-, bromo- and methyl-analogues of anilinoquinazoline have been developed [12]. These compounds show high affinity (in vitro assay at pM range for EGF tyrosine kinases) and great potency to tyrosine kinases. These compounds rapidly suppressed autophosphorylation of the epidermal growth factor (EGF) receptor at low nanomolar concentration in fibroblasts or in human epidermoid carcinoma cells and selectively blocked EGF-mediated

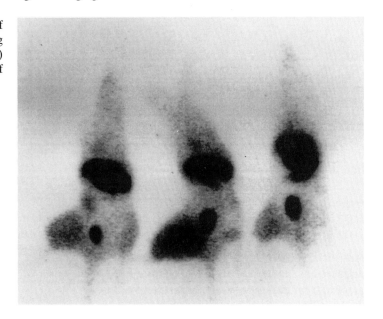

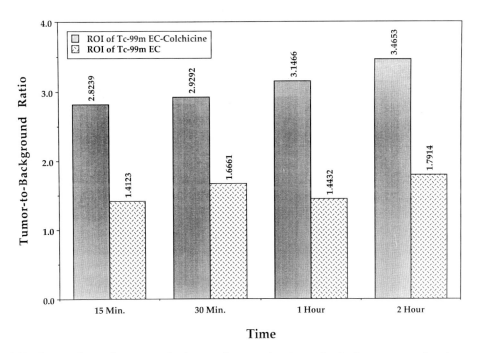

FIGURE 5.17. Comparison of tumor-to-background count density ratios in breast tumor-bearing rats with ^{99m}Tc-EC-colchicine and ^{99m}Tc-EC.

cellular processes including mitogenesis, early gene expression, and morphological transformation.

Increased tyrosine kinase activity is known to be associated with overexpression of oncogenes (e.g., HER-2/neu proto-oncogene in breast cancer). Thus, labeling tyrosine kinase inhibitors would provide a tool for understanding the physiological role of tyrosine phosphorylation in regulating tumor cell proliferation.

Gene- and Nucleic Acid-Based Approach

Advances in determining the genetic basis of diseases has made the concept of gene replacement to treat tumors increasingly attractive. For instance, P53, a key tumor suppressor gene, has proven to be an attractive target for mutation of cancer cells. P53 has been implicated in numerous cancers including breast, colon, and small cell lung cancer. Viral-based gene delivery is the most effective way to transfer genes to cells; however, concerns with immunogenic and long-term oncological effects have increased the need to develop a nonviral gene delivery system. Gene-based cancer diagnostics would offer the potential of predisposition testing, early diagnosis, and a more accurate prognosis. The detailed information is discussed in Chapter 20.

Immunological Approaches

With the exception of prostate-specific antigen (PSA), current in vitro cancer diagnostic products based on immunodiagnostics cannot identify cancer early enough for effective treatment. Therefore, the early detection of tumor antigens remains a competitive market.

Combination of cytokines and antisense have the ability to produce a strong, generalized antitumor response [13,14]. However, the cost of producing antibodies remains prohibitive. To optimize the efficiency of cancer therapy, the future trends of immunotherapy should be antibodies combined with anticancer agents (e.g., cisplatin, paclitaxel, or doxorubicin).

Tumor Angiogenesis, Metastasis, and Vascular Targeted Imaging

Angiogenesis, the proliferation of endothelial and smooth muscle cells to form new blood vessels, is an essential component of the metastatic pathway. These vessels provide the principal route by which tumor cells exit the primary tumor site and enter the circulation. For many tumors, the vascular density can provide a prognostic indicator of metastatic potential, with the highly vascular tumors having a higher incidence of metastasis than poorly vascular tumors [15–17].

Experimental research suggests that it is possible to block angiogenesis by specific inhibitory agents, and that modulation of angiogenic activity is associated with tumor regression in animals with different types of neoplasia. The promising angiosuppressive agents for clinical testing are naturally occurring inhibitors of angiogenesis (e.g., angiostatin, endostatin, platelet factor 4), specific inhibitors of endothelial cell growth (TNP-470, thalidomide, interleukin 12), agents neutralizing angiogenic peptides [antibodies to fibroblast growth factor or vascular endothelial growth factor (VEGF), suramin and analogues, tecogalan] or their receptors, agents that interfere with vascular basement membrane and extracellular matrix (metalloprotease inhibitors, angiostatic steroids), antiadhesion molecules antibodies such as antiintegrin $\alpha v\beta 3$, and miscellaneous drugs that modulate angiogenesis by diverse mechanisms of action [18–22].

The discovery of specific endothelial inhibitors such as angiostatin and endostatin not only increases our understanding of the functions of these molecules in the regulation of physiological and pathological angiogenesis but also provides an important therapeutic strategy for cancer treatment. Endostatin, a carboxyl-terminal fragment of collagen XVIII, has been shown to regress tumors in mice. Treatment of cow pulmonary artery endothelial cells by endostatin caused apoptosis (determined by annexin V-fluorescein isothiocyanate staining, caspase 3, and terminal deoxynucleotidyl transferase-mediated dUTP nick-end-labeling assay). Moreover, addition of endostatin led to a marked reduction of the Bcl-2 and Bcl-XL antiapoptotic protein, whereas Bax protein levels were unaffected. These effects were not seen in several nonendothelial cells. These findings provide important mechanistic insight into endostatin action. Measuring angiogenesis (blood vessel density) or its main regulators such as VEGF and basic fibroblast growth factor (bFGF), or the levels of apoptosis after treatment in solid tumors, provides new and sensitive markers for tumor progression, metastasis, and prognosis [20,23–27].

The identification of tumor-specific regulators of angiogenesis offers new hope. Antiangiogenesis is a strategy for starving tumors by interrupting their blood supply. The tumors are prevented from getting any bigger and even shrink in some cases. Angiogenesis is in part responsible for tumor growth and the development of metastasis. Antimitotic compounds are antiangiogenic and are known for their potential use as anticancer drugs. These compounds inhibit cell division during the mitotic phase of the cell cycle. During the biochemical process of cellular functions, such as cell division, cell motility, secretion, ciliary and flagellar movement, intracellular transport, and the maintenance of cell shape, microtubules are involved. It is known that antimitotic compounds bind with high affinity to microtubule proteins (tubulin), disrupting microtubule assembly and causing mitotic arrest of the proliferating cells. Thus, antimitotic compounds are being considered as microtubule inhibitors or as spindle poisons [28].

Many classes of antimitotic compounds control microtubule assembly and disassembly by binding to tubulin [28–32]. Compounds such as colchicinoids interact with tubulin on the colchicine-binding sites and inhibit microtubule assembly [28–30]. Among colchicinoids, colchicine is an effective antiinflammatory drug used to treat prophylaxis of acute gout. Colchicine also is used in chronic myelocytic leukemia. Although colchicinoids are potent against certain types of tumor growth, the clinical therapeutic potential is limited by the inability to separate the therapeutic and toxic effects [28]. However, colchicine may be useful as a biochemical tool to assess cellular functions.

Drugs such as TNP 470 (AGM-1470), fumagillin, heparin–steroid conjugates, ovalicin, paclitaxel [33], taxotere, and epithilone are small organic molecules that can be labeled with various isotopes. If the tumor uptake of radiolabeled antiangiogenesis agents is related to tumor vascular density, then highly vascular tumors should have more uptake than that in poorly vascular tumors. Higher uptake in tumors could be a prognostic indicator of a higher incidence of tumor metastasis.

Tumor Hypoxia Approach

Tumor cells are more sensitive to conventional radiation in the presence of oxygen than in its absence; even a small percentage of hypoxic cells within a tumor could limit the response to radiation [34–36]. Hypoxic radioresistance has been demonstrated in many animal tumors but only in few tumor types in humans [37–39]. The occurrence of hypoxia in human tumors, in most cases, has been inferred from histology findings and from animal tumor studies. In vivo demonstration of hypoxia requires tissue measurements with oxygen electrodes, and the invasiveness of these techniques has limited their clinical application.

Misonidazole (MISO) is a hypoxic cell sensitizer, and labeling MISO with different radioisotopes (e.g., ^{18}F, ^{123}I, ^{99m}Tc) may be useful for differentiating a hypoxic but metabolically active tumor from a well-oxygenated active tumor by PET or planar scintigraphy. [^{18}F]Fluoromisonidazole (FMISO) has been used with PET to evaluate tumor hypoxia. Recent studies have shown that PET, with its ability to monitor cell oxygen content through [^{18}F]FMISO, has a high potential to predict tumor response to radiation [40–47]. PET gives higher resolution without collimation; however, the cost of using PET isotopes in a clinical setting is prohibitive. Although labeling MISO with iodine was the choice, high uptake in thyroid tissue was observed. Therefore, it is desirable to develop compounds for planar scintigraphy such that the isotope is less expensive and easily available in most major medical facilities.

The assessment of tumor hypoxia by an imaging modality before radiation therapy would provide rational means of selecting patients for treatment with radiosensitizers or bioreductive drugs (e.g., tirapazamine, mitomycin C). Such selection of patients would permit more accurate treatment of patients with hypoxic tumors. It is also possible to select proper modalities of radiotherapy (neutron versus photon) by correlating a labeled tumor hypoxia marker results with tumor to background uptake ratios.

Receptor Targeting Approach

The radiolabeled ligands, such as pentetreotide and vasoactive intestinal peptide, bind to cell receptors, some of which are overexpressed on tumor cells [48–52]. Because these ligands are not immunogenic and are cleared quickly from the plasma, receptor imaging would seem to be more promising compared to antibody imaging.

Folic acid as well as antifolates such as methotrexate enter into cells via high-affinity folate receptors (glycosylphosphatidylinositol-linked membrane folate-binding protein) in addition to the classical reduced folate carrier system [53–55]. Folate receptors (FRs) are overexpressed on many neoplastic cell types (e.g., lung, breast, ovarian, cervical, colorectal, nasopharyngeal, renal adenocarcinomas, malign melanoma, and ependymomas), but are primarily expressed only in several normal differentiated tissues (e.g., choroid plexus, placenta, thyroid, and kidney) [54,56–62]. FRs have been used to deliver folate-conjugated protein toxins, drug/antisense oligonucleotides, and liposomes into tumor cells overexpressing the folate receptors [63–68]. Furthermore, bi-specific antibodies that contain anti-FR antibodies linked to anti-T-cell receptor antibodies have been used to target T cells to FR-positive tumor cells and are currently in clinical trials for ovarian carcinomas [69–73]. Similarly, this property has been inspired to develop radiolabeled folate conjugates, such as ^{67}Ga-deferoxamine-folate and ^{111}In-DTPA-folate for imaging of folate receptor-positive tumors

[74–77]. Results of limited in vitro and in vivo studies with these agents suggest that folate receptors could be a potential target for tumor imaging. Assessment of tumor folate receptors with labeled folate receptor ligands before chemotherapy would provide rational means of selecting patients for treatment with methotrexate or tomudex. Such selection of patients would permit more accurate evaluation of antifolates, because their use is limited to the patients with folate receptor overexpression who could potentially benefit from the drug.

Thymidylate Synthase and Lipid Metabolic Imaging

Thymidylate synthase (TS) is a crucial enzyme that catalyzes the reductive methylation of dUMP to dTMP. Inhibition of TS activity would lead to thymine-less death. Thus, diagnosis of TS activity has been an attractive goal for the development of antitumor agents. The antifolate proparyl dideaza folate (PDDF) is a classical inhibitor of TS at nanomolar concentration with antitumor activity [78] and may have potential use in imaging TS activity.

Choline is a small molecule that is a fragment of phosphotidyl choline. Both [18]F- and ^{11}C-choline demonstrate tumor imaging potential superior to that of PET-FDG [79].

Multidrug Resistance Markers

Diphosphine analogues were labeled with Cu-64 and demonstrated to be a P-glycoprotein substrate. Drugs such as verapamil, cholchicin, and cyclosporin A are P-glycoprotein substrates [80] that can be considered to tag with isotopes for multidrug resistance (MDR) imaging.

Peptide Imaging of Cancer

Peptides and amino acids have been successfully used in imaging of various types of tumors [81–90]. Glutamic acid-based peptide has been used as a drug carrier for cancer treatment [86–90]. It is known that the glutamate moiety of folate degraded and formed polyglutamate in vivo. The polyglutamate is then reconjugated to folate to form folyl polyglutamate, which is involved in glucose metabolism. Labeling glutamic acid peptide may be useful in differentiating the malignancy of the tumors. In this report, we evaluate ^{99m}Tc-EC-glutamic acid pentapeptide for its potential use in imaging tumors. Our data indicated ^{99m}Tc-EC-glutamic acid pentapeptide may be a promising candidate to image lung tumors. Because high uptake of amino acid is observed in viable tumor cells [81,82] imaging tumors using peptide may be able to differentiate the malignancy of the tumors.

Imaging Tumor Apoptotic Cells

Apoptosis occurs during the treatment of cancer with chemotherapy and radiation [91–95]. Annexin V is known to bind to phosphotidylserin, which is overexpressed by tumor apoptotic cells [94,95]. Assessment of apoptosis by annexin V would be useful to evaluate the efficacy of therapy such as disease progression or regression.

Conclusion

In conclusion, the ^{99m}Tc-EC-drug conjugates show potential application in molecular targeted imaging in oncology.

References

1. Brock CS, Meikle SR, Price P. Does ^{18}F-fluorodeoxyglucose metabolic imaging of tumors benefit oncology? Eur J Nucl Med 1997;24:691–705.
2. Goldsmith SJ. Receptor imaging: competitive or complementary to antibody imaging. Semin Nucl Med 1997;27:85–93.
3. Mathias CJ, Hubers D, Trump DP, et al. Synthesis of ^{99m}Tc-DTPA-folate and preliminary evaluation as a folate-receptor-targeted radiopharmaceutical. J Nucl Med 1997;38:87P (abstract).
4. Davison A, Jones AG, Orvig C, et al. A new class of oxotechnetium (+5) chelate complexes containing a TcO N_2S_2 core. Inorg Chem 1980; 20:1629–1632.
5. Verbruggen AM, Nosco DL, Van Nerom CG, et al. ^{99m}Tc-L,L-ethylenedicysteine: a renal imaging agent. I. Labeling and evaluation in animals. J Nucl Med 1992;33:551–557.
6. Van Nerom CG, Bormans GM, De Roo MJ, et al. First experience in healthy volunteers with ^{99m}Tc-L,L-ethylenedicysteine, a new renal imaging agent. Eur J Nucl Med 1993;20:738–746.
7. Surma MJ, Wiewiora J, Liniecki J. Usefulness of ^{99m}Tc-N,N'-ethylene-1-dicysteine complex for dynamic kidney investigations. Nucl Med Commun 1994;15:628–635.
8. Moran JK. ^{99m}Tc-EC and other potential new agents in renal nuclear medicine. Semin Nucl Med 1999;29:91–101.
9. Ugur O, Serdengecti M, Karacalioglu O, et al. Comparison of ^{99m}Tc-EC and ^{99m}Tc-DTPA captopril scintigraphy to diagnose renal artery stenosis. Clin Nucl Med 1999;24:553–560.
10. Ilgan S, Yang DJ, Higuchi T, et al. ^{99m}Tc-ethylenedicysteine-folate: a new tumor imaging agent. Synthesis, labeling and evaluation in animals. Cancer Biother Radiopharm 1998;13:427–435.
11. Zareneyrizi F, Yang DJ, Oh C-S, et al. Synthesis of ^{99m}Tc-ethylenedicysteine-colchicine for evaluation of antiangiogenic effect. Anti-Cancer Drugs 1999;10:685–692.
12. Fry DW, Nelson JM, Slintak V, et al. Biochemical and antiproliferative properties of 4-[ar(alk)ylamino]pyridopyrimidines, a new chemical class of potent and specific epidermal growth factor receptor tyrosine kinase inhibitor. Biochem Pharmacol 1997;54:877–887.
13. Yang SC, Fry KD, Grimm EA, et al. Successful combination immunotherapy for the generation in vivo of antitumor activity with anti-CD3, interleukin 2, and tumor necrosis factor alpha. Arch Surg 1990;125:220–225.
14. Miyake H, Tolcher A, Gleave ME. Antisense Bcl-2 oligodeoxynucleotides inhibit progression to androgen-independence after castration in the Shionogi tumor model. Cancer Res 1999; 59:4030–4034.
15. Bertolini F, Paolucci M, Peccatori F, et al. Angiogenic growth factors and endostatin in non-Hodgkin's lymphoma. Br J Haematol 1999; 106(2):504–509.
16. Gasparini G. The rationale and future potential of angiogenesis inhibitors in neoplasia. Drugs 1999;58(1):17–38.
17. Cao Y. Therapeutic potentials of angiostatin in the treatment of cancer. Haematologica 1999; 84(7):643–650.

18. Yamaguchi N, Anand-Apte B, Lee M, et al. Endostatin inhibits VEGF-induced endothelial cell migration and tumor growth independently of zinc binding. EMBO J 1999;18:4414–4423.

19. Bergers G, Javaherian K, Lo KM, et al. Effects of angiogenesis inhibitors on multistage carcinogenesis in mice. Science 1999;284(5415):808–812.

20. Dhanabal M, Ramchandran R, Waterman MJ, et al. Endostatin induces endothelial cell apoptosis. J Biol Chem 1999;274(17):11721–11726.

21. Harris AL. Anti-angiogenesis therapy and strategies for integrating it with adjuvant therapy. Recent Results Cancer Res 1998;152:341–352.

22. Moulton KS, Heller E, Konerding MA, et al. Angiogenesis inhibitors endostatin or TNP-470 reduce intimal neovascularization and plaque growth in apolipoprotein E-deficient mice. Circulation 1999;99(13):1726–1732.

23. Ramchandran R, Dhanabal M, Volk R, et al. Antiangiogenic activity of restin, NC10 domain of human collagen XV: comparison to endostatin. Biochem Biophys Res Commun 1999; 255(3):735–739.

24. Szabo S, Sandor Z. The diagnostic and prognostic value of tumor angiogenesis. Eur J Surg Suppl 1998;582:99–103.

25. O'Reilly MS, Boehm T, Shing Y, et al. Endostatin: an endogenous inhibitor of angiogenesis and tumor growth. Cell 1997;88(2):277–285.

26. Gibaldi M. Regulating angiogenesis: a new therapeutic strategy. J Clin Pharmacol 1998;38(10): 898–903.

27. Zetter BR. Angiogenesis and tumor metastasis. Annu Rev Med 1998;49:407–424.

28. Lu MC. Antimitotic agents. In: Foye WO, ed. Cancer Chemotherapeutic Agents. Washington, DC: American Chemical Society 1995;345–368.

29. Goh EL, Pircher TJ, Lobie PE. Growth hormone promotion of tubulin polymerization stabilizes the microtubule network and protects against colchicine-induced apoptosis. Endocrinology 1998;139:4364–4372.

30. Wang TH, Wang HS, Ichijo H, et al. Microtubule-interfering agents activate c-Jun N-terminal kinase/stress-activated protein kinase through both Ras and apoptosis signal-regulating kinase pathways. J Biol Chem 1998;273:4928–4936.

31. Rowinsky EK, Cazenave LA, Donehower RC. Taxol: a novel investigational antimicrotubule agent. J Natl Cancer Inst 1990;82(15):1247–1259.

32. Imbert TF. Discovery of podophyllotoxins. Biochimie (Paris) 1998;80:207–222.

33. Inoue T, Li C, Yang DJ, et al. Evaluation of ^{111}In-DTPA-paclitaxel scintigraphy to predict response on murine tumors to paclitaxel. Ann Nucl Med 1999;13(3):169–174.

34. Hall J. The oxygen effect and reoxygenation. In: Hall EJ, ed. Radiobiology for the Radiobiologist. Philadelphia: J Lippincott, 1988:137–160.

35. Bush S, Jenkins RDT, Allt WEC, et al. Definitive evidence for hypoxic cells influencing cure in cancer therapy. Br J Cancer 1978;37:302–306.

36. Gray H, Conger AD, Elbert M, et al. The concentration of oxygen dissolved in tissues at the time of irradiation as a factor in radiotherapy. Br J Radiol 1953;26:638–648.

37. Dische S. A review of hypoxic-cell radiosensitization. Int J Radiat Oncol Biol Phys 1991;20: 147–152.

38. Gatenby A, Kessler HB, Rosenblum JS, et al. Oxygen distribution in squamous cell carcinoma metastases and its relationship to outcome of radiation therapy. Int J Radiat Oncol Biol Phys 1988;14:831–838.

39. Nordsmark M. Overgaard M, Overgaard J. Pretreatment oxygenation predicts radiation response in advanced squamous cell carcinoma of the head and neck. Radiother Oncol 1996;41: 31–39.

40. Koh W-J, Rasey JS, Evans ML, et al. Imaging of hypoxia in human tumors with ^{18}F-fluoromisonidazole. Int J Radiat Oncol Biol Phys 1992;22:199–212.

41. Valk ET, Mathis CA, Prados MD, et al. Hypoxia in human gliomas: demonstration by PET with [^{18}F]fluoromisonidazole. J Nucl Med 1992;33: 2133–2137.

42. Martin V, Caldwell JH, Rasey JS, et al. Enhanced binding of the hypoxic cell marker [^{18}F]fluoromisonidazole in ischemic myocardium. J Nucl Med 1989;30:194–201.

43. Rasey S, Nelson NJ, Chin L, et al. Characterization of the binding of labeled fluoromisonidazole in cells in vitro. Radiat Res 1990;122:301–308.

44. Yang J, Wallace S, Cherif A, et al. Development of F-18-labeled fluoroerythronitroimidazole as a PET agent for imaging tumor hypoxia. Radiology 1995;194:795–800.

45. Rasey S, Koh WJ, Grieson JR, et al. Radiolabeled fluoromisonidazole as an imaging agent for tumor hypoxia. Int J Radiat Oncol Biol Phys 1989;17:985–991.

46. Hay MP, Wilson WR, Moselen JW, et al. Hypoxia-selective antitumor agents. Bis(nitroimidazolyl)alkanecarboxamides: a new class of

hypoxia-selective cytotoxins and hypoxic cell radiosensitizers. J Med Chem 1994;37:381–391.

47. Cherif A, Yang DJ, Tansey W, et al. Synthesis of [^{18}F]fluoromisonidazole. Pharm Res (NY) 1994;11:466–469.

48. Britton KE, Granowska M. Imaging of Tumors, in Tomography in Nuclear Medicine. Proceedings of an International Symposium. Vienna: IAEA, 1996:91–105.

49. Krenning EP, Kwekkeboom DJ, Bakker WH, et al. Somatostatin receptor scintigraphy with ^{111}In-DTPA-D-Phe and ^{123}I-Tyr-octretide: the Rotterdam experience with more than 1000 patients. Eur J Nucl Med 1995;7:716–731.

50. Reubi JC, Krenning EP, Lamberts SWJ, et al. In vitro detection of somatostatin receptors in human tumors. Metabolism 1992;41:104–110.

51. Goldsmith SJ, Macapinlac H, O'Brien JP. Somatostatin receptor imaging in lymphoma. Semin Nucl Med 1995;25:262–271.

52. Virgolini I, Raderer M, Kurtaran A. Vasoactive intestinal peptide (VIP) receptor imaging in the localization of intestinal adenocarcinomas and endocrine tumors. N Engl J Med 1994;331:1116–1121.

53. Westerhof GR, Jansen G, Emmerik NV, et al. Membrane transport of natural folates and antifolate compounds in murine L1210 leukemia cells: role of carrier- and receptor-mediated transport systems. Cancer Res 1991;51:5507–5513.

54. Orr RB, Kreisler AR, Kamen BA. Similarity of folate receptor expression in UMSCC 38 cells to squamous cell carcinoma differentiation markers. J Natl Cancer Inst 1995;87:299–303.

55. Hsueh CT, Dolnick BJ. Altered folate-binding protein mRNA stability in KB cells grown in folate-deficient medium. Biochem Pharmacol 1993;45:2537–2545.

56. Weitman SD, Lark RH, Coney LR, et al. Distribution of folate GP38 in normal and malignant cell lines and tissues. Cancer Res 1992;52:3396–3400.

57. Campbell IG, Jones TA, Foulkes WD, Trowsdale J. Folate-binding protein is a marker for ovarian cancer. Cancer Res 1991;51:5329–5338.

58. Weitman SD, Weinberg AG, Coney LR, et al. Cellular localization of the folate receptor: potential role in drug toxicity and folate homeostasis. Cancer Res 1992;52:6708–6711.

59. Holm J, Hansen SI, Hoier-Madsen M, et al. Folate receptor of human mammary adenocarcinoma. APMIS 1994;102:413–419.

60. Ross JF, Chaudhuri PK, Ratnam M. Differential regulation of folate receptor isoforms in normal and malignant tissue in vivo and in established cell lines. Cancer (Phila) 1994;73:2432–2443.

61. Franklin WA, Waintrub M, Edwards D, et al. New anti-lung-cancer antibody cluster 12 reacts with human folate receptors present on adenocarcinoma. Int J Cancer Suppl 1994;8:89–95.

62. Weitman SD, Frazier KM, Kamen BA. The folate receptor in central nervous system malignancies of childhood. J Neuro-Oncol 1994;21:107–112.

63. Ginobbi P, Geiser TA, Ombres D, et al. Folic acid-polylysine carrier improves efficacy of c-myc antisense oligonucleotides on human melanoma (M14) cells. Anticancer Res 1997;17:29–35.

64. Leamon CP, Low PS. Delivery of macromolecules into living cells: a method that exploits folate receptor endocytosis. Proc Natl Acad Sci USA 1991;88:5572–5576.

65. Leamon CP, Low PS. Cytotoxicity of momordin-folate conjugates in cultured human cells. J Biol Chem 1992;267:24966–24971.

66. Leamon CP, Pastan I, Low PS. Cytotoxicity of folate-pseudomonas exotoxin conjugates toward tumor cells. J Biol Chem 1993;268:24847–24854.

67. Lee RJ, Low PS. Delivery of liposomes into cultured KB cells via folate receptor-mediated endocytosis. J Biol Chem 1994;269:3198–3204.

68. Wang S, Lee RJ, Cauchon G, et al. Delivery of antisense oligodeoxyribonucleotides against the human epidermal growth factor receptor into cultured KB cells with liposomes conjugated to folate via polyethylene glycol. Proc Natl Acad Sci USA 1995;92:3318–3322.

69. Canevari S, Miotti S, Bottero F, et al. Ovarian carcinoma therapy with monoclonal antibodies. Hybridoma 1993;12:501–507.

70. Bolhuis RLH, Lamers CHJ, Goey HS, et al. Adoptive immunotherapy of ovarian carcinoma with Bs-MAb targeted lymphocytes. A multicenter study. Int J Cancer 1992;7:78–81.

71. Patrick TA, Kranz DM, van Dyke TA, et al. Folate receptors as potential therapeutic targets in choroid plexus tumors of SV40 transgenic mice. J Neuro-Oncol 1997;32:111–123.

72. Coney LR, Mezzanzanica D, Sanborn D, et al. Chimeric murine-human antibodies directed against folate binding receptor are efficient mediators of ovarian carcinoma cell killing. Cancer Res 1994;54:2448–2455.

73. Kranz DM, Patrick TA, Brigle KE, et al. Conjugates of folate and anti-T-cell-receptor antibod-

ies specifically target folate-receptor-positive tumor cells for lysis. Proc Natl Acad Sci USA 1995;92:9057–9061.

74. Mathias CJ, Wang S, Lee RJ, et al. Tumor-selective radiopharmaceutical targeting via receptor-mediated endocytosis of ^{67}Ga-deferoxamine-folate. J Nucl Med 1996;37:1003–1008.

75. Wang S, Luo J, Lantrip DA, et al. Design and synthesis of [^{111}In]DTPA-folate for use as a tumor-targeted radiopharmaceutical. Bioconjugate Chem 1997;8:673–679.

76. Wang S, Lee RJ, Mathias CJ, et al. Synthesis, purification, and tumor cell uptake of ^{67}Ga-deferoxamine-folate, a potential radiopharmaceutical for tumor imaging. Bioconjugate Chem 1996;7:56–62.

77. Mathias CJ, Wang S, Waters DJ, et al. ^{111}In-DTPA-folate as a radiopharmaceutical for targeting tumor-associated folate binding protein. J Nucl Med 1997;38:133P (abstract).

78. Gangjee A, Mavandadi F, Kisliuk RL, et al. 2-Amino-4-oxo-5-substituted-pyrrolo[2,3-d]-pyrimidines as nonclassical antifolate inhibitors of thymidylate synthase. J Med Chem 1996;39:4563–4568.

79. Hara T, Kosaka N, Kishi H, et al. PET imaging of prostate cancer using ^{11}C-choline. J Nucl Med 1998;39:990–995.

80. Demeule M, Laplante A, Sepehr-Arae A, et al. Inhibition of P-glycoprotein by cyclosporin A analogues and metabolites. Biochem Cell Biol 1999;77:47–58.

81. Wester HJ, Herz M, Weber W, et al. Synthesis and radiopharmacology of O(2-[^{18}F]fluoroethyl)-L-tyrosine for tumor imaging. J Nucl Med 1999;40:205–212.

82. Coenen HH, Stöcklin G. Evaluation of radiohalogenated amino acid analogues as potential tracers for PET and SPECT studies of protein synthesis. Radioisot Klin Forsch 1988;18:402–440.

83. Raderer M, Becherer A, Kurtaran A, et al. Comparison of iodine-123-vasoactive intestinal peptide receptor scintigraphy and ^{111}In-CFT-102 immunoscintigraphy. J Nucl Med 1996;37:1480–1487.

84. Lambert SW, Bakker WH, Reubi JC, et al. Somatostatin receptor imaging in vivo localiza-tion of tumors with a radiolabeled somatostatin analog. J Steroid Biochem Mol Biol 1990;37:1079–1082.

85. Bakker WH, Krenning EP, Breeman WA, et al. Receptor scintigraphy with a radioiodinated somatostatin analogue: radiolabeling, purification, biologic activity and in vivo application in animals. J Nucl Med 1990;31:1501–1509.

86. Stella VJ, Mathew AE. Derivatives of taxol, pharmaceutical compositions thereof and methods for preparation thereof. United States Patent 1990;4,960,790; October 2.

87. Butterfield DE, Fuji DK, Ladd DL, et al. Segmented chelating polymers as imaging and therapeutic agents. United States Patent 1998;5,730,968; March 24.

88. Piper JR, McCaleb GS, Montgomery JA. A synthetic approach to poly(glutamyl) conjugates of methotrexate. J Med Chem 1983;26:291–294.

89. Mochizuki E, Inaki Y, Takemoto K. Synthesis of polyglutamates containing 5-substituted uracil moieties. Nucleic Acids Res 1985;16:121–124.

90. Dickinson HR, Hiltner A. Biodegradation of poly(α-amino acid) hydrogel. II. In vitro. J Biomed Mater Res 1981;15:591.

91. Lennon SV, Martin SJ, Cotter TG. Dose-dependent induction of apoptosis in human tumor cell lines by widely diverging stimuli. Cell Prolif 1991;24:203–214.

92. Abrams MJ, Juweid M, Tenkate CI. ^{99m}Tc-human polyclonal IgG radiolabeled via the hydrazino nicotinamide derivative for imaging focal sites of infection in rats. J Nucl Med 1990;31:2022–2028.

93. Blankenberg FG, Katsikis PD, Tait JF, et al. In vivo detection and imaging of phosphatidylserine expression during programmed cell death. Proc Natl Acad Sci USA 1998;95:6349–6354.

94. Blankenberg FG, Katsikis PD, Tait JF, et al. Imaging of apoptosis (programmed cell death) with ^{99m}Tc annexin V. J Nucl Med 1999;40:184–191.

95. Tait JF, Smith C. Site-specific mutagenesis of annexin V: role of residues from Arg-200 to Lys-207 in phospholipid binding. Arch Biochem Biophys 1991;288:141–144.

6
Antibodies for Targeted Imaging: Properties and Radiolabeling

Noboru Oriuchi and David J. Yang

Radioimmunodetection has shown great promise as a means of whole-body imaging in patients with various malignant neoplasms. Specificity of the antibody to antigen is a distinguished property of this method. Antibodies used for imaging are being applied for radioimmunotherapy, although effective treatment of solid tumors is still difficult. Recent advances in biotechnology have made possible the production of human antibodies and could prevent immune response. In this chapter, characteristics of antibodies and their fragments and radiolabeling for radioimmunodetection are briefly summarized.

Properties of Antibodies

Antibodies consist of five types of immunoglobulin: IgG, IgM, IgA, IgE, and IgD. They bind specifically to epitopes of antigen in the foreign substance, followed by the activation of complement system. They remove foreign substances by phagocytosis and cell lysis. Therefore, antibodies themselves work as a humoral immunity and also induce chemotaxis to promote immune cells to attack invaders (cell immunity). IgG is the most common type of antibody. It consists of four components: two heavy chains, each of which weighs about 50,000 daltons, and two light chains, each weighing about 23,000 daltons. The heavy chains and the light chains are joined by disulfide bonds. IgG is functionally made up of a constant region (Fc) and a variable region (Fab). The

amino acid sequence of the Fc region is similar from one IgG to another. Fab regions determine specificity and affinity for antigen. Specificity is the ability of the antibody to bind selectively to a specific antigen. Antigen–antibody binding is tight, and a tiny difference in the structure of the antigen markedly decreases the tightness of the binding. Affinity is an index of tightness of the antibody binding to the specific antigen. Both specificity and affinity are important factors in radioimmunodetection and radioimmunotherapy.

The first application of radioiodinated polyclonal antisera was reported more than half a century ago by Pressman and Keighley [1]. Antitumor heterosera were used in the 1950s; however, radiolabeled polyclonal antibodies were accumulated in nontumor tissue, and imaging of the tumor was not significantly successful. However, clinical application of ^{131}I-labeled anti-CEA antibodies demonstrated a limited detectability in relatively large tumors [2,3].

A monoclonal antibody is produced from a hybridoma, which is a cell myeloma and B lymphocyte fused [4]. The malignant mouse myeloma cell cannot produce its own antibody, but it can be grown. The B lymphocyte is immunized by the specific antigen against which the desired antibody is to be developed. Hybridoma cells are continuously replicated and produce large quantities of an antibody. They can be grown by in vitro techniques for industrial production. The screening process to obtain a good clone is tedious and takes a long time. Recently, the phage library technique has been used for production of monoclonal antibodies. Monoclonal antibodies were used for the imaging to improve detectability because monoclonal antibodies are relatively more specific for the target and effective targeting would be expected. The first use of radiolabeled monoclonal antibodies was reported by Mach in 1981 [5]. He detected 50% of the lesions using ^{131}I-labeled anti-CEA antibody, and single photon emission computed tomography (SPECT) improved detectability. Recently, anti-CD20 monoclonal antibodies have been used to treat low-grade non-Hodgkin's lymphoma [6–10]. The results showed that anti-CD20 antibody is safe and efficacious when combined with systemic chemotherapy in treatment of indolent B-cell lymphoma. The choice of antibody is of utmost importance because the affinity and specificity of the antibody determine the tightness of antigen–antibody binding and the extent of nonspecific binding to nontarget organs.

An IgG molecule can be split by enzymatic digestion. Digestion with pepsin and papain produces $F(ab')_2$ and Fab, respectively. Two Fab' fragments are produced by splitting disulfide bonds with a reducing agent. A $F(ab')_2$ is less stable than an intact antibody. A Fab has only a single binding site (monovalent), and affinity is therefore lower than divalent molecules (Table 6.1). Recent technical advancements have made possible production of Fab fragments and single-chain Fv (scFv) fragments by *E. coli* [11].

Disulfide-bonded Fv anti-Tac monoclonal antibody (dsFv) is a genetically engineered antibody fragment. This antibody fragment penetrates tumors much faster and shows more uniform distribution than intact IgG, thereby minimizing the development of human antimurine antibody (HAMA) response. Biodistribution of this antibody labeled with ^{125}I, ^{18}F, and ^{99m}Tc-MAG$_3$ in tumor-bearing animal models showed high tumor-to-blood and tumor-to-tissue ratios [12–14]. These high uptake ratios enable radiolabeled dsFv to detect tumors that express IL-2 alpha receptors.

Kinetics of Antibodies

Distribution of antibodies within the body varies according to several factors. Disappearance of an antibody from the vascular compartment depends on the size of the fragment. Compared with the intact antibodies, fragments undergo a faster disappearance from the circulation. Renal excretion of the antibody fragments increases as the molecular weight decreases. Fab and scFv are small enough to be cleared quickly by the kidneys to reduce background radioactivity. Fragments can penetrate into a tumor faster, but their affinity to antigen is lower than intact antibody. Therefore, the peak tumor uptake of fragments is lower, but the lesion-to-background ratio is higher than intact antibody. From the clinical point of view, interaction of cells and molecules in the circulation can cause changes in pharmacokinetics and biodistribution of monoclonal antibodies [15].

Human Antimurine Antibody

Most monoclonal antibodies currently used for imaging are of mouse origin. Immune response can be evoked after administration of murine antibody, and HAMA is produced depending on the amount and species of antibody. Fragments cause less immune response. If HAMA is produced in patients, repeated use of mouse antibodies can cause changes in pharmacokinetics and adverse reaction [16]. To overcome these problems, chimeric and human antibodies

TABLE 6.1. Characteristics of antibody and fragments.

	MW (kDa)	Valence	Affinity	Blood clearance
IgG	150	Divalent	high	Slow
$F(ab')_2$	100	Divalent	high	
$F(ab')$	50	Monovalent	low	
Fab	50	Monovalent	low	
scFv	23	Monovalent	low	Fast

have been introduced. They are produced by genetic engineering and are being evaluated in clinical settings [17].

Radiolabeling of Antibodies

Iodine-131 is a radionuclide that has been used for immunoscintigraphy because ^{131}I can be labeled easily with antibodies and labeling efficiency is acceptable. Radioiodination is classified as follows: isotopic exchange, nucleophilic aromatic substitution, addition to double bonds, demetallization, and conjugation labeling. Isotopic exchange is the preparation method for many radioiodinated compounds: ^{123}I-IMP, ^{131}I-OIH, ^{131}I-MIBG, etc. Because the exchange of radioiodine for the stable iodine atom is proportional to the molar ratio of the substrate and the radioiodine, higher radiochemical yield can be achieved in exchange for lower specific activity. This labeling is suitable for many tracers for imaging when very high specific activity is not required. Electrophilic aromatic substitution is one of the best methods for radioiodination. This method is suitable for labeling monoclonal antibodies because the reactions are under mild conditions and provide high yields and efficiency. Mild oxidants such as chloramine-T, hydrogen peroxide, and lactoperoxidase are used for this reaction [18–20]. Iodine-131 has beta emission and therefore is utilized for radioimmunotherapy. The major drawbacks of ^{131}I as a radiotracer for imaging are as follows: (1) the radiation exposure is higher than with other radionuclides; (2) half-life is longer than of others; and (3) the energy of gamma rays is too high to take images of good resolution using a gamma camera. Deiodination of labeled antibodies is an inevitable characteristic of this radionuclide [21]. Iodine-123 is preferable to ^{131}I because it is suitable for imaging and radiation exposure is approximately one-third that of ^{131}I because it has no beta emission. The high production costs limit its use for routine clinical applications.

Indium-111 is widely used for radioimmunodetection. Its binding to the monoclonal antibody is easy and stable via chelates. Indium-111-labeled antibodies are suitable for imaging instead of their high uptake in the liver. The radionuclide has optimal half-life (2.8 days) for imaging with antibodies. Because direct labeling with metallic radionuclides is difficult, most metal ions need a chelating agent to be attached to the protein. Chelating agents can be covalently conjugated to the protein via bifunctional chelating agents and form a stable radionuclide–chelate protein complex. The complex must be stable in the body because instability results in high radioactivity in the nontarget organs. The bifunctional chelating agents used in the beginning are polyamino carboxylic acids, derivatives of EDTA and DTPA [22]. Macrocyclic bifunctional chelating agents—NOTA, DOTA, and TETA—have been used for conjugation to proteins [23]. They achieve sufficient stability because the nitrogen atoms and the negatively changed carboxylate oxygens favor the rate of complexation to positively charged metal ions.

Technetium-99m is an ideal radionuclide for imaging. It has excellent physical properties ($T_{1/2}$, 6.02 h; gamma emission, 140 keV) and low radiation exposure. Because of the generator production, it is easily available and inexpensive. Pertechnetate ($^{99m}TcO_4$) itself cannot bind directly to ligand. Stannous ion is mainly used as a reductant for labeling many radiopharmaceuticals for clinical use. Labeling antibodies with ^{99m}Tc involves indirect methods and direct methods. The former uses a chelator, which attaches initially to the antibody and subsequently binds the ^{99m}Tc. The latter method uses a thiol, such as 2-mercaptoethanol, which reduces disulfide bonds in the antibodies and can be stored in the freezer. Technetium labeling is then performed occasionally. Simple and stable labeling of antibodies with ^{99m}Tc can be performed by direct labeling [24]. The disadvantage of ^{99m}Tc-labeled antibodies is the short physical half-life of ^{99m}Tc relative to long biological half-life of intact antibodies. ^{99m}Tc-labeled antibodies make it possible to achieve SPECT, because a high dose can be administered to patients. The use of SPECT helps to detect lesions, even if the renal uptake of ^{99m}Tc-labeled antibody may obscure lesions in that area of the abdomen [25].

Because of the instability of ^{131}I-labeled immunoconjugates, [186]Re may be a better choice for radioimmunotherapy (RIT). The half-life of [186]Re is 3.7 days, and it has 9% gamma emission, 71% beta emission of 1.07 MeV, and 21% beta emission of 0.94 MeV. Labeling antibodies with [186]Re for RIT of cancer has been investigated [26].

Conclusion

Antibodies are not absolutely specific to the tumor target, and false-positive results are unavoidable. The sensitivity of this method is low when the lesion is very small. Gamma camera imaging has less spatial resolution than CT and MRI. Immunological reactions including allergy may occur if murine antibodies are used. Production of HAMA limits the repeated use of antibodies. However, immunoscintigraphy is more specific to the lesion than other imaging modalities. It has a complementary role in tumor detection and is advantageous for differentiating tumor recurrence from post-treatment changes.

Radioimmunotherapy has been used in clinical settings and will be developed further as a tumor-specific therapy with fewer side effects. Genetic engineering makes it possible to use phage libraries, which can produce human antibodies against virtually any antigen in vitro. The more tumor-specific antibodies will be produced, and combined application by coupling of cytotoxic drugs, cytokines, and toxins should be used to acquire effective radioimmunotherapy.

References

1. Pressman D, Keighley G. The zone of activity of antibodies as determined by the use of radioactive tracers: the zone of activity of nephrotoxic anti-kidney serum. J Immunol 1948;59:141.
2. Goldenberg DM, DeLand F, Kim E, et al. Use of radiolabeled antibodies to carcinoembryonic antigen for the detection and localization of diverse cancers by external photoscanning. N Engl J Med 1978;298:1384–1388.
3. Mach JP, Carrel S, Forni M, et al. Tumor localization of radiolabeled antibodies against carcinoembryonic antigen in patients with carcinoma: a critical evaluation. N Engl J Med 1980;303:5–10.
4. Kohler GP, Milstein C. Continuous cultures of fused cells secreting antibody of predetermined specificity. Nature (Lond) 1975;256:495–497.
5. Mach JP, Buchegger F, Forni M. Use of radiolabeled monoclonal anti-CEA antibodies for the detection of human carcinomas by external photoscanning and tomoscintigraphy. Immunol Today 1981;2:239–249.
6. Piro LD, White CA, Grillo-Lopez AJ, et al. Extended Rituximab (anti-CD20 monoclonal antibody) therapy for relapsed or refractory low-grade or follicular non-Hodgkin's lymphoma. Ann Oncol 1999;10(6):655–661.
7. Berinstein NL, Grillo-Lopez AJ, White CA, et al. Association of serum Rituximab (IDEC-C2B8) concentration and anti-tumor response in the treatment of recurrent low-grade or follicular non-Hodgkin's lymphoma. Ann Oncol 1998;9(9):995–1001.
8. Grillo-Lopez AJ, White CA, Varns C, et al. Overview of the clinical development of rituximab: first monoclonal antibody approved for the treatment of lymphoma. Semin Oncol 1999;26:66–73.
9. Czuczman MS, Grillo-Lopez AJ, White CA, et al. Treatment of patients with low-grade B-cell lymphoma with the combination of chimeric anti-CD20 monoclonal antibody and CHOP chemotherapy. J Clin Oncol 1999;17(1):268–276.
10. Witzig TE, White CA, Wiseman GA, et al. Phase I/II trial of IDEC-Y2B8 radioimmunotherapy for treatment of relapsed or refractory CD20(+) B-cell non-Hodgkin's lymphoma. J Clin Oncol 1999;17(12):3793–3803.
11. Hoogenboom HR, Marks JD, Griffiths AD, et al. Building antibodies from their genes. Immunol Rev 1992;130:41–68.
12. Yoo TM, Chang HK, Choi CW, et al. Technetium-99m labeling and biodistribution of anti-TAC disulfide-stabilized Fv fragment. J Nucl Med 1997;38(2):294–300.
13. Yokota T, Milenic DE, Whitlow M, et al. Microautoradiographic analysis of the normal organ distribution of radioiodinated single-chain Fv and other immunoglobulin forms. Cancer Res 1993;53(16):3776–3783.
14. Yokota T, Milenic DE, Whitlow M, et al. Rapid tumor penetration of a single-chain Fv and

comparison with other immunoglobulin forms. Cancer Res 1992;52(12):3402–3408.

15. Oriuchi N, Watanabe N, Kanda H, et al. Antibody-dependant difference in biodistribution of monoclonal antibodies in animal models and humans. Cancer Immunol Immunother 1998;46:311–317.

16. Shawler DL, Bartholomew RM, Smith LM, et al. Human immune response to multiple injections of murine monoclonal IgG. J Immunol 1985; 135:1530–1535.

17. Scott AM, Welt S. Antibody-based immunological therapies. Curr Opin Immunol 1997;9:717–722.

18. Hunter WM, Greenwood FC. Preparation of iodine-131-labeled human growth hormone of high specific activity. Nature (Lond) 1962;194:495–496.

19. Huber RE, Edwards LA, Carne TJ. Studies on the mechanism of the iodination of tyrosine by lactoperoxidase. J Biol Chem 1989;264:1381–1386.

20. Kung HF, Alavi A, Chang W, et al. In vivo SPECT imaging of CNS D-2 dopamine receptors: initial studies with iodine-123 IBZM in humans. J Nucl Med 1996;31:573–579.

21. Zalutsky MR, Narula AS. A method for the radiohalogenation of proteins resulting in decreased thyroid uptake of radioiodine. Appl Radiat Isot 1987;38:1051–1055.

22. Rodwell JD, Alvarez VL, Lee C, et al. Site-specific covalent modification of monoclonal antibodies: in vitro and in vivo evaluations. Proc Natl Acad Sci USA 1986;83:2632–2636.

23. Franz J, Freeman GM, Barefield EK, et al. Labeling of antibodies with ^{64}Cu using a conjugate containing a macrocyclic amine chelating agent. Nucl Med Biol 1987;14:479–484.

24. Schwarz A, Steinstrasser A. A novel approach to technetium-99m monoclonal antibodies. J Nucl Med 1987;28:721.

25. Oriuchi N, Endo K, Watanabe N, et al. Semiquantitative SPECT tumor uptake of technetium-99m-labeled anti-CEA monoclonal antibody in colorectal tumor. J Nucl Med 1995; 36:679–683.

26. Visser GW, Gerretsen M, Herscheid JD, et al. Labeling of monoclonal antibodies with rhenium-186 using the MAG3 chelate for radioimmunotherapy of cancer: a technical protocol. J Nucl Med 1993;34(11):1953–1963.

7
Radioimmunodetection of Cancer

E. Edmund Kim

Radiolabeled monoclonal antibodies have gained widespread acceptance as relatively receptor-specific radiopharmaceuticals for clinical applications. Over the past decade, several clinical trials have demonstrated the ability of radiolabeled antibodies to localize certain cancers with sensitivities and specificities comparable to and, in some instances, superior to conventional diagnostic modalities. The U.S. Food and Drug Administration (FDA) has approved four radiolabeled monoclonal antibody conjugates for human use: satumomab pendetide (OncoScint; Cytogen) for colorectal and ovarian cancer; arcitumomab (CEA-Scan; Immunomedics) for colorectal cancer; capromab pendetide (ProstaScint; Cytogen) for prostate carcinoma, and nofetumomab merpentan (Verluma; DuPont Radiopharmaceuticals) for small-cell lung carcinoma.

The field of radioimmunoscintigraphy (RIS) has benefited greatly from recent developments in immunology and tumor biology, and in radiochemistry and nuclear instrumentation. Availability of safe reagents, effective radiolabeling, and fairly large clinical trials using various antibody preparations have been achieved. Antibody imaging has also shown efficacy that is complementary, and often superior, to conventional imaging. It is insufficient for a new modality to only show adequate sensitivity and specificity for a diagnosis. For RIS to be of value, then sensitivity, specificity, and resolution of the method must translate into addition of new or important confirmatory information better than that furnished by previously avail-

able diagnostic tests [1]. Antibody imaging has the potential to significantly impact clinical cancer management by virtue of its unique ability to be truly tissue specific. While morphological studies such as computed tomography (CT), magnetic resonance imaging (MRI), and ultrasonography portray static derangement in anatomy but fail to offer any further characterization at the tissue level, antibody imaging primarily yields pathological functional information regarding the presence of cancer-related antigens at sites in question [2]. For example, anatomical imaging will fail to detect metastases within normal-sized lymph nodes and cannot differentiate local recurrence from postoperative, postradiation, or postchemotherapeutic changes [3]. Functional imaging using tumor-specific radiolabeled monoclonal antibodies (MoAbs) can detect tumors in normal-sized lymph nodes and can distinguish tumor recurrence from posttreatment changes. As with all modalities, spatial detail is limited in RIS, although this detail has been improved by using SPECT.

Basic Concepts

Antibodies are produced by the immune system following exposure to a foreign substance, known as an antigen. The antibodies are secreted by plasma cells originating from B lymphocytes in the bone marrow, lymph nodes, or spleen. These are glycoprotein molecules called immunoglobulins (Ig) that usually consist of two identical heavy and light chains linked by a disulfide bridge. Each chain is made up of a variable (V) region and a constant (C) region, known as domains. The variable region is responsible for antigenic-specific binding and the constant region for effector functions such as complement fixation and antibody-dependent cell cytotoxicity. A complex antigenic determinant will give rise to a number of immunoglobulin species known as polyclonal antibodies. Monoclonal antibodies are derived by generating a specific immunoglobulin-producing cell line after immunizing the specific species with a specific antigen to stimulate the B lymphocytes to produce antibodies. The B lymphocytes are harvested from the species and incubated with immortal myeloma cells, and the resultant hybridomas are capable of being maintained in culture and also producing large amounts of antibodies.

With the advent of recombinant DNA and gene transfection techniques, it has become possible to produce antibodies through genetic engineering, including chimeric and humanized antibodies. Through the use of these genetically engineered agents, antigen-binding specificity and affinity can be optimized. Although the molecular weight of the whole antibody is approximately 150,000 daltons, it can be fragmented into smaller units, yielding Fab' fragments (Fab' or Fab'$_2$). Fab' and Fc fragments each weigh 50,000 daltons, and a Fab'$_2$ fragment weighs approximately 100,000 daltons. The smaller the molecule, the more rapid its clearance from the blood and the easier it is for the molecule to enter the extravascular space. In some instances, the whole antibody may be more desirable because it provides increased time for scanning, especially if labeled with ^{111}In or other long-lived isotopes. Researchers have synthesized peptides that have the same amino acid sequences (16–31 compared with 1320 residues in the whole antibody) as the second or hypervariable region of the heavy chain of the parent antibody. Because of their size, they can reach sites in the body not normally accessible to the larger Mabs and are rapidly cleared from the circulation [4].

The radioisotope can interact with or be attached directly to functional groups on the surface of the Mab. The most accessible sites for drug attachment are the amino acid groups of the lysine residues and the carbohydrate moieties of the heavy-chain domains. ^{131}I or ^{123}I has been incorporated directly into the monoclonal antibody by iodination of the tyrosine residues. One can indirectly attach the radiolabel by using matrix substrate or bifunctional chelating agents after modification of the oligosaccharide moieties on the antibody molecule. Such conjugates can be labeled with a metallic radionuclide such as ^{111}In. ^{111}In has a relatively long physical half-life (3 days), which is better suited for utilization with whole antibodies in that prolonged multiple imaging can be performed.

Radioimmunodetection of Colorectal Cancer

Colorectal cancer is the third most common noncutaneous cancer in the United States, causing approximately 132,700 new cases and 57,100 yearly deaths [5]. It occurs with increasing frequency after the age of 55, and the average age of its diagnosis is 70 years of age. When detected in the early stage, the 5-year survival rate is 91% for colon cancer and 83% for rectal cancer. When it is detected after regional spread to lymph nodes, the 5-year survival rate drops to approximately 55%. Survival rates when there are distant metastases are less than 7% [6].

Approximately 15% of colorectal cancers arise in the cecum and ascending colon, 10% in the transverse colon, 5% in the descending colon, 25% in the sigmoid, and 45% in the rectum. The majority of colorectal cancers are adenocarcinomas. Metastasis may occur either by direct invasion of surrounding tissue or by way of lymphatics, blood vessels, or peritoneal implants. Recurrences are found in approximately 30% to 40% of patients (52% with rectal cancer and 40% with colon cancer) and are associated with male sex, rectal location, Duke C lesion, grade III–IV lesion, adhesion/invasion, perforation, and nondiploid status of the cancer. The liver accounts for 33% of first recurrences, and regional recurrence was seen in 21% of patients, intraabdominal recurrence in 18%, and retroperitoneal lymph node recurrence in 10% [7].

Prognosis of colorectal cancer is predicated on accurate pathological staging as well as histopathology of the primary tumor, the status of regional lymph nodes, and systemic spread. The preoperative staging includes a complete physical examination, blood count, chemistry, colonoscopy, and CT of the abdomen and pelvis. The rate of serum carcinoembryonic antigen (CEA) elevation is rapid with liver metastasis and much slower with local recurrence. Despite careful preoperative screening, additional hepatic or extrahepatic metastases are identified in 35% of patients, and intraoperative ultrasonography has been used to identify hepatic metastasis [8]. The role of immunoscintigraphy in colorectal cancer includes detection of the primary lesion, defining its extent, and finding occult metastasis [9]. The rise of serum CEA level is the common indication of RIS.

[111]In satumomab pendetide (OncoScint) was the first antibody approved by the FDA for cancer imaging. Its component antibody, B72.3, targets the glycoprotein tumor-associated glycoprotein-72 (TAG-72), which is expressed in more than 85% of colorectal cancer [10]. An indium chelator is attached to carbohydrate on the constant region of the whole antibody by a site-specific method, and the linker technology maintains the homogenous antigen affinity and binding characteristics of the antibody [11]. A whole unfragmented IgG has a biological half-life of approximately 55 h and is metabolized in the liver. The hepatocytes accumulate 15% to 20% of the injected dose. The free ^{111}In binds to serum transferrin and transferrin-like receptors in the bone marrow and gonads. The small biodegradation products are cleared by the urinary system. Following a single intravenous injection of lung satmomab pendetide, 31 of 95 patients (33%) developed positive ($\geq$400 ng/ml) human antimouse antibody (HAMA) titers [12].

There is a potential for circulating antimurine antibodies to complex with subsequently administered murine antibodies, and these immune complexes may alter the biodistribution and clearance of the antibody imaging agent and affect the imaging quality. Antibody-related adverse reactions are relatively low (6%) and include transient fever and itching [8]. ^{111}In-satmomab pendetide has undergone extensive clinical trials to demonstrate primary or recurrent colorectal, breast, ovarian, and lung cancers and to evaluate cases with rising serum tumor markers as well as equivocal lesions by conventional imaging [13]. Scintigraphy starting 24 h following the intravenous injection of ^{111}In-satmomab pendetide demonstrates prominent radioactivity in the blood pool, large vessels, bladder, bone marrow, and soft tissues, declining gradually over the following 72 to 96 h. Two imaging sessions between 96 and 144 h have been recommended for better tumor definition and enhanced lesion detection. The low level of radioactivity is usually seen in the large bowel in 50% to 60% of patients. Serial imaging is helpful in some cases.

Planar and single photon emission tomography (SPECT) (Figure 7.1) were performed and successfully identified proven cancer in 64 of 92 patients (70% sensitivity). The antibody scans were negative in 9 of 10 patients (90% specificity) [12]. False-positive findings were tubular adenomas, cystitis, or diverticulitis. Antibody imaging clearly showed superior sensitivity over conventional imaging for detection of pelvic (74% versus 57%) and extrahepatic intraabdominal disease (66% versus 34%). However, in the liver, conventional imaging proved superior to antibody imaging in sensitivity (84% versus 41%) [3]. Estimates of the overall impact of this examination on patient management has varied from moderate (beneficial or very beneficial in 26% of patients; negative or very negative in 3%) to low (beneficial or very beneficial in 2 of 15 patients; and negative or very negative in 3 of 15 patients) [14].

Arcitumomab (CEA Scan), the second RIS agent to receive FDA approval, is a radiolabeled murine monoclonal antibody Fab' fragment that targets the carcinoembryonic antigen. This antibody is labeled with [99mTc], resulting in less nonspecific hepatic uptake and

FIGURE 7.1. **A**. Axial CT image of the pelvis in a patient who had surgery for rectal cancer shows a small soft tissue density (*) adjacent to the sigmoid colon. **B**. Selected axial SPECT images of the pelvis at 48h following the injection of ^{111}In-satmomab show a focal area of moderately increased activity (*arrow*) in the left posterior pelvis, corresponding to the mass seen on CT. Biopsy confirmed a metastatic adenocarcinoma. Note curvilinear activ-ities outlining bowel loops.

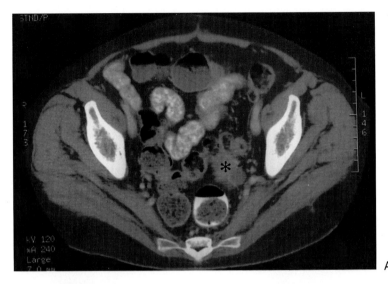

A

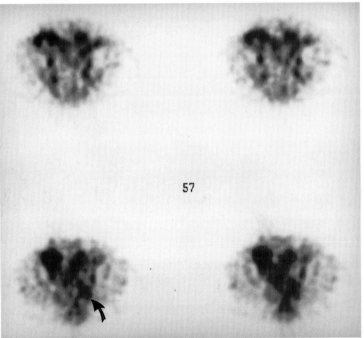

B

potentially better detection of hepatic metastases. The small fragment size (50,000 daltons) allows rapid tumor targeting, rapid clearance from blood and background tissues, and enhanced renal clearance. Tumors usually can be visualized within 2 to 4h after antibody injection (Figure 7.2). Multicenter studies have suggested a sensitivity for imaging hepatic metastases equivalent to that of conventional imaging (63% versus 64%), whereas sensitivity elsewhere in the abdomen (55% versus 32%) and pelvis (69% versus 48%) was superior [15].

Arcitumomab was more accurate than CT for predicting resectability of locally recurrent or metastatic colorectal cancer (57% versus 47%), including a subset of patients with hepatic metastases (Figure 7.3) (43% versus

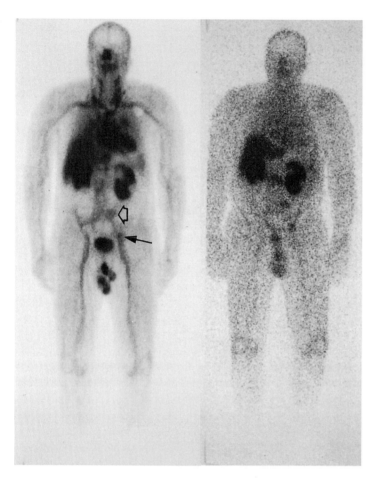

FIGURE 7.2. Anterior whole-body images at 4h (*left*) and 24h (*right*) after injection of ^{99m}Tc-arcitumomab show focal areas of moderately increased activity in the left inguinal (*closed arrow*) and iliac (*open arrowhead*) lymphatic chains in a patient who had an abdominal wall cancer. Biopsy confirmed metastatic adenocarcinomas. Note also space-occupying lesions in the left kidney as filling defects. Ultrasonography cofirmed renal cysts.

33%) [15]. Taking the surgical outcome as the final arbitrator, CT scan findings indicated that in 40 of 85 patients (47%) the cancer was resectable and in 18 of 77 patients (23%) it was nonresectable, and the CT findings ruled out the recurrence/metastases in 39 of 46 patients (85%). By comparison, CEA scans were accurate for resectable cancer in 58 of 85 patients (68%), for nonresectable cancer in 32 of 77 patients (42%), and for the absence of cancer in 34 of 46 patients (75%). The accuracy of combined CT and CEA scans were 72% in contrast to 47% by CT and 68% by CEA scan alone. However, these results do not suggest that CEA scan should replace CT; they rather complement each other [16]. The CEA scan is safe and virtually nonimmunogenic. It would be useful in detecting extrahepatic and extra-abdominal metastases. In addition, the CEA scan can also be used in conjunction with intra-operative gamma probes for more accurate localization of tumors, especially in small lymph node metastases. Probes can be utilized for better definition of tumor-free margins, particularly in the liver.

Votumumab (OncoSPECT), known also as 88BV59, is a third entry into the colorectal RIS. This ^{99m}Tc-human IgG3K antibody reacts to an altered form of cytokeratin. In occult (negative CT) metastatic colorectal cancer, ^{99m}Tc-votumumab detected 79% of surgically confirmed lesions in the pelvis and extrahepatic abdomen and 63% of hepatic metastases. In CT-positive cases, addition of RIS to CT resulted in an increase in accuracy from 28% to 63% [17]. The antibody was nonimmungenic in more than 300 subjects. ^{111}In-altumomab pentetate (ZCE025) has been relatively successful in clinical trials, but the final approval by the FDA could not be obtained.

FIGURE 7.3. (**A**) Axial CT image of the upper abdomen with oral and intravenous administration of contrast agent shows a metastatic colon canter in center of the right hepatic lobe. (**B**) Axial SPECT image using ^{99m}Tc-arcitumomab at comparable level shows markedly heterogeneous activity in the liver with focal photon-deficient lesion (*), corresponding to the mass on CT, indicating necrotic metastatic lesion.

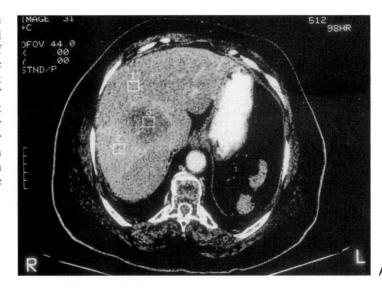

A

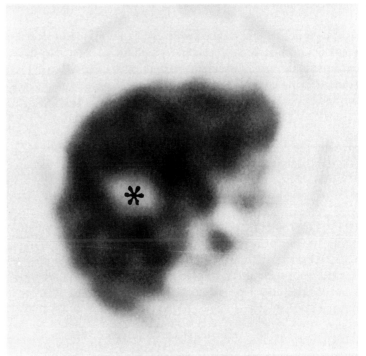

B

Radioimmunodetection of Prostate Cancer

Prostate cancer is the most common cancer in males, with 179,300 new cases in the United States, and is responsible for almost 3% of all deaths in men older than 55 years of age [5]. Its incidence is expected to increase steadily because the incidence increases with age. The widespread use of serum measurement of prostate-specific antigen (PSA) and transrectal ultrasonography will lead to an increase in the detection of prostate cancer [18]. Prostate cancer spreads by direct extension and by lymphatic and vascular routes. Lymphatic metasta-

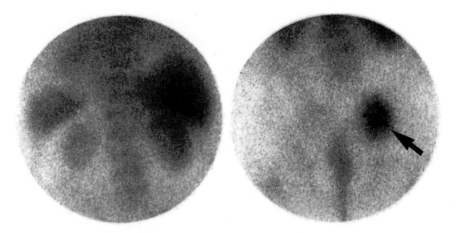

FIGURE 7.4. Posterior images of abdomen (*left*) and pelvis (*right*) using ^{111}In-anti-PAP antibody show a focal area of markedly increased activity (*arrow*) in the area of the right iliac ala.

sis is common and correlates with stage, tumor volume, and histological grades. Lymphatic or extraprostatic spread occurs in 40% to 60% of patients with clinically localized disease. The sentinel nodes are the periprostatic and obturator nodes. The tumor then invades the external iliac and hypogastric nodes before it involves the common iliac and periaortic nodes. Bilateral pelvic node involvement is not uncommon. Bone metastases were developed in 80% of patients with positive nodes compared with 30% of patients without nodal involvement [19]. Comprehensive evaluation of pelvic nodes is performed using PSA, transrectal ultrasonography, CT, and MRI. CT or MRI has detected approximately 30% to 70% of nodal metastases, and cannot detect metastases in normal-sized nodes. It does not differentiate nodal enlargement secondary to cancer, infection, or inflammation [20]. The availability of tumor-associated markers such as prostate acid phosphatase (PAP) and PSA have created antibodies against prostate cancer. Anti-PAP antibodies labeled with ^{99m}Tc and ^{111}In successfully imaged prostate cancer metastases [21], and ^{111}In-MoAb against PAP known as PAY-276 detected bone metastases in 66% of cases (Figure 7.4) [21]. ProstaScint or capromab pendetide (CYT-356 MoAb) is a murine IgG_1 reactive with the cytoplasmic membrane-rich fraction of LNCaP cells. It is not reactive with

soluble cytosol or secretory glycoproteins such as PSA or PAP. The linker-chelator glycyltyrosyl (GYK)-DTPA was conjugated to MoAb 7E-11-C5.3 to form the immunoconjugate 7E11-C5.3 GYK-DTPA. The 7E11-C5 antigen targeted seems maximally expressed in poorly differentiated and metastatic carcinomas [22].

The clinical utility of RI5 in prostate cancer includes the presurgical staging and the evaluation of suspicious recurrence. In postradical prostatectomy patients with rising PSA level, assessment of distant metastases would help determine systemic (hormonal) versus local (radiotherapy or salvage surgery) therapy [21]. In presurgical staging, MoAb was administered to 152 patients, and 40% of 64 patients with confirmed nodal metastases had at least one nodal metastasis detected by RISD (63% sensitivity) whereas CT detected only 4%. In 181 postprostatectomy patients with rising PSA and negative bone scans, RIS was positive in 108 cases including 32 with localization in the prostate fossa only, 46 in extrafossa sites, and 30 in both [23]. Babaian et al. [24] have shown 44% sensitivity and 86% specificity for detecting pelvic lymph node metastases. The primary prostate cancer was visualized by the RIS in 14 of 19 patients (74%). ProstaScint immunoscintigraphy is indicated in newly diagnosed patients with biopsy-proven prostate cancer who are at high risk for pelvic lymph node metastases. This technique circumvents many of the limitations of CT/MRI in assessing nodal metastases as well as the inability of CT/MRI to differentiate benign from malignant lymph nodes. It is also valuable in the evaluation of postprostatectomy patients who have negative or equivocal CT, MRI, or bone scans but are suspected as having recurrences on the basis of elevated or detectable PSA levels [25]. There is a potential role of radioimmunotherapy with ^{90}Y-labeled ProstaScint. This role will be most effective in patients with low tumor burden, rising PSA level after primary curative therapy, or maximal response to hormone therapy. ProstaScint can be given repeatedly because of the low (4%) incidence of adverse reactions and low (8% of HAMA-positive patients) immunogenicity [24,25].

Radioimmunodetection of Lung Cancer

Small-cell lung cancer (SCLC) comprises 20% of 171,600 new cases of lung cancer in the United States [5]. The majority (58%) of patients present with distant metastases or regional disease at the time of initial diagnosis, and overall survival is poor, ranging from 18% at 5 years if the cancer is limited to less than

2% if distant metastases are present. The primary thrust of staging of SCLC is to determine the extent of cancer, which will influence subsequent therapy. Although patients with limited cancer are treated with a combination of local radiation and systemic chemotherapy, patients with extensive cancer are palliated with intensive regimens of chemotherapy. Standard staging procedures include physical examination, chest X-ray, CT of chest, upper abdomen, and head, bone marrow aspiration or biopsy, and radionuclide bone scan.

The Fab' fragment of the pancarcinoma MoAb NR-LU-10 or nofetumomab merpentan (Verluma) is a murine IgG2b against a 40-kDa, carcinoma-associated, cell-surface-bound antigen expressed on lung as well as breast, colon, pancreas, ovary, prostate, and renal carcinomas (Figure 7.5). Labeling of the antibody (10 mg) with ^{99m}Tc was performed using pentanotate diamide dithiolate, and prominent activities are seen in the kidney, bladder, and intestinal tract as with other ^{99m}Tc Fab' fragments as the result of excretion of metabolites via the urinary and hepatobiliary tracts. The presence of radioactivity in the urinary and gastrointestinal tracts may limit the detection of tumors in the abdomen and pelvis. However, the relatively low activity in the liver may easily identify hepatic metastases. Verluma imaging was compared with conventional modalities and up-

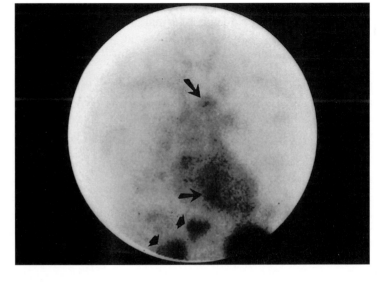

FIGURE 7.5. Anterior image of the chest at 24h following the injection of ^{99m}Tc-MoAb NR-LU-10 in a patient who had a lung cancer shows multiple metastatic lesions in the mediastinum (*arrows*) and the liver (*arrowheads*).

staged 15% of patients from limited to extensive disease. It identified 77% of the patients who had extensive disease with a positive predictive value of 94%. However, the positive predictive value in patients with limited disease was lower (70%–80%), resulting in understaging of 10% of patients [26]. Verluma imaging detected 88 of 104 primary lung lesions (85% sensitivity) and mediastinal and neck/axillary nodes (77% and 87% sensitivity, respectively); it detected 30 of 43 (70%) hepatic metastases [27].

Non-small-cell lung cancer (NSCLC) accounts for approximately 80% of the 158,900 lung cancer deaths annually in the United States [5]. Surgical resection of tumors offers possible long-term survival, and accurate staging is very important in selecting an appropriate treatment. CEA has been used to monitor lung cancers. The CEA scans were performed in 17 patients with proven NSCLC, and the combination of planar and SPECT detected 26 of 39 lesions (67% sensitivity), SPECT being most useful in improving detection of lung tumors. The study confirmed the expression of CEA in resected tumor tissue in 14 of 17 patients (82%) [28].

Radioimmunodetection of Breast and Ovarian Cancers

To date, no conventional imaging has been able to clearly differentiate a benign from malignant breast lesion until a histopathological examination occurs. Of the more than 30 million mammograms performed annually in the United States, about 20% are found ultimately to have a cancer diagnosis in 176,300 patients [5], so that 80% of about 1 million biopsies are unnecessary and produce emotional and financial burdens.

Antibody imaging of breast cancer has a potential role in analysis of the radiologically indeterminate breast mass and assessment of regional disease, as well as distant metastases. Approximately 60% to 80% of breast cancers express, although serum levels are rarely elevated in patients with primary cancer, and elevated serum CEA levels following definitive treatment tend to indicate a recurrent cancer.

Eight patients with breast cancers were targeted successfully with ^{131}I polyclonal affinity-purified goat anti-CEA antibody [29]. The antibody B72.3 was initially generated from immunization of mice from metastatic breast cancer, and TAG-72 antigen is present on 84% of invasive ductal breast carcinoma [10]. There were 14 of 14 known primary breast cancers detected by imaging using [111]In OncoScint antibody, but all 7 cases of proven axillary nodal metastases were missed [30]. In contrast, other groups using the same antibody have reported 71% sensitivity for detecting breast metastases, with 90% in the external quadrants and 43% in the internal quadrants. The sensitivity and specificity for detecting axillary lymph nodes were 91% and 78%, respectively [31]. BrE-3 is an antibody targeting a 400-kDa mucin in the human milk fat globule (HMFG) membrane, and 86% of 70 known lesions and 5 unsuspected lesions were detected by RIS using ^{111}In-BrE-3 [32]. The epidermal growth factor receptor (EGFR), a transmembrane glycoprotein with an intracellular tyrosine kinase domain, and a similar growth factor, HER-2/neu (or C-erbB-2), is overexpressed in human breast cancer. Clinical studies of ^{111}In-MoAb 225 (EGFR Ab) or ^{99m}Tc anti-HER-2/neu showed a localization of primary breast cancers as well as nodal metastases [33,34].

Breast cancer diagnosis requires an adjunctive test to mammography for the increase of diagnostic specificity while maintaining a high positive predictive value. The ^{99m}Tc sestamibi scan failed to provide the necessary accuracy and predictive values for nonpalpable lesions [35]. The CEA scan (arcitumomab) was compared to mammography in 59 patients and revealed 96% specificity, compared to 78% for mammography, with 75% and 4% positive predictive values for CEA scan and mammography, respectively. Therefore, 75% of cases would have been spared an unnecessary biopsy because of the true-negative CEA scan, whereas a definite excision or lumpectomy could occur without the biopsy because the positive prediction for cancer was higher than that of mammography [36]. Although metastatic lymph nodes have been identified with radiolabeled antibodies, some nonspecific accretion in hyperplastic nodes also has been exhibited [37]. More effort to achieve a reliable regional nodal assessment by immunoscintigraphy is needed, perhaps with different sites of injection and more dedicated cameras as well as image processing.

Ovarian cancer is the fourth leading cause of cancer deaths of women in the United States. In 1991, 25,200 new cases of ovarian cancer and 14,500 deaths occurred [5]. The median age at diagnosis is 53 years of age, and overall 5-year survival is only 38%. The ovaries do not have a peritoneal covering. Once tumor growth extends beyond the ovarian capsule, malignant cells are free to metastasize widely throughout the peritoneal cavity. Hundreds of small metastatic nodules may stud the peritoneal surface before symptoms arise. Staging of ovarian cancer is based on the findings at exploratory laparotomy, and laparotomy is not generally able to detect microscopic deposits of tumor. CT or MRI is neither sensitive nor specific enough for accurate staging, particularly in the central abdomen where more than half of metastatic lesions are located [37]. If RIS is useful in reducing unnecessary second-look surgery, considerable expense and morbidity can be avoided.

A multicenter trial of OncoScint CR/OV for ovarian cancer was performed in 108 patients, and antibody scan was more sensitive (69% versus 44%), although less specific (54% versus 79%) in 98 evaluative patients imaged by both RIS and CT. Antibody scan correctly detected tumors in 19 patients with normal CT scans. A positive RIS is not useful in differentiating a malignant from benign pelvic lesion because of the low specificity, while a negative RIS should not preclude second-look surgery because of low negative predictive value. OncoScint imaging was believed to be beneficial or very beneficial to patient care management in 27% and to have a negative or very negative effect in only 2% [38]. In 16 studies with ^{99m}Tc-88BV59 before second-look exploratory surgery, there were 7 true positives, 7 true negatives, and 2 false positives [2]. ^{99m}Tc-

labeled MoAb-170 antibody was studied in 30 ovarian cancer patients, and 26 of 33 known lesions were successfully visualized (79% sensitivity). Of 29 benign lesions, 28 showed no tracer uptake (97% specificity) [39].

Radioimmunodetection of Medullary Thyroid Cancer, Germ Cell Tumor, and Lymphoma

Medullary thyroid cancer originating in the parafollicular C-cells is uncommon and may occur as a component of multiple endocrine neoplasia (MEN) type II. Serum CEA levels often are elevated in recurrent or metastatic cancer or in patients with clinically and radiographically occult disease but elevated serum calcitonins. As many as 75% of patients present with a clinically palpable radioiodine-deficient nodule. The presence of postsurgical and postradiation changes can be a limiting factor of CT or MRI for the localization of recurrent cancer. ^{99m}Tc(V)-DMSA, ^{201}Tl-chloride, ^{99m}Tc-sestamibi, and ^{111}In-pentetreotide have been occasionally helpful but not universally reliable. Using three different antibodies directed against the same epitope of CEA, Juweid et al. [40] reported a high sensitivity for detection of known medullary thyroid cancers (76%–100% using various anti-CEA monoclonal antibodies). These antibodies, conjugated with ^{99m}Tc or ^{123}I, depicted occult lesions in seven of nine patients with elevated CEA levels. The lesions were mostly located in mediastinal or cervical lymph nodes [40]. Because of high sensitivity, ^{99m}Tc-anti-CEA antibody appears useful in the initial staging, in monitoring disease progression and therapeutic response, in localizing recurrence, and in guiding radioimmunotherapy.

B-cell lymphomas have been found to be sensitive to radioimmunotherapy (RIT) using a variety of different antibodies and therapeutic radionuclides [2]. RIS has an unique role to play in patients with hB-cell lymphomas, where it is used to assay antigen expression for biodistribution and dosimetry studies before RIT. ^{131}I-labeled Lym-1 antibody (Oncolym) and ^{131}I-labeled anti-B1 (CD20) antibody have been used as a component of the therapeutic antibody trials for radiation dosimetry [41]. ^{99m}Tc-labeled LL2 (Lymphoscan) has been developed as an independent lymphoma staging agent, over and above its use in staging before therapy with [131]I- or ^{90}Y-labeled ImmuRAIT-LL2.

Sensitivity for detecting lymphomas with ^{99m}Tc-LL2 in patients with B-cell non-Hodgkin's lymphomas was 90% for known lesions and 89% for suspected lesions. Accuracy of staging was also high for low-grade tumors [42].

Germ cell tumors account for 1% of all malignancies, but are a common malignancy of men aged 18 to 35 years. Approximately 7400

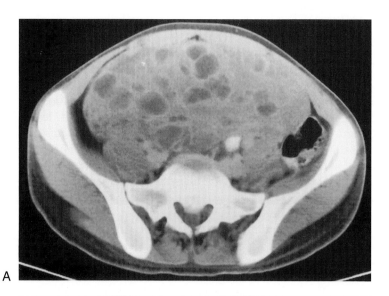

A

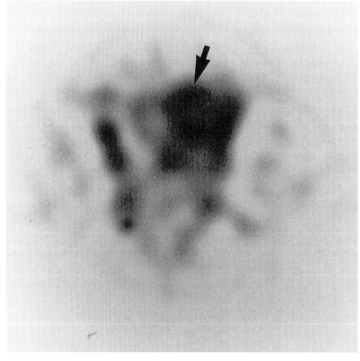

B

FIGURE 7.6. (**A**) Axial CT image of the pelvis shows a large heterogeneous mass occupying the pelvis of a patient with testicular germ cell tumor. (**B**) Selected axial image of the pelvis using ^{99m}Tc-anti-AFP Fab' at the comparable level shows moderately increased activity (*arrow*) in the left pelvis, indicating active AFP-producing tumor. Biopsy confirmed a metastatic germ cell tumor.

new cases will be diagnosed in the United States in 1999 and 300 patients will die of this disease during the year [5]. About 70% to 80% of patients generally achieve a durable complete response to cisplatin-based chemotherapy and necessary resection of residual disease. Efforts to individualize chemotherapy or minimize surgical procedures are of interest. 98% of patients with nonseminomatous germ cell tumors have elevated serum tumor markers such as alpha-fetoprotein (AFP). Falsely elevated levels may be secondary to hepatitis or hepatic injury [43]. The accuracy of CT or MRI in the evaluation of residual germ cell tumors is relatively low, and improved or complementary means of detecting residual tumors are needed [44]. Radiolabeled antibodies against AFP have been developed to localize AFP-secreting tumors [45], and preliminary data using ^{99m}Tc-anti-AFP Fab' on a limited number of patients have shown relatively high sensitivity and specificity (Figure 7.6) [46].

Conclusion

The U.S. FDA has approved four murine-based radiolabeled monoclonal antibody products for cancer evaluation with excellent safety profiles. The products have demonstrated the superiority of RIS over CT to differentiate between postsurgical scars, postradiation changes, and tumor recurrence and to identify tumor involvement in normal-sized lymph nodes. Despite the advantages of RIS, its acceptance as a clinical tool has been sporadic, possibly related to nonfocused indications, the not well documented impact on patient management or value in monitoring high-risk patients, and delayed FDA approval of repeated administration.

The challenge to RIS is to continue to translate advances in tumor biology, immunology, and recombinant engineering into optimized methods for targeting diagnostic radionuclides to tumors. New bivalent antibodies or fusion proteins incorporating two disparate functional proteins open up new vistas of radiopharmaceutical design, and the bifunctional antibodies will likely improve targeting and antibody specificity. As RIT continue to increase in effectiveness, the role of RIS in pre-RIT imaging will become further defined. If adequate resources are focused, RIS will emerge as an important and unique diagnostic method in the management of cancer patients with demonstrable clinical impact and cost-effectiveness.

References

1. Goldenberg DM, Larson SM. Radioimmunodetection in cancer identification. J Nucl Med 1992;33:803–814.
2. Zuckier LS, DeNardo GL. Trials and tribulations: oncological antibody imaging comes to the fore. Semin Nucl Med 1997;27:10–29.
3. Collier BD, Abdel-Nabi HH, Doerr RJ, et al. Immunoscintigraphy with In-111 CYT-103 in the management of colorectal carcinoma: a comparison with CT. Radiology 1992;185:179–186.
4. Serafini AN. From monoclonal antibodies to peptides and molecular recognition units. An overview. J Nucl Med 1993;34:533–536.
5. Landis SH, Murray T, Bodden S, Wingo PA. Cancer statistics, 1999. CA Cancer J Clin 1999; 49:8–31.
6. Steele GB Jr. The National Cancer Data Base report on colorectal cancer. Cancer (Phila) 1994; 74:1979–1989.
7. Galandiuk S, Wieand HS, Moertelo CG, et al. Patterns of recurrence after curative resection of carcinoma of the colon and rectum. Surg Gynecol Obstet 1992;174:27–32.
8. Doerr RJ, Kulaylat MN, Abdel-Nabi H. Imaging strategies in hepatic metastases from colorectal carcinoma. J Hepato-Biliary-Pancreatico Surg 1995;2:126–133.
9. Nabi H, Doerr RJ, Chan H-W, et al. In-111-labeled monoclonal antibody immunoscintigraphy in colorectal carcinoma: safety, sensitivity, and preliminary clinical results. Radiology 1990; 175:163–171.
10. Thor A, Ohuchi N, Szpak CA, et al. Distribution of oncofetal antigen tumor-associated glycoprotein-72 defined by monoclonal antibody B72.3. Cancer Res 1986;46:3118–3124.
11. Rodwell JD, Alvarez VL, Lee C, et al. Site-specific covalent modification of monoclonal antibodies: in vitro and in vivo evaluations. Proc Natl Acad Sci USA 1986;83:2632–2636.
12. Doerr RJ, Abdel-Nabi H, Krag D, et al. Radiolabeled antibody imaging in the management of

colorectal cancer. Results of a multicenter clinical study. Ann Surg 1991;214:118–124.

13. Markowitz A, Saleemi K, Freeman LM, et al. Role of In-111-labeled CYT-103 immunoscintigraphy in the evaluation of patients with recurrent colorectal cancer. Clin Nucl Med 1993;18: 685–700.

14. Doerr RJ, Abdel-Nabi H, Krag D, et al. Radiolabeled antibody imaging in the management of colorectal cancer. Ann Surg 1991;214:118–124.

15. Moffat FL Jr, Pinsky CM, Hammershaimb L, et al. Clinical utility of external immunoscitigraphy with the IMMU-4 Tc-99m Fab' antibody fragment in patients undergoing surgery for carcinoma of the colon and rectum. Results of a pivotal phase III trial. J Clin Oncol 1996;14: 2295–2305.

16. Hughes K, Pinsky CM, Petrelli NJ, et al. Use of carcinoembryonic antigen radioimmunodetection and computed tomography for predicting the resectability of recurrent colorectal cancer. Ann Surg 1997;226:621–631.

17. Gulec SA, Serafini AN, Moffat FL, et al. Radioimmuno-scintigraphy of colorectal carcinoma using Tc-99m human monoclonal antibody 88BV59H21-2. Cancer Res 1995;55:5774–5776.

18. Mettlin C, Jones GW, Murphy GP. Trends in prostate cancer care in the United States, 1974–1990. Observation from the patient care evaluation studies of the American College of Surgeons Commission on Cancer. Cancer J Clin 1993;43:83–91.

19. McNeil JE. Histologic differentiation, cancer volume, and pelvic lymph node metastasis in adenocarcinoma of the prostate. Cancer (Phila) 1990;66:1225–1233.

20. Golimbu M, Morales P, Al-Askaris, et al. CAT scanning in staging of prostatic cancer. Urology 1981;18:305–308.

21. Babaian RJ, Lamki LM. Radioimmunoscintigraphy of prostate cancer. Semin Nucl Med 1989; 19:309–321.

22. Schellmanner PF, Wright GL Jr. Biomolecular and clinical characteristics of PSA and other candidate prostate tumor markers. Urol Clin North Am 1993;20:597–606.

23. Burgers JK, Hinkle GH, Haseman MK. Monoclonal antibody imaging of recurrent and metastatic prostate cancer. Semin Urol 1995;13:102–112.

24. Babaian RJ, Sayer J, Podoloff DA, et al. Radioimmunoscintigraphy of pelvic lymph nodes with In-111 MoAb CTY-356. J Urol 1994;152:1952–1955.

25. Kahn D, Williams RD, Seldin DW, et al. Radioimmunoscintigraphy with In-111 CYT-356 for the detection of occult prostate cancer recurrence. J Urol 1994;152:1490–1495.

26. Breitz HB. Imaging lung cancer with radiolabeled antibodies. Semin Nucl Med 1993;23: 127–132.

27. Vansant JP. Staging lung carcinoma with Tc-99m monoclonal antibody. Clin Nucl Med 1992;17: 431–438.

28. Kramer EL, Noz, ME, Liebes L, et al. Radioimmuno-detection of non-small cell lung cancer using Tc-99m anticarcinoembryonic antigen IMMU-4 Fab' fragment. Cancer (Phila) 1994;73:890–895.

29. Goldenberg DM, Kim EE, DeLand FH, et al. Radioimmunodetection of cancer with radioactive antibodies to carcinoembryonic antigen. Cancer Res 1980;40:2984–2992.

30. Lamki LM, Buzdar AU, Singletary SE, et al. In-111 B72.3 monoclonal antibody in the detection and staging of breast cancer. J Nucl Med 1991;32:1326–1332.

31. Crippa F, Agresto R, Bombardieri E, et al. Preliminary results of preoperative axillary radioimmunoscintigraphy with In-111 B72.3 in breast cancer. Int J Oncol 1995;6:791–795.

32. Nabi H. Antibody imaging in breast cancer. Semin Nucl Med 1997;27:30–34.

33. Pauletti G, Godolphin W, Pres MF, et al. Detection and quantitation of HER-2/neu gene amplification in human breast cancer archival material using fluorescence in situ hybridization. Oncogene 1996;12:63–72.

34. Allan SM, Dean CJ, Eccles S, et al. Clinical radioimmunolocalization with a rat monoclonal antibody directed against c-erbB-2. Cell Biophys 1994;24–25:93–98.

35. Waxman AD. The role of Tc-99m methoxyisobutyliso-nitride in imaging breast cancer. Semin Nucl Med 1997;27:40–54.

36. Goldenberg DM, Nabi HA. Breast cancer imaging with radiolabeled antibodies. Semin Nucl Med 1999;24:41–48.

37. Rubin SC, Lewis JL Jr. Second-look surgery in ovarian carcinoma. Crit Rev Oncol Hematol 1988;8:75–91.

38. Surwit EA, Childers JM, Krag DN, et al. Clinical assessment of In-111 CTY-103 immunoscintigraphy in ovarian cancer. Gynecol Oncol 1993;48: 285–292.

39. Alexander C, Villena-Heinsen CE, Trampert L, et al. Radioimmunoscintigraphy of ovarian tumors with Tc-99m-labeled MoAb-170: first

clinical experiences. Eur J Nucl Med 1995; 22:645–651.

40. Juweid M, Sharkey RM, Behn T, et al. Improved detection of medullary thyroid cancer with radiolabeled antibodies to carcinoembryonic antigen. J Clin Oncol 1996;14:1209–1217.

41. Kaminski MS, Zasadny KR, Francis IR, et al. Iodine-131 anti-B1 radioimmunotherapy for B-cell lymphoma. J Clin Oncol 1996;14:1974–1981.

42. Blend MJ, Hyun H, Kozloff M, et al. Improved staging of B-cell non-Hodgkin's lymphoma patients with Tc-99m-labeled LL2 monoclonal antibody fragment. Cancer Res 1995;55:5764–5770.

43. Jadadpour N. Current status of tumor markers in testicular cancer. Eur Urol 1992;21:34–36.

44. Fossa S, Qvist H, Stenwig A, et al. Is post-chemotherapy retroperitoneal surgery necessary in patients with non-seminomatous testicular cancer and minimal residual tumor masses? J Clin Oncol 1992;10:569–573.

45. Kim EE, DeLand FH, Nelson MO, et al. Radioimmunodetection of cancer with radiolabeled antibodies to α-fetoprotein. Cancer Res 1980;40:3008–3012.

46. Kasi LP, Kim EE, Diaz M, et al. Pharmakokinetic evaluation of Tc-99m anti-AFP Fab′ in patients with germ cell tumors. J Nucl Med 1994;35:11–12 (abstract).

8
Peptide Receptor Imaging

Franklin C.L. Wong and E. Edmund Kim

Peptides are small number (<50) of units of amino acids covalently linked by the peptide bond. They are smaller in size and lower in molecular weight (<10,000 daltons) than proteins. Peptides also lack tertiary structures. Therefore, they are less prone to immunogenicity. Because target-specific imaging using monoclonal antibodies has proven elusive, imaging using biologically active peptides has raised enthusiasm among scientists and clinicians. This interest is because of the wealth of molecular recognition technology and protein biochemistry that may be applied to the diagnosis of human disease by direct visualization of the specific disease sites. This technology has become possible with the recent advances in imaging devices, protein chemistry, and the understanding of the physiological and pathological roles of protein and peptides. Advances in imaging and quantification are described elsewhere (Chapters 3 and 4) in this volume. Advances in protein chemistry have made feasible the production of small biologically active peptides, and advances in the labeling of small peptides for human imaging are also described in other chapters. This chapter concentrates on the current state of peptide imaging, especially in oncology. The additional advantages of peptide imaging in oncology include the potential for directing and monitoring of therapy.

The study of target recognition by small molecules (ligands) such as peptides evolves from the receptors studies. The idea of a receptor as a molecular entity remained elusive until 1976 when Snyder and Bennett proved its existence [1]. Until then, the evidence of ligand–receptor interaction was derived from bioassays that were technically tedious and subject to procedural and technical variances. Since 1976, the receptor methodologies have made great advances. The development of receptor technology in pharmacology, indeed, benefited from earlier studies of antibody–antigen interactions as pioneered by Yalow and Berson [2]. Despite differences in molecular weights of the ligands involved, antigen–antibody interactions, peptide–receptor interaction, and drug–receptor interactions are governed by the mass action laws.

When different molecules in aqueous solution encounter each other in close proximity they either attract, repel, pass by without any significant effect, or collide with each other. The underlying forces behind the attraction or repulsion of the moieties are governed by the hydrophobic or hydrophilic interactions, electrostatic forces, bulkiness of the entities, and hydration of the various moieties. After two molecules collide, they may remain bound for a short duration or remain bound indefinitely. This status of ligand bound to a protein is what is referred as ligand–protein binding. Such binding is governed by the affinity of the ligand toward the protein (or vice versa). In the initial phase, binding is a reversible phenomenon, that is, the ligand may leave the protein at various rates. However, with time and other events, it may occur as an irreversible event when conventional chemical reactions such as covalent bonds form between the ligand and the protein.

Such events may develop naturally, or may be triggered by other factors such as other chemicals in the vicinity or radiation-induced free radical formation and hence reaction between the ligand and the protein. Therefore, the ligand–protein interactions can be either reversible or irreversible. Furthermore, depending upon the manner in which the ligand is bound to the protein, the interaction can also be classified as noncompetitive or competitive, when other ligands with similar chemical structures may interfere with the binding itself.

In molecular pharmacology, reversible saturable competitive ligand–protein binding is the main concern because it allows the ability to study the structure–activity relationship of various analogs of the ligands and provides good rationale and explanation of the ligand–protein interactions at the molecular level. High affinity and specificity are the two key requirements for study of a ligand-binding system. Competitive irreversible bindings such as photoaffinity labeling, that is, covalent cross linking between the ligand and protein using ultraviolet light, has also been a good biochemical tool. In fact, competitive irreversible binding using tissue presentation X-ray provides an opportunity to effect in vivo receptor labeling [3]. Noncompetitive binding, whether reversible or irreversible, is typical of lower affinity but needs to be suppressed or discounted to evaluate the more biologically significant saturable competitive reversible interactions between the ligand and the protein.

The foregoing discussion only applies to the in vitro homogeneous aqueous environment, such as test tubes in the laboratory. For in vivo imaging, multiple additional factors may affect the resultant ligand binding tremendously. Venous dilution, hepatic metabolism, and the intravascular metabolism of the ligand may markedly decrease the available ligand to the tissue of interest. The vasculature and the vascular reaction to pathology or to the ligand itself may further alter the access of the ligand to the tissue. The ability of the ligand to cross the barrier between the capillary and the tissue may prevent the ligand from reaching the tissue. The internalization process of the bound ligand on the surface of the cells and subsequent metabolism in the cells may decrease the amount of the ligand to be detected from the extracorporeal imaging device. Other protein binding, whether noncompetitive or irreversible, in the intravascular compartment may decrease the availability of the ligand to the tissue of interest. The metabolism of the ligand itself in the body, whether in the serum or in the liver, may result in metabolites of the ligand released in the intravascular compartment and decrease signal-to-noise ratio because of rising background tracer activities. Last, endogenous or exogenous ligands may compete with the tracer. Therefore, the translation of in vitro ligand–protein binding studies into in vivo imaging requires careful consideration of each of these pharmacokinetic and pharmacodynamic factors. They may operate in this certainly heterogeneous environment of body fluid and tissue, in addition to permeability across the multiple biological membrane barriers.

Peptides, Receptors, and Human Disease

Receptors mediate many vital communications between extrinsic chemicals and nervous and muscular systems as demonstrated by the various types of neurotransmitter–receptor and peptide–receptor pathways. Aberrations in these types of receptors may lead to different forms of myasthenia gravis. Receptors also mediate the communication between different organs in the human body via the endocrine system. Aberrations in the receptors may lead to endocrinopathy such as Graves' disease. Additionally, receptors mediate the communication between cells and also with the cell itself through the environment via the autocrine system. Aberrations in the receptors along this system may result in uncontrolled growth of the cell lines to become tumor. Abnormalities at the receptor level, either because of altered affinity or density, may be the primary cause of the human ailment; alternatively, these could also be results of the upregulation or downregulation or interaction with other molecular entities or receptor systems within the cells. Therefore, evaluation of receptors alone does

TABLE 8.1. The main peptides and receptor systems investigated for scintigraphic targeting of human tumors.

Receptor	Receptor subtypes	Peptide	Tumor
Somatostatin	sst1/sst2/sst3/sst4/sst5	Octreotide	Endocrine-related tumors
		Pentetreotide	
Vasoactive intestinal peptide (VIP)		VIP	Intestinal adenocarcinoma
		Peptide histidine isoleucin (PHI)	
GPIIb/IIIa		RGD sequence	Melanoma
		Chemotactic peptides	

not provide the specific etiology of the human disease. Changes in receptor affinity and density may be nonspecifically correlated with disease processes, but not necessarily causally related. The study of peptides and peptide imaging may indirectly reflect receptor status on the cellular membranes and provide invaluable measures of various pathologies.

Multiple in vitro and in vivo techniques have been devised to study peptides and specific receptor systems related to human disease. In the clinical practice of oncology, elevated levels of somatostatin receptors have been found in tumors such as small-cell lung cancer, different forms of pancreatic cancers, carcinoid, meningioma, and to a lesser degree, lymphoma. With advances in receptor and peptide measurement, various peptide systems have been correlated with human cancer (Table 8.1).

Early detailed receptor imaging studies are mostly in the study of human brain diseases. For instance, the first human receptor imaging was reported on the dopamine receptors using positron emission tomography (PET) [4]. By using ^{11}C-labeled NMSP, it was found that D-2 receptors are elevated in patients with schizophrenia [5] and depression [6]. Subsequent development in single photon emission computed tomography (SPECT) tracer leads to ^{123}I-labeled IBZM for the SPECT imaging of human D-2 receptors [7]. Current peptide imaging techniques in clinical practice, nevertheless, still concentrate around the different small peptide ligands of somatostatin such as the P829 peptide labeled with ^{99m}Tc, which has been claimed to have accuracy close to that of ^{18}F-fluoro-deoxy-glucose (^{18}F-FDG) PET for the identification of lung cancer (Figure 8.1).

Prerequisites of Peptide Receptor Imaging

Eckelman outlined 16 categories of study in the development of a receptor-binding system for in vivo imaging [8]. These categories include the determination of the dissociation constant K_d for the parent compound, and in vitro displacement of the labeled compound by a non-radioactive derivative, the determination of the K_d for the radioactive derivative, the use of active and inactive stereoisomers of the radioactive derivative, and the confirmation of the animal distribution pattern of the tracer compound in humans.

The choice of a receptor system should be originally based on the in vitro binding affinity and specificity data. In general, because of the high specific activity available with radioactive ligands (up to 30 curies per millimolar per molecule) and the concern of excessive dosimetry to humans, K_d as a measure of the affinity of the ligand to the receptor should be in the range of 0.1 to 50 nM. When the affinity is too high, that is, with a very small dissociation constant or a very high association rate constant, the radioactivity determined in the target organ is independent of the receptor concentration. The rate-limiting step becomes a measure of flow rate or membrane transport rather than the ligand–receptor binding processes. With a low affinity constant, that is, when K_d is greater than 50 nM, a large amount of unbound free tracer will be in the circulation and the signal-to-noise ratio may be significantly decreased. The resultant images may become a measure of other factors such as vasculature or blood volume in the tissue of interest instead of a reflection of the receptors.

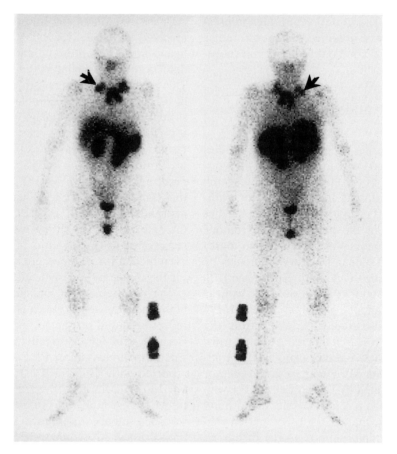

FIGURE 8.1. Whole-body anterior (*left*) and posterior (*right*) images at 4h following the injection of ^{111}In-octreotide show markedly increased activities (*arrows*) in proven metastatic neuroblastoma masses in the superior mediastinum and bilateral supraclavicular lymphatic chains. Small mass in the left adrenal gland is obscured by the intensely increased activities in the adjacent kidney and spleen.

Because the optimum condition for detection of changes in the binding occurs when the ligand-to-receptor ratio is between 0.2 and 0.8, then too much or too little tracer ligand in the vasculature will decrease the ability to detect significant alterations. The quantification of receptor–ligand interactions is beyond the scope of this chapter, but may be referred to in the reference by Vera et al. [9].

Other requirements of the ligand–receptor system for human imaging studies include the relative nontoxic nature of the tracer ligand at the dose prescribed. It also should have relatively good stability in the intravascular compartment during the imaging session. In other words, considerations for in vivo human receptor imaging start with an existing in vitro ligand–receptor binding system with additional attention to details of the pharmacokinetic characteristics such as intravascular dilution, permeability, biodistribution, metabolism, and endogenous ligand competitions.

A less preferred approach to receptor imaging is to conduct empirical studies using putative ligands. Such an approach suffers from the criticism that the interaction between the receptor and the ligand has not been characterized and therefore any findings or images may reflect the various physiological and pathological processes other than those at the receptor levels. Therefore, even though impressive images may be obtained, validation studies still have to be carried out to verify the receptor–ligand interaction.

Imaging of Peptide Receptors in Tumors

Most of the earlier receptor imaging studies were performed with the central nervous system because of the abundant basic research data on the different neurotransmitter pathways. Imaging of receptors in tumors started as a transition from the brain to brain tumors. Dopamine receptors were found to be markedly elevated in human pituitary adenomas by a PET study using [11]C-*N*-methylspiperone [10], and visualization of brain lesions as well as tumors using compounds such as ^{11}C-PK 11195 [11]. These earlier studies benefited from the abundant basic research including animal work and in vitro studies. A good example of the transition between in vitro and in vivo receptor studies is illustrated by Raderer et al. [12], who compared in vitro receptor density and affinity to the imaging characteristics of ^{123}I-labeled vasoactive intestinal peptide (VIP) in human tissue and cancer cells. He also compared the ^{123}I VIP system with indium-111-CYT-103 monoclonal antibody in vitro and in vivo imaging characteristics. This is the preferred mode of development of receptor-binding studies from in vitro to in vivo clinical studies.

In the case of PK-11195 binding to gliomas, in vitro studies found at least a 20-fold elevated receptor density on the tumor cells [13]. Ex vivo autoradiography confirmed only about a 6-fold elevated receptor density when the tissue is sectioned into thick layers and exposed to the ligand [14]. Subsequent PET images only found a 2-fold increase in the signal detected in the tumor compared with that of the surrounding brain tissues. This same experience of decreased signal-to-noise ratio from the in vitro study to the in vivo imaging is, again, confirmed in the aforementioned ^{123}I VIP study [13] with the initial tumor receptor density of 1000 fold higher by the in vitro study decreasing to a difference probably less than 10 fold in the signal detected in the tumor by an in vivo method. The explanation for this loss of signal-to-noise ratio

may be explained by the multiple factors involved in the delivery and detection of the ligand to the receptor site and the subsequent detection of the signal in the living organism. This reduction in signal-to-noise ratio will direct the search for a suitable receptor–ligand system for oncological imaging to those receptors that are markedly elevated in tumors. Using the PK-11195 as an example, a minimum of 20-fold receptor density difference is required for visualization of the receptors in the tumor using PET. When less sensitive instrumentation such as SPECT is used, as in the case of the ^{123}I VIP, the requirement of the receptor density elevation in tumors will be even higher, for instance, greater than 100 fold for the tumor to be visualized.

The requirement of high in vitro signal-to-noise receptor density ratio is not unique with receptors found on the surface of tumor cells. Because cytosolic estrogen receptors are elevated with breast cancer, PET studies have been reported with ^{18}F-labeled estrogen analogues. For 16α-F-18-fluoro-17β-estradiol, which has a target background ratio of 80:1 from in vitro studies, a signal-to-noise ratio of 2:2 is noted in breast cancer with human PET [15].

Obviously, multiple other factors such as perfusion, size of tumor, intravascular and hepatic metabolism, affinity, internalization rate of the ligand, and competition from endogenous ligands are all factors that potentially affect the threshold of the receptor density difference for the tumor to be visualized. Because in vivo quantitative evaluations of receptors requires meticulous attention to technical details, arterial blood sampling, and stringent as well as multiple time sequence of imaging sessions, they are not routinely performed in the clinical setting. Instead, optimum imaging conditions derived from the foregoing quantitative studies are typically chosen, and routine clinical imaging of receptors in oncology is performed without blood sampling.

Indium-111-Labeled Somatostatin Receptor Imaging in Oncology

Early successful imaging of human tumors involved somatostatin analogues using ^{123}I labels [16,17]. The K_d of the radioiodinated compound, ^{123}I-Tyr-octreotide, ranges between 0.5 and 1.5 nM, well within the suitable range of affinity constant for imaging [18]. The somatostatin receptor density is barely detectable in neuroendocrine tissues but markedly elevated in malignant tissues, from 80 to 2000 fmole/mg protein [19]. [111]In-[DTPA D-Phe] octreotide has been used in subsequent development of somatostatin receptor scintigraphy because of the more favorable stability and imaging characteristics in the delayed images.

Somatostatin is a peptide that exists in either a 14-amino-acid or a 28-amino-acid form. It is present in the hypothalamus, brainstem, and gastroinstestinal tract as well as in the pancreas. Somatostatin receptors are found on activated lymphocytes and cells of neuroendocrine origin such as the anterior pituitary, pancreatic islet cells, and thyroid C cells. Five subtypes of somatostatin receptors have been identified and cloned. All these subtypes exert their actions by inhibiting adenylyl cyclase activity. Subtype 2 has high affinity, or low K_d in the range of 0.1 to 1 nM, while subtypes 3 and 5 are in the 10- to 100-nM range; subtypes 1 and 4 exhibit affinity greater than 1000 nM [20]. Therefore, only subtype 2 is suitable for imaging. In fact, subtype 2 is most frequently expressed in tumors, and antiproliferative effects have been observed with activation of subtypes 1 and 2 [21].

Typically, 5 mCi of [111]In-[DTPA D-Phe] octreotide is injected intravenously and whole-body images are obtained after clearance of intravascular activities, typically at 4 h. More delayed images are obtained, typically, after 24 h. The images may further be studied by SPECT at either 4 or 24 h. It has been argued that SPECT at 4 h is adequate. Images obtained after 48 h are seldom performed and may hardly provide any additional useful information. Comparison with anatomical imaging is important to further ascertain the location of the radioactivity. Typically, a strong signal-to-background ratio is identified in the tumor sites. For instance, in a patient with neuroblastoma, suspected sites of adenopathy in the neck are confirmed to be metastatic tumor by histology (see Figure 8.1) [2].

In vivo imaging studies using [111]In-[DTPA D-Phe] octreotide have demonstrated high sensitivity of detection of tumor in most tumors of

neuroectodermal origin (Figures 8.1, 8.2). These findings are also confirmed by in vitro analysis in pituitary tumors, gastrinomas, insulinomas, paraganglioma, small-cell lung cancer, meningiomas, astrocytomas, thyroid cancers, lymphoma, and APUDomas [19]. However, sarcoidosis, rheumatoid arthritis, tuberculosis, and postradiation effects have all been reported to have elevated octreotide-avid lesions as confirmed by in vivo imaging as well as in vitro tissue analyses. Part of the explanation of the uptake of octreotide in the nonmalignant lesions may be the accumulation of activated lymphocytes in the vicinity.

[111]In-labeled octreotide has a disadvantage with beta emissions, therefore, limiting the dose of the tracer. Other somatostatin receptor imaging agents have been developed. More specific fragments of the somatostatin, technetium-labeled P829 (Figure 8.3), have been evaluated in phase II studies to achieve a dosimetry with better photon flux [22]. This agent has recently received U.S. Federal Drug Administration (FDA) approval for the evaluation of the lung [23]. Gallium-67 and Ga-68 (DFO) labeled octreotide are used to achieve better dosimetry and quantitation, respectively [22].

Conclusion

The advantage of peptide receptor imaging in oncology is that it is not a biological product and its production is not subject to animal variation as in antibody production. Furthermore, because peptides are small molecules, biodistribution is more favorable as these small molecules may be able to pass different biological barriers by mere diffusion. Peptides also lack a tertiary structure that may elicit immunological response in patients. Cost and availability are currently still constraints that limit the wide use of peptide receptor imaging. However, with more support from the basic research in receptors and the development of other alternative better and less expensive tracer, receptors may be the best example of applying basic science directly to patient care. The recent development of ^{99m}Tc-labeled p829 for the detection of lung cancer is a good example of such development.

FIGURE 8.2. (**A**) Whole-body anterior (*left*) and posterior (*right*) images at 4 h following the injection of ^{111}In-octreotide show a markedly increased activity in the large mass in right hepatic lobe, corresponding to known necrotic metastatic pancreatic islet cell tumor on CT. Note unexpected small focal areas of markedly increased activities in the left orbit (*closed arrow*) and left thigh (*open arrow*). (**B**) Coronal T_1-weighted image of the head shows a mass involving left medial rectus muscle (*).

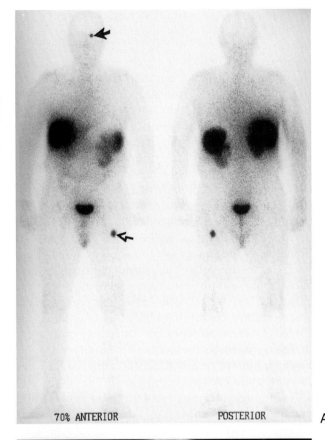

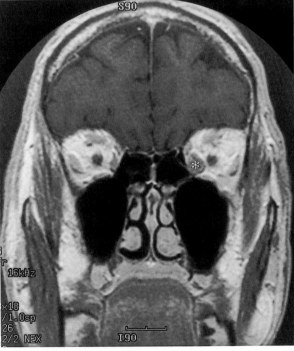

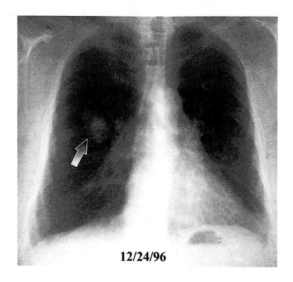

12/24/96

B.

Anterior Planar   **Posterior Planar**

R   L   L   R

Coronal SPECT slices   **Technetium Tc-99m P829**

R   L

C.

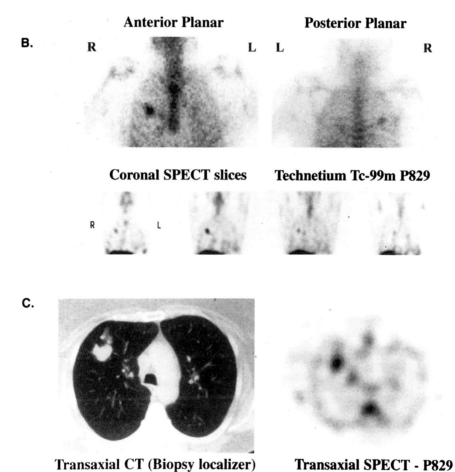

Transaxial CT (Biopsy localizer)   **Transaxial SPECT - P829**
12/24/96   **12/23/96**

FIGURE 8.3. A 42-year-old male smoker with occupational exposure to asbestos. *Top* (**A**): chest radiograph demonstrates the newly discovered solitary pulmonary nodule (SPN) in the left upper lobe. *Center* (**B**): P829 planar and SPECT images demonstrate normal P829 biodistribution with no abnormal uptake in the region of the SPN seen on chest radiography and CT scan. *Bottom* (**C**): transaxial CT scan and corresponding P829 transaxial SPECT image demonstrate no abnormal uptake in the region of the SPN. Final diagnosis: coccidioidomycosis. (From Blum et al., Chest p. 228, vol 115, 1999, with permission.)

References

1. Snyder SM, Bennett JD. Neurotransmitter receptors in the brain: biochemical identification. Annu Rev Physiol 1976;38:153–175.
2. Yalow RS, Berson SA. Basic considerations and general considerations. In: Odele WD, Daughaday WH, eds. Principles of Competitive Protein Binding Assays. Philadelphia: Lippincott, 1971:1.
3. Wong FCL, Ho B, Lu IG, et al. Affinity labeling of neuroreceptors using gamma rays. J Nucl Med 1993;34(5):26 (abstract).
4. Wagner HN, Barns HD, Dannals RJ, et al. Imaging human dopamine receptors in the human brain. Science 1983;221:1264–1266.
5. Wong DF, Wagner HN, Tune LE, et al. Positron emission tomography reveals elevated D2 dopamine receptors in drug-naive schizophrenics. Science 1986;234:1558–1562.
6. Wong DF, Pearlson G, Tune LE, et al. In vivo measurements of D2 dopamine receptor abnormalities in drug-naive and treated manic depressive patients. J Nucl Med 1987;28:611 (abstract).
7. Kung HF, Slavi A, Chang W, et al. In vivo SPECT imaging of CNS D2 dopamine receptors: initial studies with iodine-123 IBZM in humans. J Nucl Med 1990;31:573–578.
8. Eckelman WC. The testing of putative receptor binding radiotracers in vivo. In: Diksic M, Reba RD, eds. Radiopharmaceuticals and Brain Pathology Studies with PET and SPECT. Boca Raton: CRC Press, 1982:42–62.
9. Vera DR, Krohn KA, Scheibe PO, et al. Identifiability analysis of an in vivo receptor-binding radiopharmacokinetic system. IEEG Trans Biomed Eng 1985;32(5):312–322.
10. Yung BCK, Wand GS, Blevins L, et al. In vivo assessment of dopamine receptor density in pituitary macroadenoma and correlation with in vitro assay. J Nucl Med 1993;34(5):133 (abstract).
11. Junck L, Olson BS, Ciliax BJ, et al. PET imaging of human gliomas with ligands for the peripheral benzodiazepine binding sites. Ann Neurol 1989; 26:752–758.
12. Raderer M, Bechereer A, Kurtaran A, et al. Comparison of iodine-123-vasoactive intestinal peptide receptor scintigraphy and indium-111 CFT-103 immunoscintigraphy. J Nucl Med 1996; 37(9):1480–1487.
13. Starosta-Rubinstein S, Ciliax BJ, Penney JB, et al. Imaging of a glioma using peripheral benzodiazepine receptor ligands. Proc Natl Acad Sci USA 1980;84:891–895.
14. Price GW, Ahier RG, Hume SP, et al. In vivo binding to peripheral benzodiazepine binding sites in lesional rat brain: comparison between [$^{-3}$H]-P/C11194 and [^{18}F]-PK 14105 as markers for neuronal damages. J Neurochem 1990;55: 175– 185.
15. McGuire AH, Dehdashti F, Siegel BA, et al. Positron tomographic assessment of 16α-F18-fluoro-17β-estradiol uptake in metastatic breast carcinoma. J Nucl Med 1991;32:1526–1531.
16. Reubi JC, Krenning E, Lamberts SW, et al. Somatostatin receptors in malignant tissues. J Steroid Biochem Mol Biol 1990;37(6):1073–1077.
17. Lambert SW, Bakker WH, Reubi JC, Krenning EP. Somatostatin receptor imaging in vivo localization of tumors with a radiolabeled somatostatin analog. J Steroid Biochem Mol Biol 1990; 37(60):1079–1082.
18. Bakker WH, Krenning EP, Breeman WA, et al. Receptor scintigraphy with a radioiodinated somatostatin analogue: radiolabeling, purification, biologic activity and in vivo application in animals. J Nucl Med 1990;31:1501–1509.
19. Faglia G, Bazzoni N, Spado X, et al. In vivo detection of somatostatin receptors in patients with functionless pituitary xadenomas by means of a radioiodinated analog of somatostatin I-123 SD2204-090. J Clin Endocrinol Metab 1991;73:850–856.
20. Krenning EP, Kwekkeboom DJ, Panwels S, et al. Somatostatin receptor scintigraphy. Nucl Med Ann 1995;15:1–50.
21. Buscail L, Delesque N, Estéve J, et al. Stimulation of toposine phosphatase and inhibition of cell proliferation by somatostatin analogues: mediation by human somatostatin receptor subtypes SSTR1 and SSTR2. Proc Natl Acad Sci USA 1994;91:2315–2319.
22. Smith-Jones PM, Stolz B, Borms C, et al. Ga-67/Ga-68 [DFO] octreotide—a potential radiopharmaceutical for PET imaging of somatostatin receptor-positive tumors: synthesis and radiolabeling in vitro as preliminary in vivo studies. J Nucl Med 1994;35:317–325.
23. Blok D, Feitsma RIJ, Vermeij P, et al. Peptide radiopharmaceuticals in nuclear medicine. Eur J Nucl Med 1999;26:1511–1519.

9
Polymer-Based Compounds for Targeted Imaging

Chun Li and Edward F. Jackson

The ultimate aim of all targeted imaging is to achieve a large contrast enhancement at the diseased sites that offers not only anatomical but also functional and physicobiochemical information noninvasively. Thus, in this respect, targeted imaging is very similar to drug targeting where the goal is to treat the diseased condition without harming the host, that is, to achieve a large therapeutic index. Depending on the size of contrast agents, two distinct approaches can be envisaged: (1) the agent has low molecular weight (usually <1000 Da); (2) the agent has high molecular weight, or large size, and localization of the agent to the tumor is mediated by carriers that include particulate, liposomal, and macromolecular contrast agents. The latter approach can be further subclassified into passive targeting and active targeting.

Passive targeting exploits the physiological function of the targets or host system and uses their properties to advantage. One well-documented example of passive targeting is macrophage imaging agents, which utilize the efficient removal of particulate contrast agent by the cells of the reticuloendothelial system after intravenous administration [1,2]. Active targeting involves the capacity of an agent to selectively bind to specific sites within the tissue compartment (e.g., tumor versus normal) where it is concentrated and retained. In this chapter, polymer-based compounds for targeted imaging are discussed with emphasis on tumors as primary targets. The polymeric carriers may be conjugated with radionuclides, paramagnetic agents, or iodinated compounds to achieve the desirable imaging properties using different imaging modalities.

Passive Targeting

Targeting resulting from altered microvascular barriers has been the most fruitful area of targeting research in the past 10 years. Many solid tumors have disordered capillary endothelia and thus are more permeable to macromolecules than is normal tissue [3,4]. In addition, because of the paucity of lymphatics in solid tumors, macromolecules tend to persist longer in tumors than in normal tissue. This phenomenon, called the enhanced vascular permeability and retention (EPR) effect, forms the basis for selective delivery of diagnostic and chemotherapeutic agents to solid tumors using polymeric carriers. Clearly the major application of the EPR effect of macromolecules has been in cancer chemotherapy [4–8]. At present, two macromolecular polymer–drug conjugates, polystyrene-maleic anhydride copolymer-neocarzinostadin conjugate (SMANCS) and N-(2-hydroxypropyl)methacrylate copolymer-doxorubicin conjugate (HPMA-Dox), have reached the stage of clinical application [5,6]. Clinical trials of a biodegradable poly(L-glutamic acid)-paclitaxel conjugate, which has demonstrated significant antitumor efficacy in preclinical studies [7,8], were also initiated in early 1999.

Parallel to the development of macromolecular chemotherapeutic agents, the concept of using macromolecular contrast media (MMCM) to enhance contrast between the tumor lesion and surrounding tissue has been proposed and validated in experimental models and clinical studies. A variety of polymer-based contrast agents have been developed primarily for magnetic resonance imaging (MRI).

The use of paramagnetic gadolinium chelates to enhance contrast in T_1-weighted MR images has become increasingly important. These agents are capable of altering the inherent differences in spin-lattice (T_1) and spin-spin (T_2) relaxation times of water in different tissues. Almost all clinical contrast-enhanced MRI examinations are performed with the administration of low molecular weight gadolinium-containing contrast agents. After intravenous injection, these agents are rapidly distributed from intravascular to extravascular space and are rapidly cleared from the body, primarily by glomerular filtration. For example, the plasma concentration of gadopentetate dimeglumine (gadolinium diethylene triamine-pentaacetic acid, Gd-DTPA) falls by 80% just 5 min after injection with $t_{1/2}$ as short as 90 min

[9]. For some imaging applications, however, it would be desirable to have an agent that is largely retained in the intravascular space for the duration of an MRI examination.

Because macromolecules of sufficient size escape very slowly from the vascular compartment after intravenous injection, MMCM have been envisioned and tested in various studies as blood-pool agents [10]. MMCM accumulate in tumor over time in the same way as polymer–drug conjugates do when achieving enhanced therapeutic efficacy. Thus, MMCM can also have important applications in tumor diagnosis. Using albumin-(Gd-DTPA) as a prototype imaging agent, a gradual increase in magnetic resonance signal intensity within tumors over time was observed as opposed to the rapid signal intensity increase observed when low molecular weight Gd-DTPA was used [11].

In our laboratory, we synthesized and characterized a block copolymer of polyethyleneglycol-poly(L-lysine) conjugated with Gd-DTPA (Figure 9.1). Preliminary MR imaging studies demonstrated prolonged blood

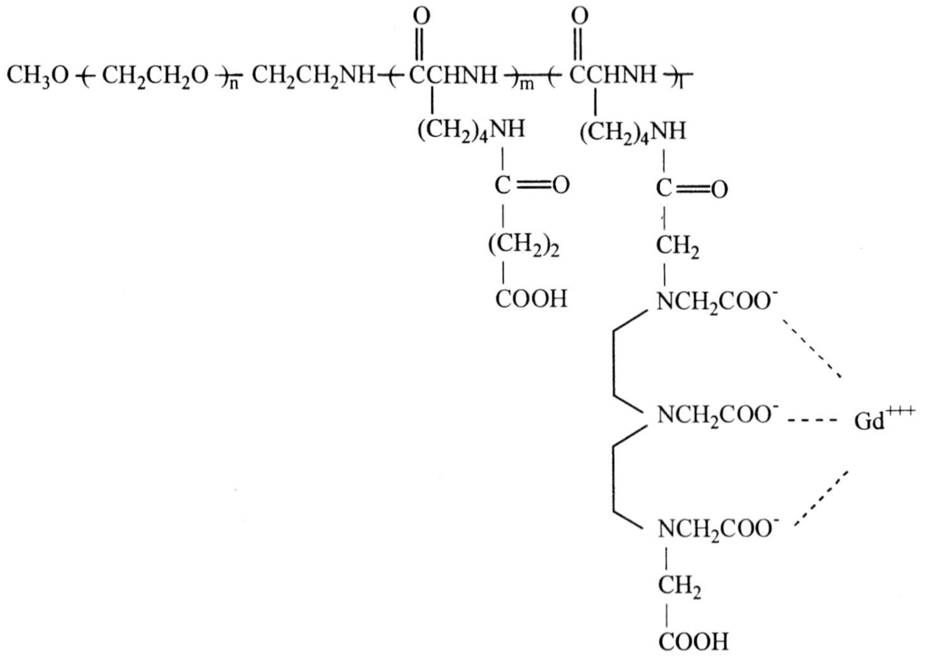

FIGURE 9.1. Structure of polyethyleneglycol-poly(L-lysine) conjugated with Gd-DTPA.

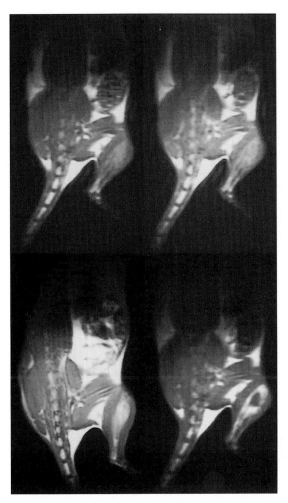

FIGURE 9.2. MRI images of a Fischer rat bearing 13762F tumor before contrast injection (*top left*), and at 1 h (*top right*) and 24 h (*bottom left*) after i.v. injection of polyethyleneglycol-poly(L-lysine)-Gd-DTPA at a dose of 0.02 mmol Gd/kg. The contrast was distributed to the center of the tumor over time. In contrast, only the rim of the tumor was delineated after bolus injection of Gd-DTPA at a dose of 0.2 mmol Gd/kg (*bottom right*).

for use in combination with other imaging modalities. Polymers have been radiolabeled with gamma-emitting radionuclides as blood-pool imaging agents for gamma scintigraphy [12], and polymer-based iodine complexes have been designed and used to prolong contrast enhancement during radiographic examinations [13–15].

MMCM Application in Lymphography

In lymphography, radiopaque or γ-emitting nuclide-labeled materials are injected subcutaneously. They are subsequently taken up into the lymphatic vessels, making them visible on X-ray or gamma camera images. However, low molecular weight materials can easily leak out of the lymphatic vessels, resulting in poor resolution and inadequate contrast enhancement of local lymph nodes. High molecular weight contrast materials would be retained within lymphatic vessels and hence higher resolution of lymph node imaging may be achieved. Frequently the tumor blocks off the lymph flow so that the delivery of contrast is not efficient. This lack of uptake of appropriately labeled agent can be used to identify tumor invasion of lymph nodes [16]. In an effort to improve the signal-to-noise ratio and improve imaging quality, T_1-type lymphotropic MRI agents have been developed. A dextran-polylysine graft copolymer labeled with Gd-DTPA has demonstrated efficient accumulation in lymph nodes after subcutaneous injection. The contrast significantly enhanced the signal intensity of normal nodes but not metastatic nodes (Figure 9.3) [17].

Development of New MMCM

In many aspects, requirements for clinically acceptable MMCM are similar to those of macromolecular chemotherapeutic agents (Table 9.1). Although progress has been made in the first four requirements involving physicochemical properties and physiological limitations, it is the acceptable toxicity profile, which is also related to degradability and immuno-

pool signal as well as accumulation and retention of the contrast material in a rat mammary 13762F tumor inoculated subcutaneously, indicating abnormal capillary leak of macromolecular contrast agent in this tumor (Figure 9.2).

In addition to applications in MR imaging, MMCM have also been developed and tested

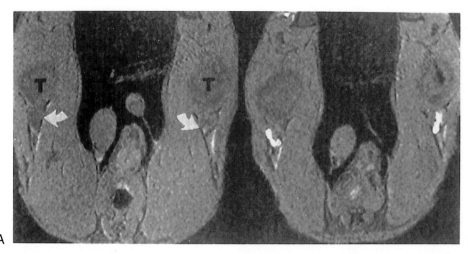

A   B

FIGURE 9.3. MR imaging of VX2 tumors (*T*), implanted into both hind legs, which have metastasized to popliteal lymph nodes (*arrows*). (**A**) Precontrast imaging. (**B**) After s.c. injection of a dextran-polylysine graft copolymer labeled with Gd-DTPA, only a portion of the popliteal lymph node is enhanced; all were histologically proven to be normal. Metastatic tumor deposits appear as nonenhancing nodal defects. (From Harika et al. Magn Reson Med 1995;33:88–92. Reprinted by permission of John Wiley & Sons, Inc.)

genicity, that proves to be the major obstacle. For any foreign material introduced into the body, a major concern is its ultimate fate via degradation and excretion. It was the awareness of this problem that originally prompted the search for materials other than polylysine-(Gd-DTPA) [18]. Further problems are the potential for immunogenicity from the polymeric carrier. This question has been addressed only in a limited way [19].

Among the various MMCM developed thus far, MMCM for MRI have received the most attention. Polylysine-(Gd-DTPA) and albumin-(Gd-DTPA) are two prototype MRI MMCM developed initially for the purpose of proof of concept. Polylysine-(Gd-DTPA) is not readily

TABLE 9.1. Requirements of clinically acceptable macromolecular contrast media (MMCM).

Stability of chelated metals
Contrast loading
Long blood circulation time
Susceptibility to removal by the reticuloendothelial
  system
Immunogenicity
Degradability
Acceptable toxicity

degradable. Small amounts of Gd (6%), which could still be measured 7 days after the injection of polylysine-(Gd-DTPA), could cause potential side effects [18]. The further development of albumin-(Gd-DTPA) is hampered by the concerns of (1) potential immunological reactivity; (2) the instability of albumin during heat sterilization; (3) problems with viral contamination of human blood products; and (4) significant uptake and prolonged retention of Gd in the liver and bone [20].

Many other macromolecular carriers containing Gd-chelates have been designed and evaluated as alternatives to polylysine-(Gd-DTPA) and albumin-(Gd-DTPA). Polymers used to graft Gd-chelates include dextran [21,22] and dendrimers [23–25]. Dendrimers are typically well-defined globular macromolecules constructed around a core unit. Highly branched macromolecules, such as dendrimers complexed with Gd ions, are attracting a lot of attention. One dendrimer-based MRI contrast agent, Gadomer-17, has a molecular weight of 17K. It is built of a central trimesoyl[benzene-1,3,5-tricarbonyl]core, contains two successive reaction steps leading to two generations of L-lysine units, and has 24 macrocyclic gadolinium(III) chelates at its surface [24]. In animal tests, Gadomer-17 appears to fulfill the essential requirement of complete elimination of the heavy metal from the body. In yet another type of synthetic polymer–metal chelate, metal chelators are incorporated into a polymer backbone. Several series of such agents have been synthesized, and their physical properties including relaxivity, metal content, viscosity, and chelate stability have been evaluated and related to polymer structural features [26,27].

Active Targeting

There are many situations in which it is desirable to achieve a degree of selectivity superior to contrast enhancement obtained by simple passive targeting. This requires more specific accumulation of a contrast agent in the target site and better lesion-to-normal-tissue contrast. The use of radiolabeled monoclonal antibodies and receptor ligands has provided a means of generating tumor-specific contrast enhancement in nuclear scintigraphy. Attempts to adapt this technology to MRI have been limited by the concentration of monoclonal antibody (mAb) that can be specifically localized to the tumor to significantly reduce the local proton relaxation times [28,29]. One strategy to overcome this problem is to use polymers that are capable of carrying a large number of chelating groups [30–32]. The polymers, capable of carrying multiple chelated ions, bind to the antibody in limited numbers, thus preserving the antigen-binding affinity. In essence, the polymers through which antibody and metal chelates are linked together serve as an amplifier for metal ions. This approach has been successfully applied to in vivo imaging of target T cells implanted in canine brain using an antibody–albumin–DTPA-Gd construct [32]. However, targeting to tumor has proven to be more difficult because tumor cells have relatively fewer antigen-binding sites.

Tumor-associated cell-surface antigens are generally found at a density of 10^5 to 10^6 sites per cell; the concentration of antigenic sites in tissue would thus be expected to fall in the range of 0.1 to 2.0 μM [29]. This fact suggests that the upper limit of achievable ligand concentration in the tumor is 2.0 μM. One approach to overcoming this limitation to achieving sufficient contrast enhancement is to find a way to increase the relaxivity of receptor ligand-targeted contrast materials. Because MR contrast agents prepared with a dendritic backbone have high relaxivities [23], Wiener et al. prepared folate-conjugated dentrimer chelates. The conjugate was able to increase the longitudinal relaxation rate of tumor cells expressing high-affinity folate receptor by 110%. This increase was inhibited by an excess of free folic acid, demonstrating the feasibility of receptor imaging in vitro [33].

Although in vivo targeting remains a challenge, some indications of success have been demonstrated. A monocloncal antibody against breast cancer cells, mAb 232/A3, has been conjugated to a gadolinium–melanin polymer. The conjugate showed substantial reduction of both T_1 and T_2 relaxation times and was expected to produce a 38% change in T_1 and a 42% change in T_2 at an mAb 323/A3–melanin conjugate concentration of 2 μM [34]. As an alternative to paramagnetically labeled antibodies, a monocloncal antibody L6 has been attached to superparamagnetic monocrystalline iron oxide nanoparticles (MION). The magnetically labeled MION-L6 conjugate demonstrated slow, antigen-specific accumulation within an intracerebral tumor [35]. These studies demonstrate that active targeting of MRI contrast media to tumor is feasible, provided that specific in vivo distribution is achieved and that sufficient paramagnetic metal ions are delivered to significantly increase the relaxation rates of the target tissue.

In addition to the ability to carry a large number of metal ions, polymers may offer additional benefits for the optimization of pharmacological properties. Negatively charged poly(L-lysine-DTPA-succinic acid) was conjugated to the Fab′ fragment of a monoclonal antimyosin antibody. When this antibody–polymer chelate conjugate was labeled with indium-111, reduced nonspecific binding was demonstrated that allowed rapid scintigraphic visualization of experimental myocardial infarction [36]. Poly (L-lysine) modified monoclonal antibody was also found to have reduced hepatic accumulation [37].

A current trend in the field of MR imaging is the use of higher magnetic field strengths for neuroimaging studies. Currently, the most commonly used field strengths for clinical imaging are in the 0.5 to 2.0 tesla range. However, there are now more than 20 MR imaging systems with field strengths at or exceeding 3 T, and one commercial vendor has recently received FDA 510K clearance for marketing a 3 T imaging system for clinical use. There are numerous advantages of such higher-field MR systems, including dramatic improvements in signal to noise in functional MR imaging studies and signal-to-noise and spectral resolution improvements in in vivo spectroscopy studies. For contrast agent studies, such higher-field systems can also offer substantial benefits and might decrease the necessary concentration of Gd necessary for measurable changes in image contrast. As the magnetic field strength increases, so do the T_1 (spin-lattice) relaxation times of the various tissues. As the T_1 relaxation times increase, the percent increase in contrast between nonenhancing tissue and enhancing tissue increases for a given concentration of Gd (assuming the T_1 and T_2 relaxivities of the agents are relatively constant or increase with field strength). Therefore, at higher field strengths, concentrations of Gd that are inadequate for providing significant increases in contrast at 1.5-T field strengths may be quite adequate at 3-T or higher field strengths. Similarly, studies that use paramagnetic contrast agents as intravascular dynamic susceptibility agents to transiently shorten the T_2^* relaxation times during "first-pass" blood volume measurements should benefit from the increased susceptibility effects that are noted at higher field strengths. The combination of targeted or macromolecular MR imaging agents discussed in this chapter and "very high field" MR systems should greatly expand our ability to more fully characterize neoplastic lesions and associated pathology as well as quantitatively monitor the effects of therapy.

MMCM in Tumor Characterization

Recent progress in molecular targets and cancer therapeutics has added a new dimension to the imaging sciences. Traditional approaches of tumor characterization by visualizing tumor location and tumor size are not necessarily sufficient to satisfy the need for monitoring free drug levels and the biological effect of the drug. MRI with MMCM may offer some assistance in more specific and probably more accurate tumor characterization. Applications of polymeric paramagnetic contrast agents include assessments of relative tissue blood volume, estimation of tissue perfusion, and detection of abnormal capillary permeability [10,38].

A fundamental concept in oncology is that the growth of solid tumors beyond a certain size is dependent on angiogenesis [39]. A reliable noninvasive in vivo assay for characterization of tumor angiogenic activity could not only be used as an in vivo tool for determining the prognostic significance of angiogenesis, but would also allow timely monitoring of the immediate and long-term effects of antiangiogenic therapy. It has been postulated that tumor angiogenesis may be assessed by the rapid (early) MRI enhancement, as demonstrated in breast carcinomas after administration of Gd-DTPA [40]. Depending on how the enhancement time curve data are interpreted, weak to moderate correlations between dynamic MRI-derived pharmacokinetic parameters and microvessel counts have been observed [40–42]. The major limitation of Gd-DTPA is that it distributes rapidly from the intravascular to the extravascular space, resulting in less than optimal quantification of vascular permeability and plasma volume.

In principle, the pharmacokinetic parameters can be measured accurately only with high molecular weight blood-pool agents that remain in the vascular space of normal tissues. Quantitative methods have been developed to estimate tissue plasma volume and vessel permeability using albumin-Gd-DTPA-enhanced MRI [43]. A recent study in a rat mammary carcinoma model showed a strong positive, but less than perfect, correlation between pharmacokinetic parameters derived from albumin-Gd-DTPA-enhanced MRI and microvessel counts, with the square of sample correlation coefficient value (R^2) of 0.85 [44]. Quantitative tumor vascular permeability and fractional plasma volume generated using albumin-Gd-DTPA were found to correlate significantly with histological tumor grade ($R^2=0.76$, $p<10^{-10}$ and $R^2=0.25$, $p<0.003$, respectively), whereas no significant correlation was found when small molecular weight Gd-DTPA was used ($R^2=0.01$, $p>0.95$ and $R^2=0.03$, $p>0.15$, respectively) [45]. Similarly, Su et al. used three contrast agents of different molecular weight [Gd-DTPA (MW 1 kDa), Gadomer-17 (35 kDa), and albumin-Gd-DTPA (70–90 kDa)] to study the imaging properties of malignant and benign breast tumors in animal models. Based on pharmacokinetic characteristics measured, they found that the intermediate-size agent Gadomer-17 could differentiate between malignant tumors of low and high grades [46]. These results validate the diagnostic potential of MMCM for the characterization of tumor angiogenic activity.

Using a radiolabeled polymeric analogue, gamma scintigraphy in normal and tumor-bearing experimental models has provided information on the tumor-targeting properties of N-(2-hydroxylpropyl)methacrylamide

copolymer-doxyrubicin conjugates and have been valuable tools in the development and understanding of these materials before phase I clinical therapeutic trials [47,48]. Thus, MMCM may be a useful tool for predicting and monitoring response to therapy with macromolecular chemotherapeutic agents. As mentioned earlier, the enhanced permeability and retention effect of macromolecules is responsible for the increased antitumor efficacy of many polymer–drug conjugates as compared to their low molecular weight parent drugs. Quantitative assessment of mice bearing murine OCa-1 ovarian tumor showed that the tumor uptake of PG-[³H]paclitaxel(TXL) over a period of 6 days is approximately fivefold higher than tumor uptake of [³H]paclitaxel [49]. This may be one of the major factors contributing to the superior antitumoral activity of PG-TXL [7]. On the other hand, if a polymer–drug conjugate is physically impeded from being distributed into the tumor, then its tumor-killing potential in vivo would be largely compromised. In an attempt to develop a suitable assay for monitoring tumor uptake of PG-TXL noninvasively, we synthesized ⁶⁷Ga-labeled poly(L-glutamic acid). As shown in Figure 9.4, tumor uptake of poly(L-glutamic

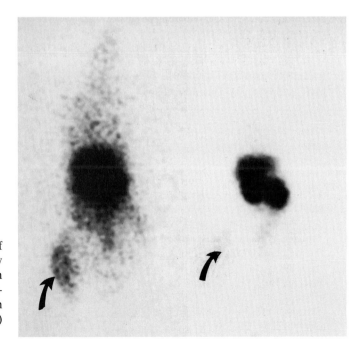

FIGURE 9.4. Gamma scintigram of Fischer rats bearing s.c. mammary 13762 tumor. *Left*: rat injected with ⁶⁷Ga-PG (molecular weight, 33 K) intravenously. *Right*: rat injected with ⁶⁷Ga-PG (molecular weight, 10 K) intravenously. *Arrows*, tumor.

acid) is a function of polymer molecular weight, suggesting that the antitumor efficacy of PG-TXL would increase with increasing PG molecular weights. Obviously, further studies using ^{67}Ga-labeled poly(L-glutamic acid) and ^{67}Ga-labeled PG-TXL to evaluate and compare their distribution to tumor in PG-TXL-responsive and PG-TXL-resistant tumor models are necessary to associate between tumor uptake of macromolecular radiotracer and responsiveness to macromolecular chemotherapy.

References

1. Li C, Kan Z-X, Yang DJ, et al. Preparation, characterization, and evaluation of ioxilan carbonate particles for computed tomography contrast enhancement of the liver. Invest Radiol 1994; 29(11):1006–1013.
2. Ivancev K, Lunderquist A, Isaksson A, et al. Clinical trials with a new iodinated lipid emulsion for computed tomography of the liver. Acta Radiol 1989;30:449–457.
3. Gerlowski LE, Jain RK. Microvascular permeability of normal and neoplastic tissues. Microvasc Res 1986;31:288–305.
4. Maeda H, Matsumura Y. Tumoritropic and lymphotropic principles of macromolecular drugs. Crit Rev Ther Drug Carrier Syst 1989;6:193–210.
5. Maeda H. SMANCS and polymer-conjugated macromolecular drugs: advantages in cancer chemotherapy. Adv Drug Delivery Rev 1991;6: 181–193.
6. Vasey PA, Kaye SB, Morrison R, et al. Phase I clinical and pharmacokinetic study of PK1 [N-(2-hydroxylpropyl)methacrylamide copolymer doxorubicin]: first member of a new class of chemotherapeutic agents-drug-polymer conjugates. Clin Cancer Res 1999;5:83–94.
7. Li C, Yu D-F, Newman RA, et al. Complete regression of well-established tumors using a novel water-soluble poly(L-glutamic acid)-paclitaxel conjugate. Cancer Res 1998;58:2404–2409.
8. Li C, Price JE, Milas L, et al. Antitumor activity of poly(L-glutamic acid)-paclitaxel on syngeneic and xenografted tumors. Clin Cancer Res 1999; 5:891–897.
9. Strich G, Hagan PL, Gerber KH, et al. Tissue distribution and magnetic resonance spin lattice relaxation effects of gadolinium-DTPA. Radiology 1985;154:723–726.
10. Brasch R. New directions in the development of MR imaging contrast media. Radiology 1992; 183:1–11.
11. Wikstrom MG, Moseley ME, White DL, et al. Contrast-enhanced MRI of tumors: comparison of Gd-DTPA and a macromolecular agent. Invest Radiol 1989;24:609–615.
12. Bogdanov AA, Callahan RJ, Wilkinson RA, et al. Synthetic copolymer kit for radionuclide blood-pool imaging. J Nucl Med 1994;35:1880–1886.
13. Bogdanov AA, Weissleder R, Brady TJ. Long circulating blood pool imaging agents. Advanced Drug Delivery Rev 1995;16:335–348.
14. Doucet D, Meyer D, Chambon C, Bonnemain B. Blood-pool X-ray contrast agents: evaluation of a new iodinated polymer. Invest Radiol 1991; 26:S53–S54.
15. Revel D, Chambon C, Havard PH, et al. Iodinated polymer as a blood-pool contrast agent: computed tomography evaluation in rabbits. Invest Radiol 1991;26:S57–S59.
16. Osborne MP, Payne JH, Richardson VJ, et al. The preoperative detection of axilliary lymph node metastases in breast cancer by isotope imaging. Br J Surg 1983;70:141–144.
17. Harika L, Weissleder R, Poss K, et al. MR lymphography with a lymphotropic T1-type MR contrast agent: Gd-DTPA-PGM. Magn Reson Med 1995;33:88–92.
18. Schumann-Giampieri G, Schmit-Wilich H, Frenzel T, et al. In vivo and in vitro evaluation of Gd-DTPA-polylysine as a macromolecular contrast agent for magnetic resonance imaging. Invest Radiol 1991;26:696–974.
19. Bagnodav AA, Weissleder R, Frank HW, et al. A new macromolecule as a contrast agent for MR angiography: preparation, properties, and animal studies. Radiology 1993;187:701–706.
20. Schmiedl U, Ogan M, Paajanen H, et al. Albumin labeled with Gd-DTPA as an intravascular, blood pool-enhancing agent for MR imaging: biodistribution and imaging studies. Radiology 1987;162:205–210.
21. Wang S-C, Wikstrom MG, White DL, et al. Evaluation of Gd-DTPA-labeled dextran as an intravascular MR contrast agent: imaging characteristics in normal rat tissues. Radiology 1990;175:483–488.
22. Rebizak R, Schaefer M, Dellacherie E. Polymeric conjugates of Gd[3+]diethylenepentaacetic acid and dextran. 2. Influence of spacer arm length and conjugate molecular mass on the paramagnetic properties and some biological parameters. Bioconjugate Chem 1998;9:94–99.

23. Wiener EC, Brechbiel MW, Brothers H, et al. Dendrimer-based metal chelates: a new class of magnetic resonance imaging contrast agents. Magn Reson Med 1994;31:1–8.

24. Weinmann HJ, Ebert W, Wagner S, et al. MR angio with special focus on blood pool agents. In: Proceedings of the IX International Workshop on Magnetic Resonance Angiography, Valencia, October 7–11, 1997, pp 335–340.

25. Adam G, Neuerburg J, Spuntrup E, et al. 24-Gadolinium-cascade-polymer: a potential blood-pool contrast agent for MR imaging. J Magn Reson Imaging 1994;4:462–466.

26. Keller KE, Henrichs PM, Hollister R, et al. High relaxivity linear Gd(DTPA)-polymer conjugates: the role of hydrophobic interactions. Magn Reson Med 1997;38:712–716.

27. Ladd DL, Hollister R, Peng X, et al. Polymeric gadolinium chelate magnetic resonance imaging contrast agents: design, synthesis, and properties. Bioconjugate Chem 1999;10:361–370.

28. Unger EC, Totty WG, Neufeld DM, et al. Magnetic resonance imaging using gadolinium labeled monocloncal antibody. Invest Radiol 1985;20:693–700.

29. Anderson-Berg WT, Strand M, Lempert TE, et al. Nuclear magnetic resonance and gamma camera tumor imaging using Gd-labeled monocloncal antibodies. J Nucl Med 1986;27:829–833.

30. Torchilin VP, Klibanov AL, Nossiff ND, et al. Monoclonal antibody modification with chelate-linked high-molecular-weight polymers: major increases in polyvalent cation binding without loss of antigen binding. Hybridoma 1987;6:229–240.

31. Shreve P, Aisen AM. Monoclonal antibodies labeled with polymeric paramagnetic ion chelates. Magn Reson Med 1986;3:336–340.

32. Kornguth SE, Turski PA, Perman WH, et al. Magnetic resonance imaging of gadolinium-labeled monocloncal antibody polymer directed at human T lymphocytes implanted in canine brain. J Neurosurg 1987;66:898–906.

33. Wiener EC, Konda S, Shadron A, et al. Targeting dendrimer-chelates to tumors and tumor cells expressing the high-affinity folate receptor. Invest Radiol 1997;32(12):748–754.

34. Orang-Khadivi K, Pierce BL, Ollom CM, et al. New magnetic resonance imaging technique for the detection of breast cancer. Breast Cancer Res Treat 1994;32:119–135.

35. Neuwelt EA, Remsen LG, McCormick CI, et al. Magnetic resonance imaging of monocrystalline iron oxide nanocompound conjugated carcinoma specific monocloncal antibody in a rodent model of intracerebral human lung cancer: the potential for knifeless diagnosis. Proc Am Assoc Cancer Res 1995;36:483.

36. Khaw BA, Kilbanov A, O'Donnell SM, et al. Gamma imaging with negatively charge-modified monoclonal antibody: modification with synthetic polymers. J Nucl Med 1991;32:1742–1751.

37. Wang TST, Fawwaz RA, Alderson PO. Reduced hepatic accumulation of radio-labeled monoclonal antibodies with indium-111 thioether-poly-L-lysine DTPA-monoclonal antibody-TP41.2F(ab')$_2$. J Nucl Med 1992;33:570–575.

38. Su MY, Muhler A, Lao X, et al. Tumor characterization with dynamic contrast-enhanced MRI using MR contrast agents of various molecular weights. Magn Reson Med 1998;39:259–269.

39. Folkman J. What is the evidence that tumors are angiogenesis dependent? J Natl Cancer Inst 1990;82:4–6.

40. Frouge C, Guinebretiere JM, Contesso G, et al. Correlation between contrast enhancement in dynamic magnetic resonance imaging of the breast and tumor angiogenesis. Invest Radiol 1994;29:1043–1049.

41. Buadu LD, Murakami J, Murayama S, et al. Breast lesions: correlation of contrast medium enhancement patterns on MR images with histopathologic findings and tumor angiogenesis. Radiology 1996;200:639–649.

42. Buckley DL, Drew PJ, Murrurakis S, et al. Microvessel density in invasive breast cancer assessed by dynamic Gd-DTPA enhanced MRI. J Magn Reson Imaging 1997;7:461–464.

43. Shames DM, Kuwatsuru R, Vexler V, et al. Measurement of capillary permeability to macromolecules by dynamic magnetic resonance imaging: a quantitative noninvasive technique. Magn Reson Med 1993;29:616–622.

44. van Dijke CF, Brasch RC, Roberts TPL, et al. Mammary carcinoma model: correlation of macromolecular contrast-enhanced MR imaging characterizations of tumor microvasculature and histologic capillary density. Radiology 1996;198:813–818.

45. Daldrup H, Shames DM, Wendland M, et al. Correlation of dynamic contrast enhanced MR imaging with histologic tumor grade: comparison of macromolecular and small-molecular contrast media. AJR 1998;171:941–949.

46. Su MY, Wang Z, Carpenter PM, et al. Characterization of N-ethyl-N-nitrosourea-induced

malignant and benign breast tumors in rats by using three MR contrast agents. J Magn Reson Imaging 1999;9920:177–186.

47. Prim MV, Perkins AC, Duncan R, et al. Targeting of N-(2-hydroxylpropyl)methacrylamide copolymer-doxyrubicin conjugate to the hepatocyte galactose-receptor in mice: visualization and quantification by gamma scintigraphy as a basis for clinical targeting studies. J Drug Targeting 1993;1:125–131.

48. Prim MV, Perkins AC, Strohalm J, et al. Gamma scintigraphy of the biodistribution of ^{123}I-labeled N-(2-hydroxylpropyl)methacrylamide copolmer-doxyrubicin conjugates in mice with transplanted melanoma and mammary carcinoma. J Drug Targeting 1996;3: 375–385.

49. Li C, Newman RA, Wu Q-P, et al. Biodistribution of paclitaxel and poly (L-glutamic-acid)-paclitaxel conjugates in mice with ovarian OCa-1 tumor. Cancer Chemother Pharmacol, in press.

10
Targeted Single Photon Emission Computed Tomography in Oncology

E. Edmund Kim and Franklin C.L. Wong

The practice of oncology is under going significant advances, and better understanding of molecular biology along with new diagnostic techniques and chemotherapeutic agents have improved the management of many cancer patients. Nuclear imaging can provide important information regarding tumor diagnosis, staging, detection of relapse or residual tumor, response to therapy, and prognosis for a variety of tumors. Currently available images have high diagnostic sensitivity, but low specificity. The use of the tomographic concept in nuclear medicine is as old as the art of radionuclide imaging itself. Single photon and positron emission tomography aim to reconstruct a three-dimensional image displaying the distribution of a radiotracer administered to a patient. Considerable attention has been given to positron emission tomography (PET) and its remarkable ability to dynamically display slices of life in various organs. It appears that the enormous expense associated with PET has kept it in academic and teaching medical centers. It is anticipated that much of the research produced at PET centers will provide the development of single photon counterparts of the positron agents. The performance of single photon emission computed tomography (SPECT) is within the capability of the community medical practice (Figure 10.1). The multipurpose nature of this equipment often makes it the best planar imaging.

The conventional tumor SPECT has gained increasing acceptance in several clinical areas, most notably gallium, thallium, and sestamibi imaging. It has become a natural step to begin to explore its quantitative capabilities. Quantitation is inherent to radionuclide methodology and has been used extensively to overcome the contribution of background activity to target organ counts as well as superimposition of extraneous tissue activity.

Gallium SPECT

Although ^{67}Ga-citrate is taken up to varying degrees by many other tumors, the staging and follow-up of lymphoma remain a predominant clinical indication for ^{67}Ga planar and SPECT studies. Gallium biologically behaves like the ferric (+3 oxidation state) ion. ^{67}Ga is produced by the cyclotron after bombardment of ^{68}Zn and decays by electron capture. It has a 78-h physical half-life and emits a spectrum of gamma rays with approximately 100, 200, 300, and 400 keV. ^{67}Ga binds to transferrin in the blood and also iron-binding proteins such as ferritin and lactoferrin. Within 24 h, 15% to 25% is excreted by the kidneys. Thereafter, clearance is slow with the colon being the major route of excretion. The biological half-life is approximately 25 days. The estimated radiation absorbed dose to the large intestine is 0.9 rads/mCi. Oral cathartics had no value in optimizing the gallium scan [1].

For tumor imaging, 8 to 10 mCi ^{67}Ga-citrate is usually used. The superior images and improved SPECT result in a clear-cut benefit–

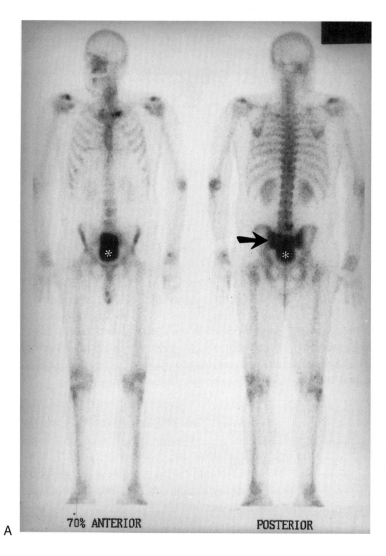

70% ANTERIOR   POSTERIOR

A

FIGURE 10.1. (**A**) Whole-body anterior (*left*) and posterior (*right*) images of nuclear bone scan using 25 mCi ^{99m}Tc-MDP (methylene diphosphate) in patient with epiglottic squamous cell cancer show focal increased activity (*arrow*) in the left sacrum overlying physiological activities in the bladder (*) and sacral ala. (**B**) Axial SPECT images of the pelvis show a ring-shaped lesion (*arrow*) in the left sacrum with peripheral increased activity, suggesting central necrosis. (**C**) T$_1$-weighted MR image of the pelvis shows a large focal area of decreased signal intensity (*) in the left sacrum, encasing the sacral neural foramen (*arrow*). Biopsy confirmed a metastatic carcinoma.

risk ratio for the high doses in cancer patients. Although 500,000 counts per view are usually adequate for whole-body imaging, 1,000,000 counts are generally needed for imaging organs of normally high uptake such as the liver. The larger dose also permits delayed imaging when more background has cleared. High-quality SPECT can be obtained at 48, 72, and often 96 h. Chest and abdominal SPECT are routinely performed for areas of clinical concern. Serial abdominal images are useful in the differentiation of normal bowel activity and a suspicious gallium-avid lesion. ^{67}Ga-citrate normally localizes in the liver, spleen, bone, bone marrow, and lacrimal, salivary, and mammary glands. Thymic uptake can occur, especially with thymic hyperplasia after therapy. Multiple transfusions have shown increased renal, bladder, or bone localization of ^{67}Ga and decreased liver and colon activity [2]. Although tumor uptake is maximal within 24 h of injection, physiological clearance results in an improved target-to-background count density ratio on more delayed imaging at 48 to 72 h.

The mechanism of ^{67}Ga localization is incompletely understood. After binding to transferrin, it enters the tumor extracellular fluid space via the leaky capillary endothelium of the tumor. ^{67}Ga is bound to the tumor cell surface by transferrin receptors and then transported

FIGURE 10.1. *Continued*

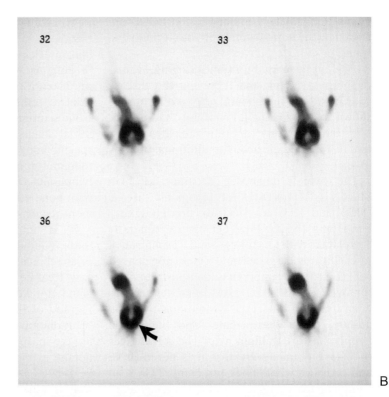

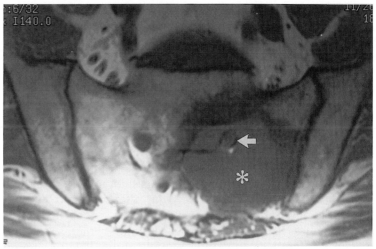

into the cell. It localizes intracellularly in the lysosomes of growing or viable tumor cells, not in necrotic tumor or fibrosis [3,4].

The ability of ^{67}Ga to detect tumors depends on several factors. Tumors less than 2 cm in size are not reliably detected, and tumors larger than 5 cm are sometimes poorly seen by planar imaging because of central necrosis. Superficial lesions are easier to detect than deep ones. SPECT usually allows detection of smaller and more centrally located tumors. ^{99m}Tc-sulfur colloid liver–spleen scan is helpful for diagnosing hepatoma in conjunction with ^{67}Ga scan because cold lesions with filling defects on colloid scan fill in on the ^{67}Ga scan. SPECT is particularly useful in the evaluation of a mediastinal, hilar, or midline lesion that is obscured by the normal uptake in the sternum and spine.

[67]Ga has been used for tumor staging, evaluating tumor extent, and following the disease course and the therapeutic response in tumors shown to be ^{67}Ga avid. Persistent ^{67}Ga uptake after the cessation of therapy indicates persistent disease and the need for additional therapy [3,4].

The overall diagnostic accuracy of ^{67}Ga SPECT is about 90% for Hodgkin's disease (HD) and 55% to 85% for non-Hodgkin's lymphoma (NHL) [5]. [67]Ga avidity generally correlates with histology and proliferative rate. Diffuse large-cell and small noncleaved cell (Burkitt's) lymphomas demonstrate ^{67}Ga uptake (Figure 10.2). Low ^{67}Ga avidity has been found in low-grade lymphomas by some authors. Most intermediate- and high-grade lymphomas are gallium avid. The advantages of ^{67}Ga for staging are that it is noninvasive and provides whole-body screening. [67]Ga scan complements CT and can affect management by altering staging. [67]Ga scan altered radiation treatment in 12% of patients and in 31% when CT and ^{67}Ga results were combined. [67]Ga scan has a role in restaging with 75% to 100% sensitivities and 75% to 95% specificities because CT or MRI has limited ability to distinguish residual active tumor from fibrotic mass [5,6].

The ^{67}Ga scan can provide useful prognostic information. Ablation of ^{67}Ga uptake by radiotherapy or chemotherapy is a predictor of therapeutic response (Figure 10.3). Persistent ^{67}Ga uptake may indicate the need for alternative therapy. Serial ^{67}Ga scans can predict lymphoma-free and overall survival, information not available from clinical and other imaging parameters. The negative predictive values for CT and ^{67}Ga scans were greater than 80% for HD and NHL. However, the positive predictive values for ^{67}Ga scan for HD and NHL were 80% and 73%, compared with 29% and 35%, respectively for CT [7]. In patients after bone marrow transplant for diffuse aggressive NHL, ^{67}Ga SPECT at day 100 post transplant was highly predictive of eventual outcome and was more predictive than CT.

[67]Ga scan is useful for monitoring therapeutic response (Figure 10.4). Persistent ^{67}Ga uptake halfway through the course of chemotherapy in patients with diffuse large-cell lymphoma predicted a poor outcome, either by failure to achieve remission or by subsequent relapse. Bone scintigraphy may not be necessary in the initial staging of lymphoma unless there are specific bony symptoms. [67]Ga scan can be used to monitor response of bony involvement of lymphoma to treatment and is more reliable than bone scintigraphy for following the treatment response.

It is important to recognize common therapy-induced changes to facilitate appropriate clinical management and avoid unnecessary treatment or additional testing. Salivary gland uptake is often increased after radiotherapy of the neck or mediastinum because of radiation sialadenitis, and the increased uptake may be persistent beyond 1 year. [67]Ga uptake in the mediastinum after therapy may be related to rebound thymus in children as well as adults. Bilateral hilar uptake of ^{67}Ga is more readily identified and remains undetermined and challenged [8]. If the uptake appears before treatment and CT is negative, the uptake is probably of no clinical significance. When the uptake is new after treatment, the reactive hyperplasia of lymph nodes can be considered if it is fairly symmetrical and has no greater intensity than that of the sternum. [201]Tl has been proposed to aid in the differentiation of benign and malignant nodes. Diffuse lung uptake [9] may be seen during or after chemotherapy, and probably represents inflammation caused by the chemotherapeutic agent with lung toxicity. It may be seen after radiation therapy to the chest. Areas of bone remodeling following trauma may also be noted with ^{67}Ga, which is a weak bone scan agent.

CT has been the primary imaging modality for staging lung cancer, and the detection of hilar and mediastinal involvement is critical for determining operability, prognosis, and appropriate treatment. The high spatial resolution of CT makes it a sensitive screening modality, but tumor can present in normal-sized nodes. The overall sensitivity of ^{67}Ga for the detection of lung cancer is reported to be 85% to 90%, but

FIGURE 10.2. (**A**) T$_1$-weighted coronal MR image of the head following injection of Gd-DTPA shows contrast-enhanced lesion (*) in the right basal ganglia in patient who previously received radiation therapy for known large-cell lymphoma in the brain. (**B**) Selected coronal SPECT images of the head at 48h following injection of ^{67}Ga-citrate show focal area of markedly increased activity (*arrow*) in the right basal ganglia area. Biopsy confirmed recurrent lymphoma.

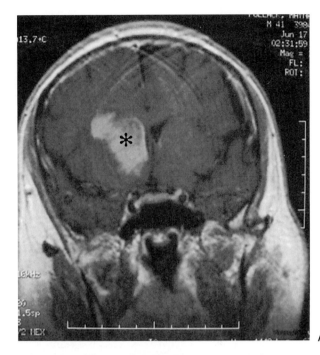

A

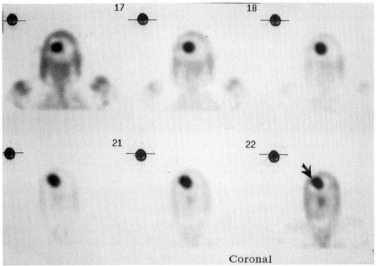

Coronal

B

diagnostic accuracy appears suboptimal for preoperative staging. There is no clear-cut role of ^{67}Ga scan in the detection of metastatic lung cancer [10,11]. Hepatocellular carcinoma is frequently multifocal in patients with hepatic cirrhosis. [67]Ga can be useful for differentiating hepatoma from regenerating nodules or metastatic adenocarcinomas because approximately 90% of hepatomas are gallium avid [12]; most malignant melanomas and metastases are gallium avid. With ^{67}Ga SPECT, the overall sensitivity and specificity for detecting metastatic melanoma are reported to be 82% and 99%, respectively [13]. Most soft tissue sarcomas are also ^{67}Ga avid with a 93% sensitivity for detecting primary lesions, local recurrence, and metastatic lesions. Tumor grade generally predicts ^{67}Ga uptake, and thus low-grade

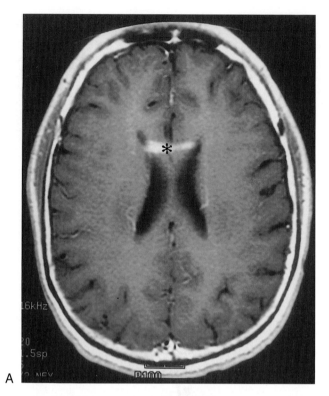

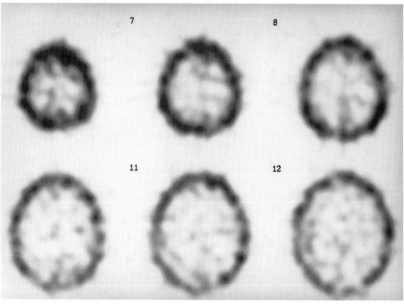

FIGURE 10.3. (**A**) Postcontrast T_1-weighted axial MR image of the head shows a bandlike enhanced lesion (*) in the anterior body of corpus callosum in lymphoma patient who previously received brain irradi- ation. (**B**) Selected transaxial SPECT images of the head at 48 h following injection of ^{67}Ga-citrate show no focal increased activity in the area of corpus callosum, indicating no active lymphomatous lesion.

FIGURE 10.4. (**A**) Frontal view of chest X-ray shows persistent mass lesion (*) in the medial aspect of right lung overlying right hilum and cardiac border in a patient with lymphoma. (**B**) Selected coronal SPECT images of the chest at 48 h following the injection of ^{67}Ga-citrate show a large lymphoma lesion in the right lung with a necrotic cavity in the middle portion shown as a donut-shaped area of increased activity (*arrow*).

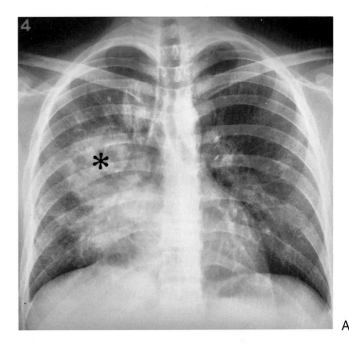

A

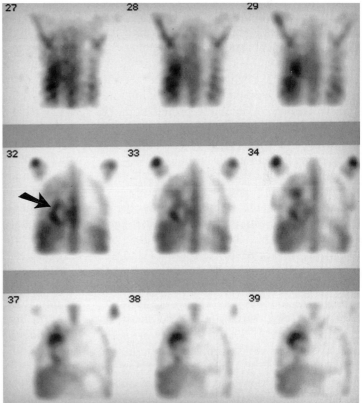

B

liposarcomas are typically associated with a higher false-negative rate. The ^{67}Ga-positive site that becomes negative after therapy is indicative of a favorable clinical response [14,15].

Thallium SPECT

Thallium-201 has been used since the 1970s to evaluate myocardial perfusion. Much of the initial tumor work was done for the evaluation of thyroid masses to differentiate benign and malignant nodules. [201]Tl was subsequently used to diagnose various tumors including malignant brain tumor and parathyroid adenoma. [201]Tl is handled by cells similarly to potassium and is concentrated by the sodium potassium adenosine triphosphatase (ATPase) pump within cell membranes. There is also a cotransport system that transports potassium and sodium as well as chloride. The former is inhibited by ouabain and the latter by furosemide. The third mechanism has been attributed to a calcium-dependent ion channel system. [201]Tl accumulates in viable tumor, less in connective tissue, and to a negligible level in necrotic tissue. It mainly exists in the free form in tumor fluid, and the minor amount is protein bound in the nuclear, mitochondrial, and microsomal fractions. Other possible factors influencing ^{201}Tl uptake by tumor cells are blood flow, vascular immaturity caused by leakage, cell membrane permeability, and tumor type [16].

[201]Tl is a metallic element and decays by electron capture with a half-life of 73 h. It emits a cluster of X-rays between 69 and 83 keV (94%) and γ-rays of 167 keV (10%) and 135 keV (3%). It is distributed in proportion to regional blood flow, and excreted primarily through the kidneys. The kidney is the target organ, receiving 3.6 rads/mCi. The heart receives only 3% to 5% of the dose, with the majority in the liver, spleen, muscle, brain, and kidneys. There is no consensus regarding the optimal imaging time, and 20 to 60 min or 1 to 4 h has been proposed. There is normal uptake of ^{201}Tl in the lacrimal and salivary glands, thyroid, myocardium, liver, spleen, kidneys, and muscles. Normal myocardial uptake may be a problem in evaluating lung and breast cancer,

and variable bowel activity may also be a problem in evaluating abdominal cancer. The majority of tumors show variable washout of approximately 25% [201]Tl uptake over 2 h, but some tumors may show a continuous uptake over the same period. Quantification of ^{201}Tl uptake in lesions has been proposed to increase sensitivity and specificity for detection of malignancy and determination of tumor grade [17]. However, ratios vary according to the definition of the region, region size, uniformity within the lesion, and location.

Multiple studies have shown the clinical application of ^{201}Tl for the evaluation of brain tumors [16,17]. The ^{201}Tl uptake in gliomas has been correlated well with the tumor grade and valuable for evaluating therapeutic effectiveness (Figure 10.5). [201]Tl can determine viability of residual tumor when CT or MRI cannot differentiate from posttreatment changes. The results are similar to those achieved with ^{18}F FDG PET scan [18]. [201]Tl has also been used to differentiate cerebral lymphoma from toxoplasmosis as it is taken up by lymphomas but not in infections [19]. Several studies have investigated the use of ^{201}Tl for thyroid cancer after thyroidectomy [20]. A significant advantage is that the patient can continue taking thyroid hormone therapy. The clinical role for ^{201}Tl is in localizing the site of recurrent thyroid cancer when ^{131}I scan is negative but serum thyroglobulin level is elevated because ^{201}Tl is not specific for thyroid cancer. [201]Tl has been successfully used to detect primary lung cancer as well as hilar and mediastinal metastases. It is useful in differentiating malignant from benign lung masses [21].

[201]Tl uptake is usually greater than that with ^{67}Ga-citrate, and it is rarely taken up by inflammatory lesions. [201]Tl showed 97% sensitivity for detecting breast cancer and 38% for breast adenoma [22]. Fibrocystic breast disease revealed no ^{201}Tl uptake. The smallest detectable lesion was about 1 cm on 15 to 30-min images. [201]Tl scan may be useful in patients with indeterminate lesions on mammography to minimize unnecessary biopsies. [201]Tl may be more accurate than ^{99m}Tc-MDP or ^{67}Ga-citrate in determining the extent of primary bone tumors and is valuable for assessing the

FIGURE 10.5. (**A**) Postcontrast T$_1$-weighted transaxial image of the head shows an enhanced focal lesion (*) in right frontal brain of patient who previously received radiation therapy for anaplastic astrocytoma. (**B**) Selected coronal (*left upper*), sagittal (*right upper*), and axial (*left lower*) SPECT images using ^{201}Tl-chloride show focal lesion with markedly increased activity in the right frontal brain (*arrow*), indicating active recurrent malignant brain tumor that was confirmed by biopsy.

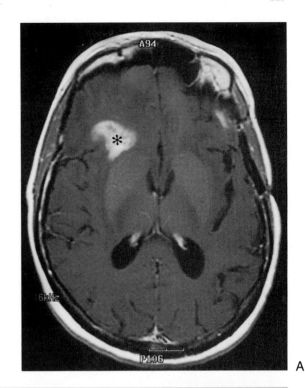

A

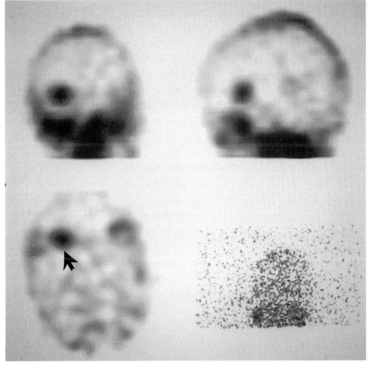

B

therapeutic response [23]. [201]Tl is often positive for Kaposi's sarcoma whereas ^{67}Ga is usually negative [24]. However, nuclear imaging has not generally been found to be adequately specific for purposes of clinical management. There is overlap between benign and malignant lesions using visual and quantitative techniques.

Sestamibi or Tetrofosmin SPECT

[99m]Tc-sestamibi or tetrofosmin is a myocardial perfusion agent like ^{201}Tl and has tumor imaging capability. Its ^{99m}Tc label would suggest that it may have some imaging advantage of [201]Tl. However, it has disadvantages similar to those associated with ^{201}Tl scan for lung and breast images. Its uptake by the heart and soft tissues and its hepatobiliary clearance pose problems. Sestamibi or tetrofosmin is a cationic lipophilic molecule, and its uptake by tumors has not been clearly understood. Proposed mechanisms are extrapolated from studies of myocardial cell uptake. Unlike ^{201}Tl, sestamibi uptake is not related to the sodium/potassium ATPase pump. Its normal uptake is into tissues with negative plasma membrane potential and with relatively high mitochondrial content such as heart, liver, kidney, and skeletal muscle [25]. Malignant tissues share these properties, and its retention is related to mitochondrial metabolism and membrane potential. Calcium in the +2 state causes sestamibi release at levels that are above the concentration in the normal cytosol. With irreversible ischemia, extracellular calcium enters the cell and floods the mitochondria such that sestamibi is not retained.

Sestamibi or tetrofosmin is a substrate for P glycoprotein (Pgp), which is a 170-kD a plasma membrane lipoprotein encoded by the human multidrug resistance (MDR) gene. It functions as a cellular efflux pump for many cytotoxic agents such as chemotherapeutics. Expression of the MDR gene has been shown to modulate the transport of daunorubicin, doxorubicin, paclitaxel, and vinblastine. Increased Pgp expression has been found in nearly all cancers, and is correlated with a poor prognosis in some

cancers, possibly due to decreased efficacy of chemotherapeutics. Multidrug resistance modifiers that block the transport activity of Pgp are being investigated to improve chemotherapeutic effectiveness. Sestamibi or tetrofosmin appears to be transported out of tumor cells like many chemotherapeutic agents, and its accumulation is inversely proportional to the level of Pgp expression. Sestamibi or tetrofosmin may provide an in vivo functional assay of Pgp activity in tumors because Pgp expression and function are not always correlated in tumors. It may have a clinical role in assessment of chemotherapy and effectiveness of MDR modulator early in the course of patient management in addition to its scintigraphic utility [25].

Sestamibi has been used for evaluation of brain tumors. In a comparison of ^{99m}Tc-sestamibi and ^{201}Tl in 19 children, the spectrum of tumor avidity was similar for the two tracers [26]. Because tumor-to-background count-density ratios were higher for sestamibi, sestamibi may have an advantage for the identification of tumor boundaries. However, there is an uptake of sestamibi in normal choroid plexus that cannot be blocked by perchlorate administration. Choroid plexus activity is a limitation when the paraventricular region is the area of interest. A multicenter trial involving 673 patients with palpable and nonpalpable breast lesions found 85% sensitivity and 81% specificity by ^{99m}Tc-sestamibi [27]. Sensitivity and specificity for the subgroup of nonpalpable lesions were 55% and 72%, respectively. False-positive sestamibi uptake has been found in some benign processes such as fibroadenoma or fibrocystic disease. Areas in which sestamibi may prove advantageous include the dense breast, breasts with scarring, evaluation of the axilla, and patients with adenocarcinoma of an axillary node with no identified breast primary (Figure 10.6) [28]. Similar to ^{201}Tl, ^{99m}Tc-sestamibi has been used to assess the response of osteosarcoma during neoadjuvant treatment (Figure 10.7) and to predict tumor response [29,30]. Evaluation of skeletal lesions in the trunk may be compromised by physiological activity in the heart, gastrointestinal tract, or bladder.

FIGURE 10.6. Anterior (*left*) and posterior (*right*) whole-body images using ^{99m}Tc-sestamibi show a focal area of moderately increased activity (*arrow*) in the right axillary lymphatic chain in patient who had right mastectomy for adenocarcinoma. Biopsy confirmed metastatic adenocarcinoma.

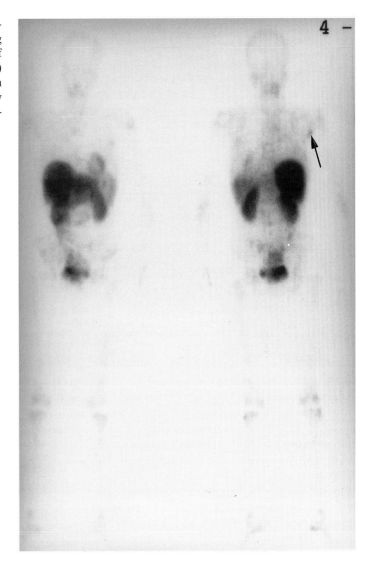

There is considerable controversy regarding the use of preoperative studies to localize parathyroid abnormalities prior to a primary neck exploration. Preoperative localization procedures usually are indicated in patients with previous neck surgery or with recurrent disease or prior surgical failure. There is no general consensus as to the preferred imaging procedure. Most parathyroid adenomas and hyperplastic parathyroid glands accumulate sestamibi more avidly than normal thyroid, and some may be identified on the early image as a hot spot against the background activity in the neck and chest [31]. Most demonstrate washout that is slower than the thyroid, such that the abnormal parathyroid tissue becomes more prominent on delayed images. However, some adenomas show washout of sestamibi similar to the thyroid. False-positive results may occur because of uptake in thyroid adenoma, carcinoma, or Hürthle cell tumor [32].

Conclusion

The clinical role for ^{67}Ga SPECT has been established for lymphoma and hepatoma. Other gallium-avid tumors have been investi-

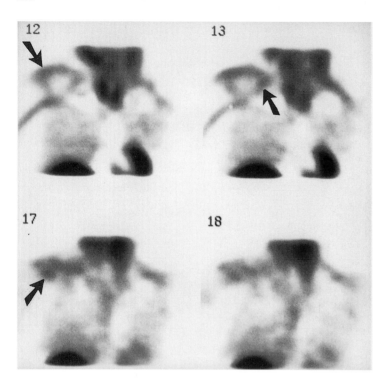

FIGURE 10.7. Selected coronal SPECT images of neck and chest using ^{99m}Tc-sestamibi in a patient with osteogenic sarcoma in the right distal clavicle show moderately increased activity (*arrows*) in the periphery of known sarcoma and also right brachial plexus. Biopsy confirmed sarcoma involvement.

gated, such as lung cancer and melanoma, but clinical utility has not been established as firmly. ^{201}Tl has an established role in the evaluation of malignancies such as brain tumors, low-grade lymphoma, osteosarcoma, and Kaposi sarcoma. Although ^{201}Tl scan can demonstrate uptake in lung, breast, and thyroid carcinoma, its clinical utility is not firmly established. ^{99m}Tc-sestamibi has been used clinically in evaluating parathyroid adenoma, breast cancer, osteosarcoma, and brain tumor. SPECT removes from the diagnostic image unwanted activity that originates from in front and behind the tomographic plane of medical interest, and allows one to examine with greater contrast and anatomical clarity.

References

1. Silberstein EB, Fernando-Ulloa M, Hall J. Are oral cathartics of value in optimizing the gallium scan? J Nucl Med 1981;22:424–427.
2. Engelstad B, Luk SS, Hattner RS. Altered Ga-67 citrate distribution in patients with multiple red blood cell transfusions. AJR 1982;139:755–759.
3. McLaughlin AF, Magee MA, Greenough R, et al. Current role of gallium scanning in the management of lymphoma. Eur J Nucl Med 1990;16:755–771.
4. Front D, Israel O. The role of Ga-67 scintigraphy in evaluating the results of therapy of lymphoma patients. Semin Nucl Med 1995;25:60–71.
5. Front D, Ben-Haim S, Israel O, et al. Lymphoma: predictive value of Ga-67 scintigraphy after treatment. Radiology 1992;182:359–363.
6. Kostakoglu L, Yeh SD, Portlock C, et al. Validation of gallium-67 citrate single photon emission tomography in biopsy-confirmed residual Hodgkin's disease in the mediastinum. J Nucl Med 1992;33:345–350.
7. Sanrock D, Iastoria S, Magrath IT, et al. The role of gallium-67 tumor scintigraphy in patients with small non-cleaved cell lymphoma. Eur J Nucl Med 1993;20:119–122.
8. Champion PE, Groshar D, Hooper IIR, et al. Does gallium uptake in the pulmonary hila predict involvement by non-Hodgkin's lymphoma. Nucl Med Commun 1992;13:730–737.
9. Bar-Shalom R, Israel O, Haim N, et al. Diffuse lung uptake of Ga-67 after treatment of lymphoma: is it of clinical importance? Radiology 1996;199:473–476.

10. Abdel-Dayem HM, Scott AN, Macapinlac H, et al. Tracer imaging in lung cancer. Eur J Nucl Med 1994;21:57–81.

11. Kwekkeboom DJ, Kho GS, Lamberts SW, et al. The value of octreotide scintigraphy in patients with lung cancer. Eur J Nucl Med 1994;21: 1106–1113.

12. Sostre S, Villagra D, Morales ME, et al. Dual-tracer scintigraphy and subtraction studies in the diagnosis of hepatocellular carcinoma. Cancer (Phila) 1988;61:670–672.

13. Beckerman C, Hoffer PB, Bitran JD. The role of gallium-67 in clinical evaluation of cancer. Semin Nucl Med 1984;14:296–322.

14. Front D, Bar-Shalom R, Israel O. The continuing clinical role of gallium-67 scintigraphy in the age of receptor imaging. Semin Nucl Med 1997;27: 68–74.

15. Kaplan WD, Jochelson MS, Herman TS, et al. Ga-67 imaging: a predictor of residual tumor viability and clinical outcome in patients with diffuse large cell lymphoma. J Clin Oncol 1990;8:1966–1970.

16. Carvalho PA, Schwartz RB, Alexander E, et al. Detection of recurrent gliomas with quantitative thallium-201/Tc-99m HMPAO SPECT. J Neurosurg 1992;77:565–570.

17. Dierckx TA, Martin JJ, Dobbeleir A, et al. Sensitivity and specificity of Tl-201 SPECT in the functional detection and differential diagnosis of brain tumors. Eur J Nucl Med 1994;21:621–633.

18. Kahn D, Follett KA, Bushnell DL, et al. Diagnosis of recurrent brain tumor: value of Tl-201 SPECT vs. F-18 FDG PET. AJR 1994;163: 1459–1465.

19. O'Malley JP, Ziessman HA, Kumar PN, et al. Diagnosis of intracranial lymphoma in patients with AIDS: value of Tl-201 SPECT. AJR 1994; 163:417–421.

20. Lorberboym M, Murthy S, Cechanick JI, et al. Thallium-201 and iodine-131 scintigraphy in differentiated thyroid carcinoma. J Nucl Med 1996;37:1487–1491.

21. Matsuno S, Tanabe M, Kawasaki Y, et al. Effectiveness of planar image and SPECT of Tl-201 compared with Ga-67 in patients with primary lung cancer. Eur J Nucl Med 1992; 19:86–95.

22. Waxman AD, Ramanna L, Memsic LD, et al. Tl-201 scintigraphy in the evaluation of mass abnormalities of the breast. J Nucl Med 1993; 34:18–23.

23. Ohtomo K, Terni S, Yodoyama R, et al. Tl-201 scintigraphy to assess effect of chemotherapy in osteosarcoma. J Nucl Med 1996;37:1444–1448.

24. Abdel-Dayem HM, Bag R, DiFabrizio L, et al. Evaluation of sequential thallium and gallium scans of the chest in AIDS patients. J Nucl Med 1996;37:1662–1667.

25. Rao VV, Chiu ML, Kronauge JF, Pwinica-Worms D. Expression of recombinant human multidrug resistance P-glycoprotein in insect cells confers decreased accumulation of Tc-99m sestamibi. J Nucl Med 1994;35:510–515.

26. O'Tuama LA, Treves ST, Larar JN, et al. Tl-201 versus Tc-99m MIBI SPECT in evaluation of childhood brain tumors. J Nucl Med 1993; 34:1045–1051.

27. Khalkhali I, Cutrone JA, Mena IG, et al. Scintimammography: the complementary role of Tc-99m sestamibi prone breast imaging for the diagnosis of breast carcinoma. Radiology 1995; 196:421–426.

28. Waxman AD. The role of Tc-99m methoxy-isobutylisonitrile in imaging breast cancer. Semin Nucl Med 1997;27:40–54.

29. Taki J, Sumiya H, Tsuchiya H, et al. Evaluating benign and malignant bone and soft tissue lesions with Tc-99m MIBI scintigraphy. J Nucl Med 1997;38:501–506.

30. Soderlund V, Johnson C, Bauer HCF, et al. Comparison of Tc-99m MIBI and Tc-99m tetrofosmin uptake by musculoskeletal sarcomas. J Nucl Med 1997;38:682–686.

31. Irvin GL, Prudhomme DL, Deriso GT, et al. A new approach to parathyroidectomy. Ann Surg 1994;219:579–581.

32. Aigner RM, Fueger GF, Nicoletti R. Parathyroid scintigraphy: comparison of Tc-99m MIBI and Tc-99m tetrofosmin studies. Eur J Nucl Med 1996;23:693–696.

11
Targeted Positron Emission Tomography in Oncology

E. Edmund Kim and Franklin C.L. Wong

Positron emission tomography (PET) is a technology that provides functional imaging data of target organ perfusion and metabolism. PET has made it possible to visualize the mind, to detect viable myocardial tissue, and to assess the biomedical behavior of tumors [1–3]. Being aware of PET applications may allow physicians not only to obtain quick and correct diagnoses, but also to make cost-effective clinical decisions for patient treatment or follow-up.

Although the PET scanner is a very complex system, its fundamental physics is the utilization of annihilation coincidence detection. When a PET radiotracer is produced, the tracer is then chemically bound to a compound such as fluro-2-deoxyglucose. After injection of the radiopharmaceutical intravenously, the radiation is emitted from the tracer in the form of positrons (also called antimatter electrons). These positrons travel a short distance and collide into free electrons in tissue, and then annihilation takes place. Each event of annihilation produces two 511-keV photons, which are emitted in opposite directions, approximately 180° to each other with the energy being equivalent to the mass of colliding positron and electron. The photons are intercepted by an array of detectors that encircle the region of interest of the patient's body. A coincidence in the output signals of two detectors is taken as being from a single decay event. An annihilation event must have taken place somewhere along the line joining two detectors. Positrons travel 1 to 2 mm before colliding into orbital electrons, and thus the site of annihilation usually is 1 to 2 mm

away from the site of the positron emission. Reconstruction of the tomographic image, which is nothing more than the drawing of all these lines, is made by a computer using the backprojection technique. The probability of detecting these accidental coincidences increases as the time window is widened or the radioactivity in the PET scanner increases. The coincidence time window usually is set at 5 to 20 nanoseconds (ns). The best spatial resolution in PET scanning is about 2 mm (4–7 mm for the present scanners).

PET with ^{18}F-FDG has dominated metabolic imaging studies of cancer during the last two decades, based on the hypothesis of aerobic glycolysis in cancer. Glucose metabolism reflects cellular energetics in tumors. The value of ^{18}F-FDG for staging tumors and differentiating recurrent tumor from fibrosis is widely accepted [4]. Cancer is a multifaceted disease process, often involving loss of regulation, abnormal metabolism of substrates, changes in cellular membranes, and increased and uncontrolled cellular proliferation.

Cancer is a disease of altered enzymology associated with loss of regulation of growth. Radiopharmaceuticals are also being developed that characterize tumor biochemistry and measure tumor growth at the level of DNA replication and protein synthesis. The hormonal status of tumors is being characterized by PET, as are factors such as hypoxia that influence response of a tumor therapy. PET is being used to observe the pharmacokinetics of drugs including antibodies. These radiopharmaceuticals are intended to study metabolic differences between normal, malignant, and treated tissue and to determine how these differences might lead to more useful strategies for differentiating tissues based on biochemical characteristics. Some tumors acquire much of their energy from mitochondrial metabolism of substrates, and labeling of such substrates could provide important information on tumor metabolism and how it changes with therapy. Damage to chromosomal DNA renders clonogenic death, but can leave surviving mitochondria that continue to metabolize energy substrates.

Tracers of protein synthesis have been advanced as markers of biosynthesis. The methods using labeled amino acids are complex with many potential pitfalls. The general limitation to measuring protein synthesis from amino acids stems from their secondary metabolism and their dilution into unknown pool sizes of intracellular amino acids and their acylated tRNAs [5]. Imaging the presence and extent of estrogen and progesterone receptors should be useful in predicting the hormonal response of breast cancer and in monitoring response to hormonal therapy. Because hypoxia may limit response to radiation therapy, a convenient regional measure of hypoxia would be useful in individualizing therapy. Image registration refers to the spatial matching or merging of two or more images from the same or different imaging modalities. The most widely used correlative imaging application has involved the registration of PET or SPECT images for measuring function with high-resolution MR or CT images of anatomy. The registration of correlative images provides a useful approach to combine the best sensitivities and specificities of complementary procedures to detect, locate, monitor, and measure pathological and other physical changes.

Clinical Applications

Technical Features

The basic principles of PET and SPECT are based on the detection of photons emitted from the patient. The continuing development of new and specific diagnostic and therapeutic tracers is the unique adaptive feature of PET. The intravenous administration of radiopharmaceuticals closely mimics endogenous compounds. The most commonly used PET radiotracer for tumor imaging is the glucose analog 2-^{18}F-fluoro-2-deoxy-D-glucose (FDG). FDG-PET has been shown to be of particular value in many different types of cancer, especially brain, lung, breast, and gastrointestinal cancers and malignant melanoma [6]. Neoplastic cells exhibit increased glucose use compared with normal tissues. It has been shown that transformation of some cell lines is associated with increased cellular activity of hexokinase, reduced cellular activity of glucose-6-phosphatase, and a greater concentration of glucose transporter protein. Marked overexpression of the GLUT-1 glucose transporter has been reported in breast cancer [7]. Like glucose, FDG is a substrate for the first enzyme of glycolysis, hexokinase, and is phosphorylated intracellularly to FDG-6-phosphate. However, because FDG lacks a hydroxyl group in the two-position, FDG-6-phosphate is not a substrate for either the second enzyme of glycolysis, glucose-6-phosphate isomerase, or for other intracellular metabolic pathways. In addition, FDG-6-phosphate does not diffuse out of the cell, but remains trapped within the cell.

There are several important issues for successful whole-body FDG PET of oncological patients. The patient should have fasted for at least 4h before injection of 10 to 15mCi of FDG. The fasting blood glucose should not exceed 130mg/dl. Because FDG activity in the urinary system can result in artifacts, intravenous hydration using 1500ml 0.9% saline over 2h and also injection of 20mg furosemide 20min after FDG administration are recommended. The placement of a Foley catheter in the bladder is also recommended. Attenuation correction is required for quantitative or semiquantitative assessment of trace uptake. Attenuation correction using the segmentation technique employs a short (2-min) postinjection transmission scan to generate attenuation-coefficient maps [8].

In addition to qualitative visual inspection of FDG uptake, semiquantitative methods are used such as ratio of tumor to normal tissue uptake or standardized uptake value (SUV). The SUV is a decay-corrected measurement of activity per unit volume of tissue (mCi/ml) adjusted for administered activity per unit of body weight (mCi/kg) or lean body mass [9]. Semiquantitative methods are most useful for longitudinal comparison studies, such as for determination of tumor response to therapy. The Patlak graphical approach provides an estimate of the net FDG phosphorylation rate constant (ml/min/g). To obtain the glucose metabolic rate, knowledge of the lumped constant (ratio of net extraction of natural glucose to the net extraction of FDG) is needed.

Lung Cancer

The prevalence of lung cancer is increasing globally, and it claims approximately 170,000 lives each year in the United States [10]. The overall 5-year survival of patients with lung cancer is approximately 14% despite aggressive treatments [11]. Patients who have lung cancer often present with solitary pulmonary nodules, and approximately one-third of these solitary pulmonary nodules in persons 35 years of age or older are malignant. Chest radiography, computed tomography (CT), and magnetic resonance imaging (MRI) provide morphological information, but they cannot accurately characterize abnormalities as benign or malignant. The diagnosis of lung cancer has required tissue obtained by sputum cytology, bronchoscopy, needle biopsy, thoracoscopy, or open lung biopsy. It has been reported that more than 50% of radiographically indeterminate lesions resected at thoracoscopy were benign [11]. Small-cell lung cancer accounts for 17% to 29% of all cases of lung cancer and is mostly peripheral. Squamous cell carcinoma now accounts for 30% of all lung cancers and arises frequently in the proximal segmental bronchi. Large-cell carcinoma is the least common type of non-small-cell lung cancer (NSCLC).

The lymphatic drainage follows the bronchoarterial branching pattern, and the lymphatic channels coalesce into draining lymph nodes. Lower lobe lymphatics drain into the posterior mediastinum and ultimately to the subcarinal lymphatic nodes. Right upper lobe lymphatics drain into the superior mediastinum whereas left upper lobe lymphatics run along the great vessels in the anterior mediastinum and along the main bronchus into the superior mediastinum. Metastatic lymphatic spread of lung cancer follows these lymphatic channels with tumor involving bronchopulmonary (N1), mediastinal (N2–3), and supraclavicular (N3) lymph nodes. Lymphatic spread to the pleural surface can occur in peripheral tumors. Any lymph node larger than 1 cm in diameter is considered abnormal. The most accurate method of staging the superior mediastinal lymph nodes is mediastinoscopy. Video-assisted thoracoscopy has been used to excise peripheral nodules. Unsuspected involvement is frequently found changing the stage of lung cancer. CT can detect metastases to the liver and adrenal glands. Bone scans have been advocated in clinical stage III disease. Sputum cytologis is positive in 80% of central tumors. Percutaneous fine-needle aspiration biopsy is usually performed using CT guidance, and the positive yield is 95%, and bronchoscopy provides greater than 90% diagnostic yield [11,12].

Approximately 130,000 patients are identified with solitary lung nodules each year in the United States [8]. Stability in the size of the nodule for 2 years or more is indicative of a benign nodule. If the nodule is not definitely benign by its characteristics on CT, then further evaluation is required [12].

Multiple studies have shown the utility of FDG-PET in characterizing pulmonary nodules (Figure 11.1), and the reported sensitivity and specificity of FDG-PET in differentiating benign from malignant have been 100% and 89%, respectively, using a standard uptake ratio (SUR) value of 2.5 or greater as indicating malignancy [13]. It has been noted that the mean SUR of malignant lesions (5.9 ± 2.7) was significantly different from benign lesions (2.0 ± 1.7) [14]. There was no correlation between lesion diameter and FDG uptake as measured by the SUR. However, a significant correlation was found between SUR and lesion doubling time [15]. Tuberculous pneumonia, cryptococcosis, histoplasmosis, aspergillosis, and other infections may have substantial FDG uptake

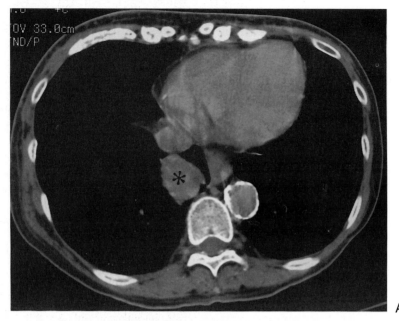

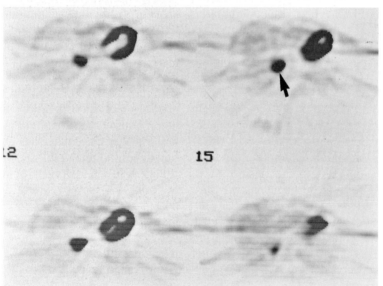

FIGURE 11.1. (**A**) Axial CT image of the chest at the level of the heart shows a mass (*) in the right lower lung adjacent to the esophagus. (**B**) Selected axial PET images using ^{18}F-FDG show a focal area of markedly increased activity (*arrow*) in the right lower lung posteromedially, indicating malignant lesion. Surgery confirmed an adenocarcinoma.

and SUR values in the abnormal range. However, most chronic inflammatory processes and most acute infectious processes do not have significant FDG uptake.

A recent study has documented a relationship between the amount of FDG uptake and prognosis in patients with lung cancer. Of the 118 patients with SUR alone less than 10, a median survival of 24.6 months was found, whereas 37 patients with SUR value of 10 or more had a significant shorter median survival, 11.4 months [8]. Nodules with increased FDG uptake require a biopsy, and the cost savings of FDG-PET results from the prevention of unnecessary thoracotomies. CT and MRI in staging of NSCLC showed a sensitivity of 52% and 48% and a specificity of 69% and 64%, respectively [16]. FDG-PET is more accurate than CT in the detection of malignant mediastinal nodes (81% versus 52%) [17]. The sensitivity and specificity for hilar/lobar lymph node metastases using PET were 73% and 76%, and for CT, 27% and 86%, respectively [18]. The PET had 100% sensitivity and 80% specificity of CT-detected adrenal metastases of NSCLC [19]. The sensitivity of FDG-PET for the detection of distant metastases from lung cancer was 100% with specificity of 94% and accuracy of 96%. FDG-PET correctly modified the stage of the disease in 34% of patients and changed the therapeutic strategy in more than 20% [20].

Lesions with higher tumor to muscle count density ratios of FDG uptake responded better to treatment than those with lower ratio. The decrease in FDG uptake after therapy correlated with a partial response to therapy (Figure 11.2). The relapse rate was higher in lesions with higher uptake ratios either before or after therapy [21]. The PET was more accurate than CT in predicting the downstaging that occurred with induction chemotherapy. The PET obtained after induction chemotherapy was predictive of clinical outcome. Using SUR greater than 2.5 to indicate malignancy, FDG-PET had a sensitivity of 97% and a specificity of 100% for the detection of persistent or recurrent lung cancer [22]. In another study after therapy for lung cancer, 100% sensitivity and 62% specificity were reported [23]. CT and PET strategy showed a saving of $1154 per patient compared with the alternate strategy of CT alone. The major advantage of FDG-PET is the cost savings that result when a patient with unresectable disease does not undergo an unnecessary surgery [24].

Breast Cancer

Breast cancer is the most common malignancy in women, with an estimated incidence in the United States of 176,300 cases in 1999 [10].

Approximately one-third of women who develop this disease will die of disseminated breast cancer. In most patients, the initial diagnosis of breast cancer is made by physician examination or mammography. Much of the improvement in the early detection of breast cancer has been attributed to recent significant progress in mammographic technique and the use of ultrasonography [25]. However, it is of limited value in women with dense breasts or with breast implants, for early detection of tumor recurrence after surgery, and for monitoring response to therapy.

PET of the breast offers physiological information and can act as an adjunct to conventional imaging. It is available at a limited number of sites with high cost and limited resolution. FDG-PET is both sensitive (66%–96%) and specific (83%–100%) in detecting primary cancers and for differentiating breast cancers from benign lesions (Figure 11.3) [26,27]. False-positive results can occur in patients with breast abscess, mastitis, or early after biopsy, surgery, or radiation therapy [28]. The majority of false-negative results occurred with tumor diameter less than 1 cm [29]. Slowly growing or well-differentiated tubular carcinoma and ductal carcinoma in situ often have less FDG uptake than does the usual invasive ductal carcinoma [30]. Radiodense breasts found in younger women, or women undergoing hormone therapy, breast augmentation, or conserving therapy for breast cancer, reduced mammmographic sensitivity for detection of breast cancer. FDG-PET appears to be particularly useful and may obviate the biopsy [31]. Approximately 60% of patients with breast cancer have regional nodal metastasis at initial diagnosis, and the axillary lymph nodes are involved in 40% of patients with breast cancer. Multicenter trials reported a high sensitivity (96%) and specificity (96%) for detecting axillary nodal metastasis in patients with breast cancer. Overall sensitivity of 79% and specificity of 96% for detection of axillary nodal involvement have also been reported [32]. However, PET is unable to detect micrometastasis to lymph nodes, producing false-negative PET results [33].

FIGURE 11.2. (**A**) Axial CT image of the chest at the level of the aortic arch shows a residual mass (*arrow*) along the right chest wall following chemotherapy. (**B**) Selected axial PET images of the upper chest show a markedly increased uptake of ^{18}F-FDG (*arrow*) along the right chest wall, suggesting residual malignant tumor. Biopsy confirmed a malignant fibrous histiocytoma (MFH).

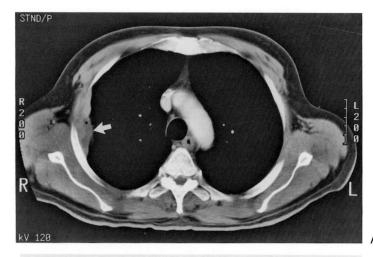

A

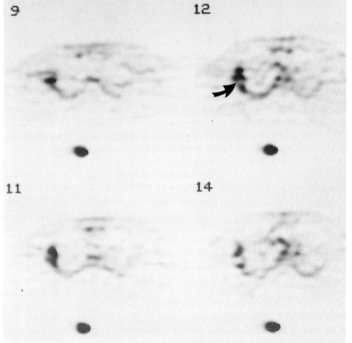

B

Many reports have suggested that PET is more sensitive than conventional staging methods at detecting true extent of the disease and often reveals unsuspected metastatic disease [32]. FDG-PET can reveal unsuspected metastatic disease in patients with breast cancer (Figure 11.4) [28]. After therapy, the amount of tumor FDG uptake reflects the number of viable tumor cells present and possible also the glucose metabolic rate of the individual tumor cells [33]. A substantial decrease in tumor metabolism was noted early in the course of effective chemotherapy [34]. Only 55% to 60% of patients with ER+ breast cancer respond to hormonal therapy, and conversely 5% to 10% of patients with ER-disease respond to such treatment [35]. It has been found that 16α-^{18}F-fluoro-17β-estradiol (FES) has been success-

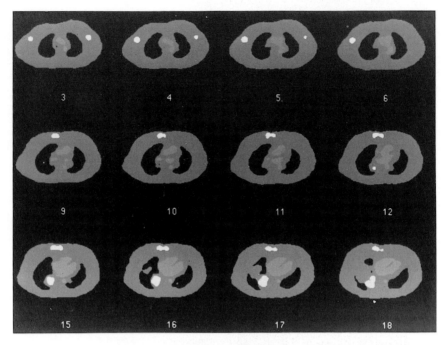

FIGURE 11.3. Transaxial PET images of the chest superimposed with transmission images show focal areas of markedly increased uptake of ^{18}F-FDG in the bilateral breast tails (*upper row*). Note also metastatic lesions involving sternum (*middle* and *lower rows*) and right lung base medially (*lower row*). Biopsy confirmed primary and metastatic breast adenocarcinomas.

fully used to image ER+ breast cancers and to accurately determine the ER status of these tumors. FES-PET has been shown to be highly sensitive (93%) for detection of ER+ metastatic foci in patients with known metastatic breast cancer [36,37]. FES accumulation within metastatic lesions decreased following institution of tamoxifen therapy. There was no significant relationship between FDG uptake and either ER status or FES uptake. The mean SUV for FDG in ER+ tumors was 4.0 ± 2.1 and for EDR− tumors was 4.5 ± 3.0 [38]. The median survival of patients with FES disease was 21.6 months while the median survival had not yet been achieved in FES+ patients at a median follow-up interval of 22 months [39]. The clinical flare reaction is seen in 5% to 20% of patients with ER+ metastatic breast cancer and generally occurs within 7 to 10 days after institution of antiestrogen therapy. Clinically and radiographically, the flare reaction is indistinguishable from progression of disease. It is assumed that this phenomenon is due to temporary

agonist effects of the antiestrogen agent on the tumor and is predictive of subsequent response to antiestrogen therapy in 80% of patients [40]. Presumably, both estrogen and tamoxifen initially result in increased cell proliferation and glucose metabolism and thus increased FDG uptake. It is possible that increased FDG uptake seen early during a course of tamoxifen therapy (metabolic flare) may reflect an agonist effect of the drug on ERs and indicate the likelihood of therapeutic response. Response to tamoxifen was correctly predicted by the presence of metabolic flare and the degree of ER blockade [41].

Head and Neck Cancer

Head and neck cancers comprise 2% to 3% of all tumors diagnosed in the United States [10], and the majority of these are squamous cell carcinomas that originate in mucosal structures. Such tumors are easily accessible by means of physical examination and biopsy. MRI or CT

FIGURE 11.4. Axial CT images of the lower chest (*upper*) shows a sclerotic lesion (*) in the sternum extending into right parasternal soft tissue in patient who had a left mastectomy for cancer. Axial PET image of the chest at the comparable level (*lower*) shows a markedly increased uptake of F-18 FDG, indicating malignant lesion (*arrow*). Biopsy confirmed metastatic breast cancer.

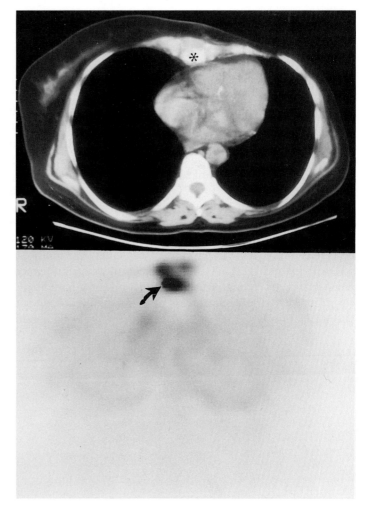

provides detailed morphological information, such as destruction of normal fascial planes and tumor infiltration into deep structures. The local recurrence of head and neck cancers depends on multiple factors including location, stage, and histological findings. Recurrence can occur in as many as 50% of patients with head and neck cancer. FDG-PET enabled correct identification of 22 (88%) of the 25 primary lesions and corresponded with the pathological finding for cervical node disease in 22 (81%) of 27 specimen [42]. CT or MRI enabled identification of 21 (88%) of 24 primary lesions, and corresponded with the pathological findings in 21 (81%) of 27 neck specimens. FDG-PET cannot replace CT or MRI in the initial workup

of these patients because it lacks the anatomical clarity needed for therapeutic planning.

After surgery, normal anatomical structures can be extensively distorted. This distortion can render CT, MRI, and physical examination unreliable because of the edema and fibrosis often present after treatment. One of the complications of radiation therapy is tissue necrosis. After radiotherapy, biopsy of the radiation necrosis can actually precipitate progressive necrosis and lead to complications. FDG-PET was found to be effective in the posttherapy setting. Radiation therapy caused little or no change in the normal pattern of FDG uptake in the head and neck [42]. There was slightly increased soft tissue uptake, particularly muscle, in the early postirradiation period. Residual or recurrent tumor appears much the same as it does in pretherapy studies as intense sharply delineated FDG uptake that is typically asymmetrical. Normal structures are usually symmetrical from side to side, and the posterior laryngeal uptake may be caused by stressed vocal muscles. The sensitivity and specificity of FDG-PET for the detection of recurrence after radiation therapy of laryngeal cancer were 80% and 81%, respectively, compared with 58% and 100% for CT (Figure 11.5) [42]. False-negative studies were found at 1 month after completing therapy, possibly because of suppression of FG uptake by radiation or decreased number of viable tumor cells. FDG-PET also yielded a sensitivity and specificity of 88% and 100%, respectively, by others for the detection of recurrent head and neck cancers after surgery and irradiation [43].

Metastatic cervical adenopathy of unknown primary origin poses a diagnostic challenge of considerable clinical consequence in patients with head and neck cancer. Location of the primary site in these patients enables direction of surgical excision, radiation therapy or both, thereby improving the outcome and avoiding the unwanted adverse reactions (Figure 11.6). Primary tumors of the head and neck manifesting as metastatic adenopathy may remain occult in approximately 3% to 6% of patients [44]. Biopsies performed without accompanying imaging studies usually have a yield of only 10% [42]. It has been found that FDG-PET allows effective localization of the unknown primary site of origin in metastatic head and neck cancer and can contribute substantially to patient care. In 12 of 15 patients with metastatic cervical adenopathy of unknown primary origin, a focus of increased FDEG uptake with

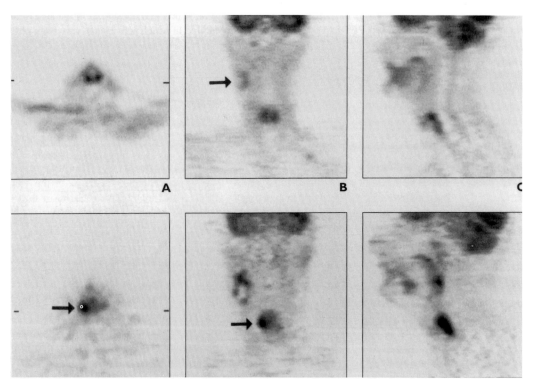

FIGURE 11.5. Selected axial (**A**), coronal (**B**), and midsagittal (**C**) PET images of the neck using ^{18}F-FDG show focal areas of slightly increased activity in the metastatic right cervical node (*arrow* in **B**) in patients with right tonsilar cancer (*upper*) and right laryngeal cancer (*arrows* in *lower* **A**, **B**). (From Keyes et al. [42] with permission of *AJR*.)

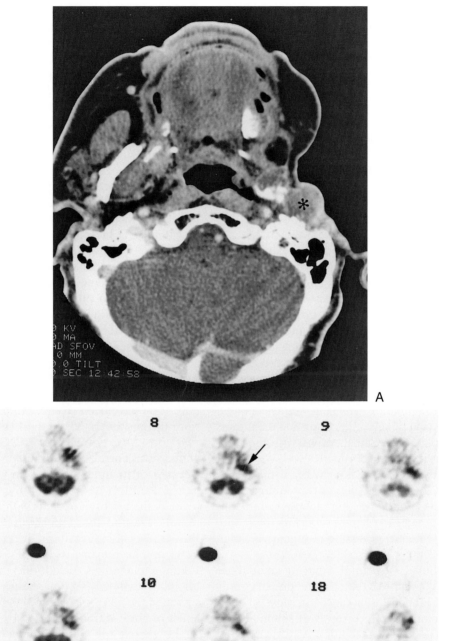

FIGURE 11.6. (**A**) Axial CT image of skull base shows a contrast-enhanced nodule (*) in the left preauricular upper neck in patient who had surgery and radiation therapy for squamous carcinoma. (**B**) Selected axial PET images of skull base show moderately increased uptake of ^{18}F-FDG (*arrow*) in the left skull base corresponding to nodular lesion seen on CT. Biopsy confirmed recurrent squamous carcinoma.

directed biopsy of these sites led to confirmation of a primary carcinoma in 9 patients [44]. Squamous cell tumors arising below the level of the nasopharynx have a high association with secondary primary tumors of the upper aerodigestive tract. Head and neck cancers can also metastasize, and these metastases in the lung can be difficult to differentiate from second primary lesions. FDG-PET has shown high sensitivity not only for tumors arising in the head and neck but also for tumors in the lung and esophagus [45].

Brain Tumors

In the study of patients with brain tumors, anatomical changes that are clinically significant occur starting at sizes of millimeters (mm), and the pathological processes occurs at submillimolar concentration. In fact, genetic aberrations and early subcellular injuries occur at subpicomolar ranges. Before imaging studies became available, these events were usually identified on autopsy or by surgical biopsy, followed by histochemistry and detailed microscopic examination. Imaging studies analyze the chemical signals of the brain and the tumors and display these signals, along with their differences, in spatial coordinates with good resolution. Evaluation of human brain tumors by imaging techniques therefore requires good spatial resolution of the anatomical details as well as sensitive signals reflecting the pathological processes occurring at organic, cellular, and subcellular levels.

Traditional structural imaging modalities such as CT and MRI remain the primary study tools of human brain cancer because of their superior resolution, currently at submillimeter levels. The spatial resolution of CT and MRI are an order of magnitude better than the current PET resolution of 5 to 8 mm. Together with contrast-enhancement techniques, CT or MRI provides visualization of anatomical as well as gross physiological aberrations, such as tumor mass, edema, and rupture of blood–brain barriers. These anatomical and gross pathological changes occur at the molar and millimolar ranges. The use of CT and MRI are limited by their current abilities to detect cellular or molecular alterations at concentrations below millimolar levels. However, current PET technologies detect molecular changes from molar to subpicomolar ranges and are the only imaging modalities to fill the large void left by CT or MRI, that is, the cellular and subcellular events at the millimolar to picomolar levels.

The study of human brain tumors using PET started in the 1970s. Gross pathology at the vascular level, such as perfusion abnormalities, was reported with ^{15}O-water PET [46]. Breakdown of blood–brain barriers were reported by ^{68}Ga-PET [47]. Differential vascular responses between vessels in tumor versus brain were reported under adenosine pharmacological stimulation using ^{15}O-water PET [48]. Vascular response to physiological stimulation in patients with brain tumors to identify motor or sensory representation in brain parenchyma has been used as a clinical tool for presurgical planning [49]. Down to the cellular and subcellular levels, the study of tumor regional perfusion, oxygen consumption, and glucose utilization have been reported in the literature since the late 1970s [50]. In the 1980s, increased ^{18}F-fluoro-2-deoxy-D-glucose (FDG) uptake in gliomas was correlated with tumor grades [51]. Because of its uptake by the normal cerebral cortex, ^{18}F-FDG has remained the main tracer to study the brains of patients with and without tumors. Despite the popular use of FDG in PET studies of brain tumors, the mechanism of FDG uptake remains to be fully understood. Likely explanations include increased hexose kinase activities [52], increased uptake by surrounding macrophages [53], and increased levels of glucose transporters [54].

The search for specific tumor markers in imaging continues, with increasing emphasis on tumor-specific molecules such as essential amino acids (e.g., L-methionine) [55], nucleotides (thymidine) [56], dopamine D-2 receptors [57], and peripheral benzodiazepine receptors [58]. Because of the stringent technical requirements, most of these studies were conducted from a research perspective; the clinical use of this expensive PET technology, which is not widely available, often demands different considerations.

Tumor grading and staging remains an important task of the clinical oncologist. There are earlier reports on correlation of glioma grades with ^{18}F-FDG-PET. However, the acceptance of this notion varies. Often PET is not used to grade human brain tumor.

Because of limited availability of the short-lived tracers, which require a nearby cyclotron and rapid synthesis as well as quality assurance, clinical PET is available only to large academic medical centers. Furthermore, because of the inferior spatial resolution, PET is best positioned to study the brain tumor patients for whom CT and MRI offer little help. In fact, owing to improved early diagnosis and treatment, brain tumor patients have improved survival rates and, ironically, they have proved difficult for CT or MRI to evaluate. Because either the tumor or the treatment or both have altered the architecture of normal brain parenchyma, grossly abnormal CT or MRI

signals such as contrast enhancement often remain, regardless of whether there is recurrent tumor. PET remains most useful in the differentiation of recurrent brain tumor from posttreatment necrosis (Figure 11.7).

The most frequently used tracer in clinical PET is ^{18}F-FDG. When used to study patients with brain tumors, it posts a technical challenge. The tumor is expected to have higher uptake (and hence contrast) than the surrounding tissue (Figure 11.7). However, the gray matter in normal human cerebral cortex already has higher FDG uptake than the white matter [59]. The contrast of the signal from the tumor versus the signal from the brain is thus decreased, leading to possible lowered sensitivity. This problem may be overcome by the following technically simple schemes. First, the location of the hypermetabolic tumor helps to identify tumors in the hypometabolic white matter. Second, comparison with prior studies may find a lesion with increasing uptake. Third, coregistration with anatomical imaging, such as

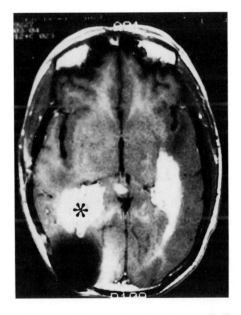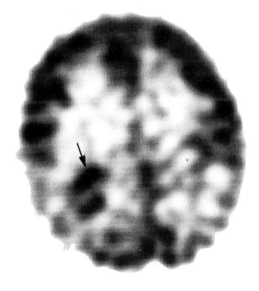

FIGURE 11.7. Axial T$_2$-weighted MR image (*left*) of the head shows a hyperintense mass (*) anterior to the surgical changes in the right posterosuperior temporal lobe. Axial PET image (*right*) at the comparable level shows a donut-shaped increased uptake of ^{18}F-FDG (*arrow*), indicating malignant lesion. Biopsy confirmed a recurrent oligodendroglioma.

MRI, will reveal the exact locations of the lesions. Finally, presentation of the images in stand uptake value (SUV) or other semiquantitative parameters help to assess the contrast of the signals.

To be clinically useful, the results of the PET study should have direct impact on the treatment plans. Most PET studies of brain tumors are concerned with primary brain tumor, that is, gliomas, because the findings may direct the subsequent treatment plans, such as continuing chemotherapy, further surgery, or observation. Other tumors, such as meningiomas and metastases, have only been scantily reported because the treatment plans are directed by surgery for meningioma. In the case of metastases, therapy is directed by the treatment of the primary tumor. Furthermore, PET of both meningiomas and metastases are reported to have variable uptake of FDG. Therefore, the usefulness of FDG-PET in the routine clinical evaluation of brain tumors other than gliomas remains to be established. Although glioma refers to a group of brain tumors of varying grade, and there is an apparent trend of higher uptake with higher grade, there are very few studies further delineating the FDG uptake of the various gliomas.

There is a unique place for PET in the differentiation of recurrent tumor versus posttreatment necrosis because MRI of these posttreatment patients often reveals persistent contrast enhancement. However, necrotic tissues often have little FDG uptake, whereas tumors exhibit marked uptake. It has been found that FDG uptake by brain and tumor may slightly increase immediately after radiation treatment, only to return to normal and then become subnormal in a few weeks [59]. Furthermore, surgery and systemic steroid did not produce any significant FDG-uptake change during the next few days. Because the chronic effects of radiation treatment on the normal brain are depressed perfusion and metabolism, the posttreatment effects are expected to enhance the tumor contrast on FDG-PET scans. This change will add to the ability to detect tumors in the brain, which has a known high uptake of FDG. There is an argument that there are many micrometastases in a

patient with primary glioma and, therefore, distinction of tumor versus no tumor may not be very important because tumors are already spread throughout the entire brain, including the posttreatment necrotic tissues. One recent study has shown that the FDG uptake in the evaluation of posttreatment necrosis versus residual tumor is indeed important for the clinical management of brain tumor patients [60].

Although ^{11}C-methionine PET is mostly restricted to research studies, it is most promising as an alternative to ^{18}F-FDG-PET because there is minimal background activity in the brain and, therefore, the lesions stand out with good contrast. This technology is, however, limited by the requirement of very short synthesis time because of the short half-life of ^{11}C (20 min). Occasionally, posttreatment necrosis also exhibits high uptake of the tracer.

Melanoma and Lymphoma

Cutaneous malignant melanoma is a common tumor, and 44,200 new cases will be diagnosed in 1999 in the United States [10]. Tumor thickness is the most important prognostic factor. Surgical excision is curative for early primary melanoma, but there has been no effective treatment for advanced metastatic disease. The production of melanin starts by conversion of L-tyrosine to L-dihydroxyphenylalanine by tyrosinase, and methionine is a precursor of S-adenosyl-L-methionine, the principal methyl group donor for melanin synthesis. FDG-PET showed an overall accuracy of 100%, detecting 7 of 7 metastatic lesions and correctly predicting 13 of 13 negative lymph node regions in a small study for staging of metastatic melanoma [61]. For detection of intraabdominal, visceral, and lymph node metastases, FDG-PET sensitivity was also 100% (15 of 15). PET detected three metastatic foci which were later noted respectively on CT. However, two metastatic foci were seen only on follow-up CT several months later. The PET sensitivity was lower than CT for detecting tiny pulmonary lesions, probably because of respiratory motion or prior treatment. All 22 malignant melanomas larger than 1.5 cm in diameter were visualized (100%

sensitivity), and 22 of 27 lesions of any size (81% sensitivity) were detected with PET using ^{11}C-methionine (Figure 11.8) [62]. There were no false-positive findings.

Clinically, there are two non-Hodgkin's lymphoma (NHL) groups based on the histological grading. Low-grade NHL is usually considered to be incurable, but it often progresses slowly. Some low-grade tumors may have a more aggressive course and some tumors may transform into high-grade NHL. These patients have a poor prognosis. High-grade NHL has aggressive tumors with high proliferation rates, but its treatment has a curative intention. The transformation of low-grade to high-grade NHL may occur unpredictably, sometimes requiring multiple tissue samplings. All 23 NHL lesions detected by CT or MRI were clearly visualized by PET using ^{18}F-FDG or ^{11}C-methionine [63]. The FDG uptake values were significantly

higher for high-grade than low-grade NHL, whereas such significant difference was seen for ^{11}C-methionine uptake values. This discrimination was apparently better when transport rate calculation was used instead of SUV or mass influx estimations. However, Leskinen-Kallio et al. [64] found that ^{11}C-methionine was better for identifying tumors than ^{18}F-FDG, but ^{18}F-FDG was superior in predicting malignant grade. This discrepancy may be related to the different method to draw a mean region of interest for the viable tumor area. The accuracy of FDG-PET in thoracoabdominal lymphoma compared with that of CT in 16 patients with lymphoma. There was no lesion missed by PET, and PET detected 5 lesions that were not seen on CT. No difference of FDG uptake between low- and intermediate-grade lymphoma was found [65]. Staging using whole-body PET was concordant with conventional staging in 14

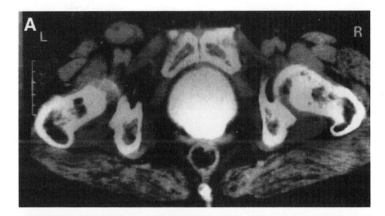

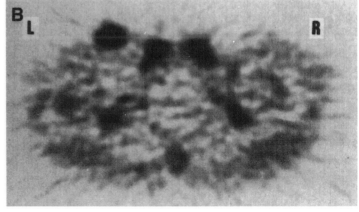

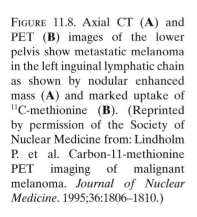

FIGURE 11.8. Axial CT (**A**) and PET (**B**) images of the lower pelvis show metastatic melanoma in the left inguinal lymphatic chain as shown by nodular enhanced mass (**A**) and marked uptake of ^{11}C-methionine (**B**). (Reprinted by permission of the Society of Nuclear Medicine from: Lindholm P. et al. Carbon-11-methionine PET imaging of malignant melanoma. *Journal of Nuclear Medicine*. 1995;36:1806–1810.)

of 17 patients, better than conventional staging in 3 patients, and poorer in 1 patient [4]. The actual total cost for conventional staging was $66,292 whereas the cost for PET was $36,250.

Gastrointestinal Cancers

Several authors have demonstrated the high sensitivity and specificity, usually greater than 90%, of 2-[^{18}F]-fluoro-2-deoxy-D-glucose positron emission tomography (^{9}FDG-PET) in detection of a variety of tumors, including primary and metastatic hepatic cancers (Figure 11.9) [66]. FDG-PET using modern scanners has the ability to depict small (5–7 mm in diameter) tumors by virtue of increased metabolic rate. Whole-body FDG-PET in a recent report [66] depicted all known intraluminal carcinomas in 37 patients, including 2 in situ carcinomas (100% sensitivity), but 4 false-positive findings (3 with inflammatory bowel disease, 1 after recent polypectomy) were noted. In these studies, they obtained specificity of 43% (3 of 7 patients), and 90% positive-predictive value (37 of 41 patients) as well as 100% negative-predictive value (3 of 3 patients). No FDG accumulation was noted in 35 hyperplastic polyps. FDG-PET depicted lymph node metastases in 4 of 14 patients (29% sensitivity) and

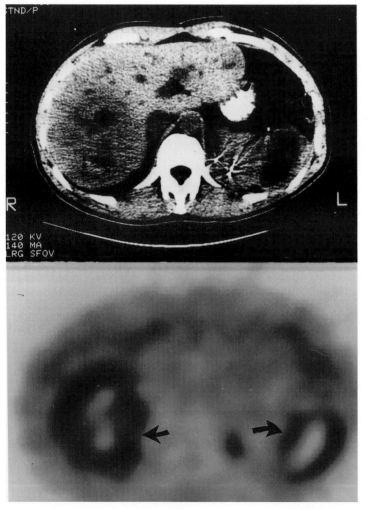

FIGURE 11.9. Axial CT (*top*) image of upper abdomen shows metastatic leiomyosarcoma involving right hepatic lobe and spleen. Axial PET (*bottom*) image at the comparable level shows ring-shaped increased uptake of ^{18}F-FDG, indicating malignant lesions with central necrosis (*arrows*).

hepatic metastases in 7 of 8 patients (88% sensitivity). CT sensitivities for detecting lymph node and hepatic metastases were 29% and 38%, respectively. FDG-PET and CT correctly depicted the absence of hepatic metastases in 35 and 32 patients, respectively (100% and 97% specificity, respectively). These results are in agreement with those reported previously by others [67].

The low sensitivity of FDG-PET to accurately detect lymph node metastases is not significantly different from the sensitivity of CT, and the limited resolution of FDG-PET is probably a problem for small metastatic nodes. The ability of FDG-PET to detect subclinical hepatic metastases not appreciated at preoperative CT and undetected during surgical exploration could have a direct effect on surgical approach and patient management. If confirmed in a large number of patients, FDG-PET could replace CT as the first screening procedure in routine liver evaluation, and save at least $445 per patient [67]. ^{18}F-FDG-PET was more accurate (92%) than CT and CT portography (78% and 80%, respectively) in detecting hepatic metastases and more accurate than CT for extrahepatic metastases (92% and 71%, respectively) in 52 colorectal cancer patients with 166 suspicious lesions [68]. Outside the liver, FDG-PET was especially helpful in detecting nodal metastases and differentiating local recurrence from posttreatment changes.

Many studies conclude that FDG-PET should be considered as a screening method in staging patients considered for resection of metastases. The PET findings should guide the performance, increase specificity of CT and CT portography, and help to identify patients with resectable disease. PET may also be useful in the evaluation of therapeutic responses for malignant tumors in the abdomen. The limitations of PET include the lack of detection of some tiny metastases and possible false positives in lesions containing activated macrophages. Although PET has been increasingly used to obtain quantitative data about the metabolism of malignant lesions, little is known about the use of radiolabeled drugs.

PET has been helpful in differentiating recurrent tumor from scar. In 33 patients with recurrent colorectal cancer, all tumors except 1 showed high FDG uptake, whereas FDG uptake was low in the scar area. PET accurately characterized areas of residual or recurrent rectosigmoid cancer in 17 patients (Figure 11.10) [69]. FDG uptake in recurrent rectal cancer does not decrease significantly within 3 months of radiation therapy [70]. FDG uptake resulting from radiation therapy is probably due to an inflammatory reaction. Only 5 patients who were thought to have a palliative response had a decrease of FDG uptake in 6 months [71]. PET was more sensitive than carcinoembryonic antigen (CEA) measurements for determining tumor recurrence. In contrast to FDG, radiolabeled cytostatic drugs provide a direct measurement of the distribution of a chemotherapeutic agent in the target area. Therefore, chemotherapy management can be optimized either using metabolic studies with FDG or cytostatic agents [69]. Dynamic PET and ^{18}F-fluorouracil (FU) were used in patients with hepatic metastases from colorectal cancer to examine the pharmacokinetics of the drug up to 120 min after intravenous and intraarterial injection of the same dose of FU. Dynamic PET studies lasting up to 5 min with ^{15}O-labeled water were performed immediately before the FU study. Hepatic metastases from colorectal cancer reached the highest ^{18}F-FU concentrations after intraarterial administration, with a maximum standard uptake value of 18.75 for the FU influx and 5.03 for FU trapping [72]. Cluster analysis revealed a group of metastases with a nonperfusion-dependent FU transport using the intravenous application, and most of them did not show any enhancement of ^{18}F-FU after the intraarterial application.

In examination of 106 patients with unclear pancreatic masses by ^{18}F-FDG, 63 of the 74 (85%) were identified to have pancreatic carcinoma by PET. PET revealed chronic pancreatitis in 27 of 32 (84%), and it was possible to exclude malignancy. False-negative results (10 of 11) were obtained in patients with elevated serum glucose levels, and five false positives in patients with pancreatic inflammation. There-

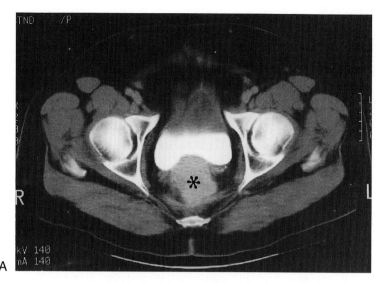

A

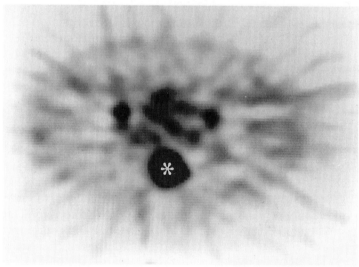

B

FIGURE 11.10. (**A**) Axial CT of lower pelvis shows a mass (*) in the presacral space in patient who had rectal cancer. (**B**) Selected axial image at the comparable level shows markedly increased uptake of ^{18}F-FDG (*) in the presacral space, indicating malignant lesion. Biopsy confirmed recurrent carcinoma.

fore, PET showed an overall sensitivity of 85%, a specificity of 84%, a negative-predictive value of 71%, and a positive-predictive value of 93% [73].

Accumulation of [1-^{11}C]acetate by the pancreas allows rapid metabolic imaging using PET, and may be a useful metabolic probe for the study of pancreatic disease. The normal pancreas demonstrates prompt uptake of [1-^{11}C] acetate with maximal activity achieved in less than 5 min. Moderately reduced [1-^{11}C]acetate uptake was observed in acute pancreatitis, and pancreatic adenocarcinoma revealed no significant uptake of [1-^{11}C]acetate [74]. FDG-PET imaging of gastroenteropancreatic (GEP) tumors demonstrated increased glucose metabolism only in less differentiated GEP tumors with high proliferative activity and metastasizing medullary thyroid cancer associated with rapidly increasing CEA levels [75]. It was recommended that FDG-PET should be performed for the imaging of neuroendocrine tumors only if somatostatin receptor scintigraphy is negative.

Conclusion

The current applications of PET in clinical oncology have been in differentiating and characterizing indeterminate lesions, differentiating recurrent cancers from posttreatment changes, staging and evaluating the extent of cancer, and monitoring the success or failure of treatments (Figure 11.11). Future developments in medicine may use the unique imaging capabilities of PET not only in diagnostic imaging but also in basic drug development and in monitoring or evaluating the eligibility of patients for new therapies such as gene therapy. PET provides biochemical and molecular information, and plays a very important role in understanding the biology of cancer as well as assisting the development of new treatments with better cost-effectiveness for the management of cancer patients.

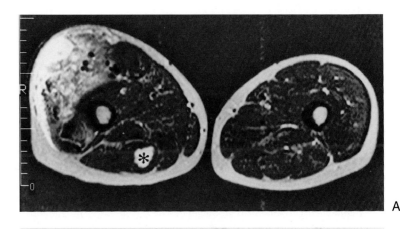

A

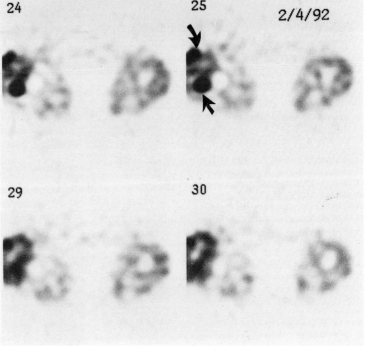

FIGURE 11.11. (**A**) Axial post-contrast T_1-weighted image of bilateral midthigh shows a diffusely enhanced lesion in the anterolateral compartment of right thigh. Note also the small hemorrhagic lesion (*) in the right semitendinosus muscle. (**B**) Selected axial PET images at the comparable level show markedly heterogeneous uptake of ^{18}F-FDG in the anterolateral portion of right thigh (*arrows*). Note no significant activity in the hemorrhagic lesion in the right semitendinosus muscle. Biopsy confirmed recurrent MFH.

B

References

1. Raichle ME. Visualizing the mind. Sci Am 1994; 270:51–64.
2. Soufer R, Dey HM, Lawson AJ, et al. Relationship between reverse redistribution on planar thallium scintigraphy and regional myocardial viability. A correlative PET study. J Nucl Med 1995;36:180–187.
3. Braams JW, Prium J, Freling NJM, et al. Detection of lymph node metastases of squamous cell cancer of the head and neck with FDG-PET and MRI. J Nucl Med 1995;36:211–226.
4. Hoh CK, Swchiepers C, Seltzer MA, et al. PET in oncology: will it replace the other modalities? Semin Nucl Med 1997;27:94–106.
5. Ishiwata K, Kubota K, Murakami M, et al. Re-evaluation of amino acid PET studies: can the protein synthesis rates in brain and tumor tissues be measured in vivo? J Nucl Med 1993;34:1936–1943.
6. Rigo P, Paulus P, Kaschten BJ, et al. Oncological applications of positron emission tomography with F-18 fluorodeoxyglucose. Eur J Nucl Med 1996;23:1641–1674.
7. Brown BS, Wahl RL. Overexpression of Glut-1-glucose transporter in human breast cancer: an immunohistochemical study. Cancer (Phila) 1993;72:2979–2985.
8. Flanagan FL, Dehdashti F, Siegel BA. PET in breast cancer. Semin Nucl Med 1998;28:290–302.
9. Zasadny K, Wahl RL. Standardized uptake valves of normal tissues at PET with 2-F-18-fluro-2-deoxy-D-glucose: variations with body weight and a method for correction. Radiology 1993;189:847–850.
10. Landis SH, Murray T, Bolden S, Wingo PA. Cancer statistics, 1999. CA Cancer J Clin 1999;49:8–31.
11. Mack MJ, Hazelrigg SR, Landreneau RJ, et al. Thoracoscopy for the diagnosis of the indeterminate solitary pulmonary nodule. Ann Thorac Surg 1993;56:825–832.
12. Kuriyama K, Tateishi R, Doi O, et al. Prevalence of air bronchogram in small peripheral carcinoma of the lung on the thin-section CT: comparison with benign tumors. AJR 1991;156:921–924.
13. Patz EF, Lowe VJ, Hoffman JM, et al. Focal pulmonary abnormalities: evaluation with F-18 fluorodeoxyglucose PET scanning. Radiology 1993; 188:487–490.
14. Duhaylongsod FG, Lowe VJ, Patz EF, et al. Detection of primary and recurrent lung cancer by means of F-18 fluorodeoxyglucose PET. J Thorac Cardiovasc Surg 1995;110:130–140.
15. Duhaylongsod FG, Lowe VJ, Patz EF, et al. Lung tumor growth correlates with glucose metabolism measured by FDG-PET. Ann Thorac Surg 1995;60:1348–1352.
16. Webb WR, Gatsonis C, Zerhouni EA, et al. CT and MRI in staging non-small cell bronchogenic carcinoma: report of the radiologic diagnostic oncology group. Radiology 1991;178: 705–713.
17. Wahl RL, Quint LE, Greenough RL, et al. Staging of mediastinal non-small cell lung cancer with FDG PET, CT and fusion images: preliminary prospective evaluation. Radiology 1994; 191:371–377.
18. Patz ER, Lowe VG, Goodman PC, et al. Thoracic nodal staging with PET with F-18 FDG in patients with bronchogenic carcinoma. Chest 1994;108:1617–1621.
19. Erasmus JJ, Patz EF, McAdams HP, et al. Evaluation of adrenal masses in patients with bronchogenic carcinoma using FDG-PET. AJR 1997; 168:1357–1360.
20. Bury T, Dowlete A, Corhay JL, et al. Whole-body F-18 FDG in the staging of non-small cell lung cancer. Eur Respir J 1997;10:2529–2534.
21. Ichija Y, Kuwabara Y, Sasaki M, et al. A clinical evaluation of FDG-PET to assess the response in radiation therapy for bronchogenic carcinoma. Ann Nucl Med 1996;10:193–200.
22. Patz EF, Lowe VJ, Hoffman JM, et al. Persistent or recurrent bronchogenic carcinoma: detection with PET and F-18 FDG. Radiology 1994;191: 379–382.
23. Inoue T, Kim EE, Komaki R, et al. Detecting recurrent or residual lung cancer with FDG PET. J Nucl Med 1995;36:788–793.
24. Gambhir SS, Hoh CG, Phelps ME, et al. Decision tree sensitivity analysis for cost-effectiveness of FDG PET in the staging and management of non-small cell lung carcinoma. J Nucl Med 1996;37:1428–1436.
25. Tabar L, Faggerberg G, Chen HH, et al. Efficacy of breast cancer screening by age: new results from Swedish two-country trial. Cancer (Phila) 1995;75:2507–2514.
26. Nieweg OE, Kim EE, Wong WH, et al. Positron emission tomography with F-128 deoxyglucose in the detection and staging of breast cancer. Cancer (Phila) 1993;71:3920–3925.
27. Scheidhauer K, Scharl A, Pietrzyk K, et al. Quantitative F-18 FDG PET in primary breast cancer. Eur J Nucl Med 1996;23:618–623.

28. Hoh K, Hawkins RA, Glaspy JA, et al. Cancer detection with whole-body PET using F-18 fluoro-2-deoxy-D-glucose. J Comput Assist Tomogr 1993;17:582–589.

29. Avil N, Dose F, Bense S, et al. Metabolic characterization of breast tumors with PET using F-18 fluorodeoxyglucose. J Clin Oncol 1996;14:1848–1857.

30. Tse NY, Hoh K, Hawkins RA, et al. The application of PET with fluorodeoxyglucose to the evaluation of breast disease. Ann Surg 1992; 216:27–34.

31. Wahl RL, Helvic MA, Chang AE, et al. Detection of breast cancer in women after augmentation mammoplasty using F-18 deoxyglucose PET. J Nucl Med 1994;35:872–875.

32. Avil N, Dose J, Jäniicke F, et al. Assessment of axillary lymph node involvement in breast patients with PET using radiolabeled 2-F-18-fluoro-2-deoxy-D-glucose. J Natl Cancer Inst 1996;88:1204–1209.

33. Adler LP, Crowe JP, Al-Kaisi NK, et al. Evaluation of breast masses and axillary lymph nodes with F-18 radiolabeled 2-F-18-fluoro-2-deoxy-D-glucose PET. Radiology 1993;187:743–750.

34. Haberkorn U, Reinhardt M, Strauss LG, et al. Metabolic design of combination therapy: use of enhanced fluorodeoxyglucose uptake caused by chemotherapy. J Nucl Med 1992;33:1981–1987.

35. Bassa P, Kim EE, Inoue T, et al. Evaluation of preoperative chemotherapy using PET with F-18 FDG in breast cancer. J Nucl Med 1996;37:931–938.

36. Ravdin PM, Green S, Dorr TM, et al. Prognostic significance of progesterone receptor levels in estrogen receptor positive patients with metastatic breast cancer treated with tamoxifen. J Clin Oncol 1992;10:1284–1291.

37. McGuire AH, Dehdashti F, Siegel BA, et al. Positron tomographic assessment of 16α-F-18-fluoro-17β-estradiol uptake in metastatic breast carcinoma. J Nucl Med 1991;32:1526–1531.

38. Dehdashti F, Mortimer JE, Siegel BA, et al. Positron tomographic assessment of estrogen receptors in breast cancer. Comparison with FDG-PET and in vitro receptor assays. J Nucl Med 1995;36:1766–1774.

39. Mortimer JE, Dehdashti F, Siegel BA, et al. Clinical correlation of FDG and FES-PET imaging with estrogen receptor and response to systemic therapy. Clin Cancer Res 1996;2:933–939.

40. Vogel CL, Schoenfelder J, Shemano I, et al. Worsening bone scan in the evaluation of antitumor response during hormonal therapy of breast cancer. J Clin Oncol 1995;13:1123–1128.

41. Dehdashti F, Flanagan FL, Siegel BA. PET assessment of metabolic flare in advanced breast cancer. Radiology 1997;205:220–225.

42. Keyes JW Jr, Watson NE Jr, Williams DW III, et al. FDG PET in head and neck cancer. AJR 1997;169:1663–1669.

43. Anzai Y, Carroll WR, Quint DJ, et al. Recurrence of head and neck cancer after surgery or irradiation: prospective comparison of 2-deoxy-F-18-fluoro-D-glucose PET and MRI diagnoses. Radiology 1996;200:135–141.

44. Assar OS, Fischbein NJ, Caputo GR, et al. Metastatic head and neck cancer: role and usefulness of AFDG PET in locating occult primary tumors. Radiology 1999;210:177–181.

45. Flanagan FL, Dehdashti F, Siegel BA, et al. Staging of esophageal cancer with F-18 FDG PET. AJR 1997;168:417–424.

46. Ito M, Lammertsma AA, Wise RSJ, et al. Measurement of regional cerebral blood flow and oxygen utilization in patients with cerebral tumors using ^{15}O and positron emission tomography: analytical techniques and preliminary results. Neuroradiology 1982;23:63–74.

47. Yamamoto YL, Thompson CJ, Meyer E, et al. Dynamic positron emission tomography for study of cerebral hemodynamics in a cross section of the head using positron-emitting ^{68}Ga-EDTA and ^{77}Kr. J Comp Assist Tomogr 1977;1:43.

48. Baba T, Fukui M, Takeshita I, et al. Selective enhancement of intratumoral blood flow in malignant gliomas using intra-arterial adenosine triphosphate. J Neurosurg 1990;72(6):907–911.

49. Nariai T, Senda M, Ishii K, et al. Three-dimensional imaging of cortical structure, function and glioma for tumor resection. J Nucl Med 1997;38(10):1563–1568.

50. Rhodes CG, Wise RJS, Gibbs JM, et al. In vivo disturbance of the oxidative metabolism of glucose in human cerebral gliomas. Ann Neurol 1982;14:614–626.

51. Di Chiro G, De La Paz RL, Brooks RA, et al. Glucose utilization of cerebral gliomas measured by ^{18}F-fluorodeoxyglucose and PET. Neurology 1982;32:1323–1329.

52. Weber G. Enzymology of cancer cells I. N Engl J Med 1977;296:486–493.

53. Kubota R, Kubota K, Yamada S, et al. Active and passive mechanisms of [fluorine-18] fluorodeoxyglucose uptake by proliferating and

prenecrotic cancer cells in vivo: a microautoradiographic study. J Nucl Med 1994;35:1067–1075.

54. Fulham MJ, Melisi JW, Nishimiya J, et al. Neuroimaging of juvenile pilocytic astrocytomas: an enigma. Radiology 1994;189(1):221–225.

55. Derlon J-M, Bourdet C, Bustany P, et al. [^{11}C] L-Methionine uptake in gliomas. Neurosurgery (Baltim) 1989;25(5):720–728.

56. Conti PS, Hilton J, Wong DF, et al. High performance liquid chromatography of carbon-11-labeled compounds. J Nucl Med 1994;21(8):1045–1051.

57. Yung BCK, Wand GS, Blevins L, et al. In vivo assessment of dopamine receptor density in pituitary macroadenoma and correlation with in vitro assay. J Nucl Med 1993;34(5):133.

58. Pappata S, Cornu P, Samson Y, et al. PET study of carbon-11-PK-11195 binding to peripheral type benzodiazepine sites in glioblastoma: a case report. J Nucl Med 1991;32(8):1608–1610.

59. Lichtor J, Dohrmann GJ. Oxidative metabolism and glycolysis in benign brain tumors. J Neurosurg 1987;67:336–340.

60. Valk PE, Budinger TF, Levin VA, et al. PET of malignant cerebral tumors after interstitial brachytherapy. J Neurosurg 1988;69:830–838.

61. Gritters LS, Francis IR, Zasadny KR, et al. Initial assessment of positron emission tomography using 2-F-18 fluoro-2-deoxy-D-glucose in the imaging of malignant melanoma. J Nucl Med 1993;34:1420–1427.

62. Lindholm P, Leskinen S, Någren K, et al. Carbon-11 methionine PET of malignant melanoma. J Nucl Med 1995;36:1806–1810.

63. Rodriguez M, Rehn S, Sundström C, Glimelius B. Predicting malignant grade with PET in non-Hodgkin's lymphoma. J Nucl Med 1995;36:1790–1796.

64. Leskinen-Kallio S, Ruotsalainen U, Någren K, et al. Uptake of C-11 methionine and F-18 FDG in non-Hodgkin's lymphoma: a PET study. J Nucl Med 1991;32:1211–1218.

65. Newman JS, Francis LR, Kaminski ME, et al. Imaging of lymphoma with PET using F-18 FDG. Correlation with CT. Radiology 1994;190:111–116.

66. Abdel-Nabi H, Doerr RJ, Lammonica DM, et al. Staging of primary colorectal carcinomas with fluorine-18-fluorodeoxyglucose whole-body PET: correlation with histopathologic and CT findings. Radiology 1998;206:755–760.

67. Falk PM, Gupa NC, Thorson AG. Positron emission tomography for preoperative staging of colorectal carcinoma. Dis Colon Rectum 1994;37:153–156.

68. Powers TA, Wright JK Jr, Chapman WC, et al. Staging recurrent metastatic colorectal carcinoma with PET. J Nucl Med 1997;38:1196–1201.

69. Strauss LG, Conti PS. The applications of PET in clinical oncology. J Nucl Med 1991;32:623–648.

70. Haberkorn U, Strauss LG, Dimitrakopoulou A. PET studies of fluorodeoxyglucose metabolism in patients with recurrent colorectal tumors receiving radiotherapy. J Nucl Med 1991;32:1485–1490.

71. Haberkorn U, Reinhardt M, Strauss LG. Metafluorodeoxyglucose uptake caused by chemotherapy. J Nucl Med 1992;33:2981–2987.

72. Dimitrakopoulou-Strauss LG, Schlag P, Hohenberger P, et al. Intravenous and intra-arterial oxygen-15 labeled water and fluorine-15 labeled fluorouracil in patients with liver metastases from colorectal carcinoma. J Nucl Med 1998;39:465–473.

73. Zinny M, Bares R, Fab J, et al. Fluorine-18-fluorodeoxyglucose positron emission tomography in the differential diagnosis of pancreatic carcinoma: a report of 106 cases. Eur J Nucl Med 1997;24:678–682.

74. Shreve PD, Gross MD. Imaging of the pancreas and related disease with PET carbon-11 acetate. J Nucl Med 1997;38:1305–1310.

75. Adams S, Baum R, Rink T, et al. Limited value of fluorine-18 fluorodeoxyglucose positron emission tomography for the imaging of neuroendocrine tumors. Eur J Nucl Med 1998;25:79–83.

12
Targeted Magnetic Resonance Imaging Contrast Agents

E. Edmund Kim

Magnetic resonance (MR) contrast agents have been used to improve detection of lesions (better contrast-to-noise ratio) or to improve their characterization by changing tissue signal intensity. The more specific the accumulation of a contrast agent within the target tissue, the better the lesion-to-tissue contrast. Ideally, the target should be an organ of sufficient size with a large number of specific binding sites and also have a high blood flow. Target-specific molecules are called vectors, and "the carrier" means a compound-containing vector. Typical carrier systems include antibodies, proteins, peptides, polysaccharides, cells, and liposomes.

Development of targeted contrast agents for receptor, metabolic, and functional MRI (magnetic resonance imaging) requires magnetic labels that have a high magnetic susceptibility and also the ability to be attachable to carrier molecules. In a typical targeting, the carrier-magnetic label unit would preserve its integrity, escape rapid metabolism, and selectively recognize and associate with the target. It is obvious that target selectivity and receptor or antigen specificity are the most important issues if functional MRI is to be established.

Metal iron chelates (paramagnetic), stable free radicals (paramagnetic), and colloidal iron oxides (superparamagnetic) have been used as contrast agents. Gd(III), Mn(III), Mn(II), Fe(II), and Dy(III) are paramagnetic ions in decreasing order of R_1 relaxicity, and they must be chelated because of toxicity following an intravenous administration. Chelation decreases proton relaxation due to inhibited

access of protons to the paramagnetic ion [1]. Tissue concentrations of 10^{-4} M metal ion, much higher than needed for radiopharmaceuticals (10^{-10} M), must be achieved to be effective in increasing MR signal intensity [1]. Tissue concentrations of monoclonal antibody are usually in the nanomolar range. Metal ion chelates result in an R_1 relaxivity of 3 to 6 mM s^{-1} in water (37°C, 0.5–1 T). R_1 relaxivities for Gd polychelates are usually 2 to 3 times higher per gadolinium molecule [2] and usually 40 to 220 times higher per mole of target-specific molecule [3]. Multiple ion chelates have been clustered on polymers such as polylysine, dextran, or human serum albumin [1,2]. These polymers usually contain 5 to 100 paramagnetic ions. Free radical labels consist of nitroxide moieties that achieve their paramagnetic effect through individual unpaired electrons [4]. Free radicals undergo reduction to magnetically ineffectual diamagnetic species, and the relaxivity is lower when compared with paramagnetic metal ions [4]. Most iron oxides have substantially higher R_1 and R_2 relaxivities and magnetic susceptibility. However, they are not well suited for targeting because of their rapid extraction by phagocytic cells in liver and spleen [5]. Prototypes of monoclonal iron oxide nanoparticles (MION) were developed as a universal label for immunospecific and receptor-specific MR contrast agents. This label has a long blood half-life (several hours in rats) and can leave the vascular space because of its small size. This label can be detected at very low tissue concentrations (<20 nmol Fe/g tissue) because of its superparamagnetic behavior [6]. Conjugation of this label to proteins is typically done through partial oxidation of dextran and linkage to amino groups on proteins or through the use of bifunctional cross-linkers.

Target-Specific Vectors and Carriers

Monoclonal antibodies targeted to pathological tissue have been labeled with radionuclides, superparamagnetic iron oxides, or paramagnetic polylanthanides. Magnetically labeled antibodies have faced problems similar to those of their radiolabeled counterparts such as low concentration of antibody localized within pathological tissue, scarcity of the target antigen itself, and low specificity in vivo [7]. Antitumoral monoclonal antibodies to MION have shown efficient accumulation in tumors. The antibody (L6) recognizes an epitope located on a tumor-associated cell-surface glycoprotein expressed by lung, breast, colon, and ovarian carcinomas [8]. MION-labeled antimyosin antibody has been used to detect regions of myocardial infarction [9]. MRI clearly demonstrated accumulation of the immunoconjugate at the infarcted myocardium with higher spatial resolution when compared with scintigraphy. Lanthanide chelates are usually assembled on carrier molecules before the latter are attached to the antibody, and such antibody complexes labeled with polylysine-$(DTPA-Gd)_n$ have been used for tumor detection of MRI [1].

Several proteins and peptides have been used as potential targeting agents for MRI. Asialoglycoproteins (ASG) and asialofetuin (ASF) have been studied to target hepatocytes because of their high affinity to ASG receptors, and animal MRI has shown selective accumulation of MION-ASF within normal hepatocytes [10]. ASG receptor activity has been demonstrated in normal liver, focal nodular hyperplasia, adenoma, and cirrhotic liver. Neither primary hepatic tumors (hepatoma, hemangioma) nor metastatic tumors (colon, renal cell cancer) have shown any significant uptake of receptor agents [11]. Wheat germ

agglutinin (WGA), a lectin, when attached to MION localizes within neurons and can be used to detect slow neuronal transport. Significant uptake and transport by damaged axons in the sciatic nerve could be visualized by MRI [12]. Cholecystokinin (CCK) has been attached to monocrystalline iron oxide and the CCK–MION complex has been utilized to improve detection of pancreas cancer by MRI. CCK does bind to normal pancreas acinar cells and is subsequently transported to the endoplasmic reticulum. However, CCK does not bind to pancreatic cancer cells, and CCK-MION uptake is competitively inhibited with CCK receptor antagonist such as proglumide [13]. The conjugation product, MION-streptavidin-biotin-secretin, has been shown to contain one to two secretins per MION particle with a high affinity for pancreatic acini, similar to unconjugated secretin [6].

A variety of polysaccharides have been used to coat magnetic particles or to synthesize paramagnetic macromolecular agents. Most dextran-stabilized iron oxide particles are efficiently extracted from the blood pool by the reticuloendothelial system (RES) and are thus clinically used as contrast agents for liver and spleen [14]. Small iron oxides (9USPIO, MION, AMI-227) with long blood half-life accumulate in considerable amounts in lymph nodes by direct extravasation within capillaries in lymph nodes or by clearance of lymphatic fluid once the particles reach the tissue interstitium [15,16]. Dextran-coated polylysine (PL) graft copolymer labeled with Gd-DTPA, known as polyglucose-associated macromolecule (9-PGM) accumulates in lymph nodes after subcutaneous injection and significantly enhances the signal intensity of normal nodes but not metastatic nodes [17]. It has also been shown that, after intravenous injection of PGM-Gd-DTPA ($10\,\mu mol\,Gd/kg$), approximately 25% of the injected dose accumulates in rat lymph nodes [17]. Arabinogalacton (AG) is a natural polysaccharide exhibiting specificity for asialoglycoprotein receptors on hepatocytes. Animal studies have shown an improved hepatoma to background signal intensity ratio using polysaccharide AG [18]. Recent advances in polymer chemistry have facilitated the development of magnetically labeled macromolecular polymers. Polylysine (PL) with higher (480 kDa) molecular weight has shown longer (7h) blood half-lives, whereas short (36kDa) chain polylysines show a more rapid excretion (2h). PL-Gd-DTPA has been shown to localize rat adrenal glands [19], and targeted MRI of adrenal gland has been attempted with a Gd-cholesterol analogue [20]. Methoxypolyethylene glycol (9-MPEG)-PL-Gd-DTPA has been used to assess tumor neovascularity, a parameter to correlate with the malignant potential of tumor [21].

Liposomes are artificial lipid vesicles of nano-to-micrometer scale and were developed as a target vehicle for delivering drugs. Magnetic labels have been either encapsulated within or incorporated into the lipid bilayer of liposomes. During the vascular distribution phase, magnetic liposomes act as blood pool agents. As they become trapped by phagocytic cells, they also have been exploited as contrast agents for the liver and spleen [22].

Researchers have taken advantage of the ability of white blood cells to bind or internalize magnetic labels and thus transport them to their cellular destination. T cells can be labeled with superparamagnetic iron oxide by endocytosis [23]. Successful labeling of human phagocytic cells has been reported by various techniques including iron oxide encapsulated into liposomes, dextran-coated iron oxides, and cell-surface labeling with PL-MION [24]. Such labeled cells potentially offer an opportunity to track the migration of different cell types in vivo by MRI.

MR Contrast Agents

The MR image is rich with inherent contrast from numerous tissues, and relative tissue contrast can be manipulated by changing the device variables. MR images represent the macroscopic behavior of the water proton, which must have molar concentrations to provide sufficient signal. Therefore, the MR contrast agent must influence a large fraction of these resident water protons. The elements that determine MR contrast are numerous, and the process of prescribing the imaging protocol that produces the best image in a given clinical setting is often complex. Contrast agents influence image contrast indirectly to the extent that T_1 or T_2 relaxation times of tissues are affected. Relaxation stimulated by proton interactions with other biomolecules for routine MRI is indistinguishable from that caused by contrast agents.

Contrast-enhanced MRI has been restricted to the use of gadolinium-based interstitial contrast agents for clinical studies for the past decade (Figure 12.1). Two new agents, Mn-DPDP and ferumoxides, with specific cellular uptake have been approved for routine hepatic studies. A wide range of new agents are under clinical development, and many of these are likely to be introduced for clinical use in the next several years (Table 12.1). Gadolinium has an excellent safety profile and has been very useful for detection and characterization of many diseases. Within a very short period of time it is rapidly filtered into the larger extracellular space, similar to iodine-based contrast agents. T_1-weighted gradient-echo pulse sequences with short acquisition times are employed for most applications. The new contrast agents have much longer periods of enhancement duration. Each of the agents is tailored for specific clinical applications.

There are several classification for the MRI contrast agents. The agents are routinely classified as either paramagnetic or superparamagnetic. Paramagnetic agents have unpaired electrons, and the relaxation effect is proportional to the square of the magnetic moment of the paramagnetic. Superparamagnetic agents have a much larger magnetic moment than paramagnetic chelates. The gadolinium chelates, which shorten tissue and blood T_1 are referred to as T_1 agents. The reticuloendothelial system (RES) agents, which shorten tissue T_2, are referred to as T_2 agents. At low doses, some of the RES agents have a T_1-shortening effect, whereas at higher doses they shorten T_2. The agents are practically divided into four categories: extracellular agents, RES agents, hepatobiliary agents, and blood-pool agents.

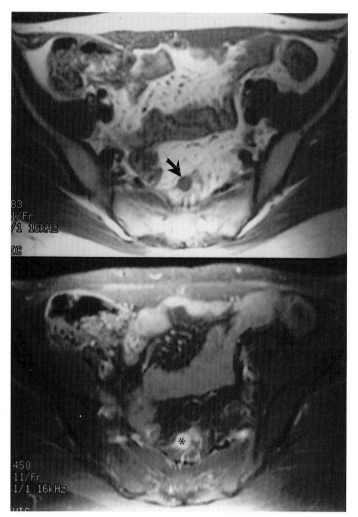

FIGURE 12.1. Axial T_1-weighted MR images of the pelvis before the injection of Gd-DTPA (*top*) shows a small nodule with low signal intensity (*arrow*) in the presacral space. Fat-suppressed T_1-weighted image at the comparable level after injection of Fd-DTPA shows significant contrast enhancement of the lesion (*). Surgery confirmed recurrent ovarian carcinoma.

TABLE 12.1. MRI contrast agents.

Agents	Names	Applications
RES	AMI-25 (Feridex, Endorem)	Liver imaging
	(Combidex)	Liver, lymph node, vascular imaging
	SHU-555A (Resovist)	Liver imaging
Hepatobiliary	Mn-DPDP (Teslascan)	Liver imaging
	Gd-EOB-DTPA (Eovist)	Liver imaging
	Gd-BOPTA (MultiHance)	Liver imaging
Blood-pool	MS-325	Vascular imaging
	Gd-DTPA-dextran	Vascular imaging
	Gd-DTPA-cascade-polymer	Vascular imaging
Extracellular	Gd-DTPA, Gd-DOTA	Dynamic MRI

Extracellular Agents

Gadolinium diethylenetriaminepentaacetate (Gd-DTPA) and Gd tetraazacyclododecanetetraacetate (Gd-DOTA) are initially distributed in the intravascular space but are then rapidly filtered through the capillaries into the extracellular space, similar to the water-soluble iodine-containing contrast agents. Nonionic Gd-containing agents such as gadodiamide, gadobutrol, and dadoteridol with a similar biodistribution have been introduced (Figure 12.2). Because of the rapid equilibrium of these agents in the interstitial space both of normal tissue, such as liver, and of tumors, the utilization of pulse sequences with high temporal resolution such as fast gradient-echo sequences is necessary after intravenous bolus injection so the dynamic imaging can capture the rapid changes in contrast agent distribution and makes the best use of the extremely narrow imaging window. Dynamic Gd-enhanced MRI has been shown not only to improve the distinction between benign and malignant lesions but also to achieve a specific diagnosis in many focal hepatic lesions [25].

Reticuloendothelial System Agents

The RES agents are iron oxide-based particles and specifically target cells of the RES, cell-surface receptors, or the blood pool. They form particles of different sizes and have been referred as superparamagnetic iron oxides (SPIO, >50 nm) and ultrasmall superparamagnetic iron oxides (USPIO, <50 nm). Two SPIOs, ferumoxides (AMI-25, feridex) and resovist (SAHU-555A), and one USPIO (AMI-227) are undergoing clinical trials [26,27]. These agents are superparamagnetic and create a rapid dephasing of proton spins. They produce a dose-dependent decrease in signal intensity on both T_1- and T_2-weighted images. About 80% of an AMI-25 dose is taken up by the Kupffer cells, 6% by the spleen, and a small amount by the bone marrow in a normally functioning liver. Owing to its small particle size, AMI-227 is not immediately recognized by the RES and has a longer blood half-life of 8 to 10 min [28].

Thus, AMI-227 is accumulated in lymph nodes after being cleared by the mononuclear phagocytic system or drained by lymphatic fluid. It may be useful in MR angiography, lymphocyte marking, and receptor imaging targeted to other organs. A normal liver loses significant signal intensity on T_2-weighted

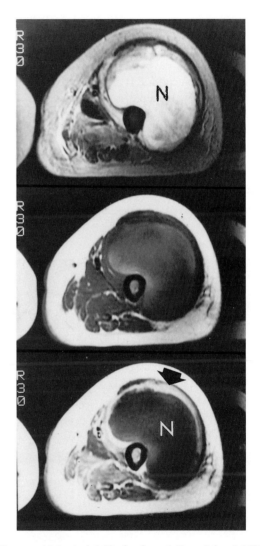

FIGURE 12.2. Axial T_2 (*top*) and T_1-weighted MR images of left thigh before (*middle*) and after (*bottom*) injection of Gd-gadodiamide show a large malignant fibrous histiocytoma with large central necrosis (*N*). Note contrast enhancement (arrow) in the periphery of the tumor.

images, and the difference in enhancement increases the lesion-to-liver contrast-to-noise ratio (CNR). Focal nodular hyperplasia (FNH), hepatic adenoma, and hepatocellular carcinoma (HCC) may uptake the agent leading to signal loss.

Hepatic hemangiomas also demonstrate signal changes on T_1- and T_2-weighted imaging because of residual blood-pool effect, and metastases do not show signal changes [26] (Figure 12.3). AMI-25-enhanced T_2-weighted images depicted additional hepatic lesions in 27% of patients as compared with unenhanced MRI and 40% of patients as compared with contrast-enhanced CT. It also has greater detection capability for hepatic malignancies as compared with spiral CT [29]. However, there have been contradictory reports that spiral CT during arterial portography (CTAP) is still more sensitive than ferumoxide-enhanced MRI in patients who are to undergo liver resection. SHU-555A has a similar blood half-life but has

a smaller particle size than AMI-25 (60 nm versus 80–160 nm, respectively) [30]. Bolus administration of SHU-555A potentially enables dynamic MRI, similar to that performed with the gadolinium chelates [31]. It has been compared with Gd-DTPA-enhanced MRI and found to have superior lesion detection capabilities [32]. AMI-227 is not immediately recognized by the RES because of its small size, and has a blood half-life of about 200 min [27]. It remains in the blood long enough to accumulate in lymph nodes [33]. Normal lymph nodes accumulate the agent and become darker on T_2-weighted images. Nodes replaced by tumor cells will not take up as much of the agent and remain high in signal intensity [33]. This characteristic is also useful for performing MR angiography. Because the vessels become hyperintense to liver parenchyma on T_2-weighted images, they become distinguishable from solid tumors [34]. It has been reported that ring enhancement after administration of

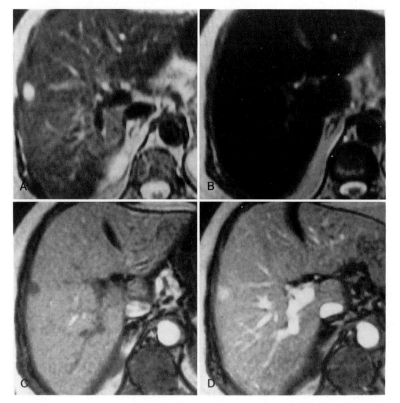

FIGURE 12.3. Hemangioma of the liver before and after injection of AMI-227 on predose T_2 (**A**), postdose T_2 (**B**), predose T_1 (**C**), and postdose T_1 (**D**) weighted images. Note that hemangioma has completely disappeared on postdose T_2 image (**B**) whereas it has changed contrast character from hypointense (**C**) to hyperintense (**D**) on T_1 images. (From Petersein J. et al. [26], with permission.)

AMI-227 is a finding seen more often with malignant lesions (62% versus 14%) than benign lesions [35].

Hepatobiliary Agents

The hepatobiliary agents are actively taken up by hepatocytes and produce T_1 shortening of the liver. Manganese(II)-N,N^1-dipyridoxyleth-ylene diamine-N,N^1-diacetate 5,5'-bis (phosphate) (Mn-DPDP) has been used for routine clinical use, and Gd-ethoxybenzyl-diethylene-triaminepentaacetic acid (EEOB-DTPA) as well as Gd-benzyloxypropionictetraacetate dimeglumine (BOPTA-Dimeg) are paramagnetic agents in clinical trials and increase lesion conspicuity with higher liver-to-lesion contrast [36]. Mn-DPDP is not entirely specific for hepatocytes and has been shown to enhance the pancreas, kidneys, adrenal gland [36], and tumors of endocrine origin [37]. As an agent targeted to hepatocytes, there is potential to characterize tumors of hepatocellular origin. Tumors of hepatocellular origin demonstrate enhancement of any type, but a peripheral enhancement was most common [38]. Well-differentiated hepatoma showed greater enhancement than poorly differentiated hepatoma [39]. It has been reported that each of three adenomas demonstrated at least 40% enhancement on post-Mn-DPDP images, whereas two metastases enhanced not at all or only 12% [39].

Gd-EOB-DTPA and Gd-BOPTA/Dimeg are paramagnetic MR contrast agents that are selectively taken up and secreted into the bile by hepatocytes [40]. Therefore, the signal intensity of normal hepatocytes is increased on T_1-weighted images, and the contrast between hepatocytes and focal liver lesions is enhanced. The agents are rapidly distributed into the extracellular fluid after injection, and a portion of them becomes bound to plasma proteins while the remainder is either taken up by hepatocytes or undergoes renal filtration and excretion. The optimal imaging time post contrast for delayed scans appears to be 25 to 40 min post injection with Gd-EOB-DTPA as compared with 60 to 120 min post injection of Gd-BOPTA [41].

Blood-Pool Agents

Following infusion of the gadolinium chelates, optimal arterial enhancement occurs within the first minute, which is followed by increased venous and interstitial enhancement. Blood-pool agents are specifically designed to remain in the blood pool for a prolonged period of time. MS-325 is formed by substitution of a Gd-DTPA with a diphenylcyclohexyl phosphate group. Following intravenous injection, 80% to 96% of the agents binds reversibly to human serum albumin in plasma [42]. Therefore, the gadolinium is retained within the intravascular compartment, and it also has a relaxivity 6 to 10 times that of Gd-DTPA [43]. Gd-DTPA-polylysine, Gd-DTPA-dextran, Gd-DTPA-cascade polymer, and Gd-DTPA-albumin have also been developed. They may serve as markers of perfusion and abnormal vascular permeability [44]. The USPIO and AMI-227 have also been used as MR blood-pool agents.

Conclusion

The use of target-specific MR contrast agents can dramatically improve information obtained by MRI. Various components of target-specific MR contrast agents including various carriers as well as magnetic labels have been utilized for clinical applications. Contrasted MRI for clinical studies has been expanded from the use of Gd-based interstitial agents to the specific cellular agents. Clinicians performing MRI studies will have an increasing array of pharmaceutical agents that can be tailored to specific clinical problems.

References

1. Wang SC, Wikström MG, White DL, et al. Evaluation of Gd-DTPA-labeled dextran as an intravascular MR contrast agent. Radiology 1990;175:483–488.
2. Voxler VS, Clement O, Schmitt-Willich H, et al. Effect of varying the molecular weight of the MR contrast agent Gd-DTPA-polylysine on blood pharmacokinetics and enhancement patterns. J Magn Reson Imaging 1994;4:381–388.

3. Brasch RC. New directions in the development of MR imaging contrast media. Radiology 1992; 183:1–11.

4. Leander P. Liver-specific contrast media for MRI and CT experimental studies. Acta Radiol Suppl 1995;396:1–36.

5. Weissleder R, Papisov M. Pharmaceutical iron oxides for MRI. J Magn Reson Imaging 1992; 4:1–6.

6. Shen T, Weissleder R, Papisov M, et al. Monocrystalline iron oxide nanocompounds (MION). Magn Reson Med 1993;29:599–604.

7. Orang-Khadivi K, Pierce BL, Ollom CM, et al. New magnetic resonance imaging techniques for the detection of breast cancer. Breast Cancer Res Treat 1994;32:119–135.

8. Stenzel-Johnson PR, Yelton D, Bajorath J, et al. Identification of residues in the monoclonal antibody L6 important for binding to its tumor antigen. Biochemistry 1994;33:14400–14406.

9. Weissleder R, Lee AS, Khaw BA. Antimyosin-labeled monocrystalline iron oxide allows detection of myocardial infract. Radiology 1991;181: 245–249.

10. Schaffer BK, Linder C, Papisov M, et al. MION-ASF: biokinetics of an MR receptor agent. Magn Reson Imaging 1993;11:411–417.

11. Reimer P, Weissleder R, Wittenberg J, et al. Receptor-directed contrast agents for MRI. Radiology 1992;182:565–569.

12. van Everdingen KJ, Enochs WS, Bhide PG, et al. Determinants of in vivo MRI of slow axonal transport. Radiology 1994;193:485–591.

13. Reimer P, Weissleder R, Shen T, et al. Pancreatic receptors: initial feasibility studies with a target contrast agent for MRI. Radiology 1994;193: 527–531.

14. Weissleder R, Papisov M. Pharmaceutical oxides for MRI. Rev Magn Reson Med 1992;4:1–20.

15. Weissleder R, Heautot JF, Schaffer BK, et al. MR lymphography. Radiology 1994;191:225–230.

16. Vassallo P, Matei C, Heston WD, et al. AMI-227-enhanced MR lymphography: usefulness for differentiating reactive from tumor-bearing lymph nodes. Radiology 1994;193:501–506.

17. Harika L, Weissleder R, Poss K, et al. MR lymphography with a lymphotropic T1-type MR contrast agent: Gd-DTPA-PGM. Magn Reson Med 1995;33:88–92.

18. Reimer P, Weissleder R, Brady TJ, et al. Experimental hepatocellular carcinoma: MR receptor imaging. Radiology 1991;180:641–645.

19. Weissleder R, Wang YM, Papisov M, et al. Polymeric contrast agents for MRI of adrenal glands. J Magn Reson Imaging 1993;3:93–97.

20. Mühler A, Platzek J, Radüchel B, et al. Characterization of a Gd-cholesterol derivative as an organ specific contrast agent of adrenal imaging. J Magn Reson Imaging 1995;5:7–10.

21. Weidner N, Folkman J, Pozza F, et al. Tumor angiogenesis: a new significant and independent prognostic indicator in early-stage breast carcinoma. J Natl Cancer Inst 1992;84:1875–1887.

22. Niesman MR, Bacic GG, Wright SM, et al. Liposome encapsulated $MnCl_2$ as a liver specific contrast agent for MRI. Invest Radiol 1990;25: 545–551.

23. Yeh T, Zhang W, Ilstad ST, et al. Intracellular labeling of T-cells with superparamagnetic contrast agents. Magn Reson Med 1993;30:617–625.

24. Bulte JWM, Ma LD, Magin RL, et al. Selective MRI of labeled human peripheral blood mononuclear cells by liposome mediated incorporation of dextran-magnetite particles. Magn Reson Med 1993;29:32–37.

25. Mahfouz A-E, Hamm B. Contrast agents. MRI Clin North Am 1997;5:223–240.

26. Petersein J, Saini S, Weissleder R. Iron oxide-based reticuloendothelial contrast agents for MRI. MRI Clin North Am 1996;4:53–60.

27. Weissleder R, Reimer P, Lee AS, et al. MR receptor imaging: ultrasmall iron oxide particles targeted to asialoglycoprotein receptors. AJR 1990;155:1161–1167.

28. Weissleder R, Elizondo G, Wittenberg J, et al. Ultrasmall superparamagnetic iron oxide: characterization of a new class of contrast agents for MRI. Radiology 1990;175:489–493.

29. Ros PR, Freeny PC, Harms SE, et al. Hepatic MRI with ferumoxides: a multicenter clinical trial of the safety and efficacy in the detection of focal hepatic lesions. Radiology 1995;196:481–488.

30. Kopp AF, Laniado M, Dammann F, et al. MRI of the liver with Resovist: safety, efficacy and pharmacodynamic properties. Radiology 1997;204: 749–756.

31. Shamsi K, Balzer T, Saini S, et al. Superparamagnetic iron oxide particles (SH U 555A): evaluation of efficacy in three doses for hepatic MRI. Radiology 1998;206:365–371.

32. Vogl TJ, Hammerstingl R, Schwartz W, et al. Superparamagnetic iron oxide-enhanced versus Gd-enhanced MRI for differential diagnosis of focal liver lesions. Radiology 1996;198:881–887.

33. Weissleder R, Elizondo G, Wittenberg J, et al. Ultrasmall superparamagnetic iron oxide (USPIO): an intravenous contrast agent for assessing lymph nodes with MRI. Radiology 1990;175:494–498.

34. Saini S, Edelman RR, Sharma P, et al. Blood-pool MR contrast material for detection and characterization of focal hepatic lesions: initial clinical experience with ultrasmall superparamagnetic iron oxide (AMI-227). AJR 1995;164:1147–1152.

35. Mergo PJ, Helmberger T, Nicolas AI. Ring enhancement in ultrasmall superparamagnetic iron oxide MRI: a potential new sign for characterization of liver lesions. AJR 1996;166:379–384.

36. Mitchell DG, Outwater EK, Matteucci T, et al. Adrenal gland enhancement at MRI with Mn-DPDP. Radiology 1995;194:783–787.

37. Wang C, Ahlstrom H, Eriksson B, et al. Uptake of mangafodipir trisodium in liver metastases from endocrine tumors. J Magn Reson Imaging 1998;8:682–686.

38. Rofsky NM, Weinref JC, Bernardin ME, et al. Hepatocellular tumors: characterization with Mn-DPDP-enhanced MRI. Radiology 1993;188:53–59.

39. Murakami T, Baron RL, Peterson MS, et al. Hepatocellular carcinoma: MRI with mangafodipir trisodium (Mn-DPDP). Radiology 1996;200:69–77.

40. Oksendal AN, Hals PA. Biodistribution and toxicity of MRI contrast media. J Magn Reson Imaging 1998;3:157–165.

41. Runge VM. A comparison of two MR hepatobiliary gadolinium chelates: Gd-BOPTA and Gd-EOB-DTPA. J Comput Asst Tomogr 1998;22:643–650.

42. Lauffer RB, Parmelee DJ, Dunham SU, et al. MS-325: albumin-targeted contrast agent for MR angiography. Radiology 1998;207:529–538.

43. Grist TM, Korosec FR, Peters DC, et al. Steady-state and dynamic MR angiography with MS-325: initial experience in humans. Radiology 1998;207:539–544.

44. Schmiedl U, Sievers RE, Brasch RC, et al. Acute myocardial ischemia and reperfusion: MRI with albumin-Gd-DTPA. Radiology 1989;170:351–356.

13
Magnetic Resonance Characteristics of Tumors

E. Edmund Kim

Dynamic Contrast Magnetic Resonance Imaging

Dynamic magnetic resonance imaging (MRI) with rapid sequential image acquisition after bolus injection of gadolinium-diethylene tri-aminepentaacetic acid (Gd-DTPA) can be used to differentiate benign from malignant lesions. Approximately 84% of malignant tumors exhibited slope values (the slope of the contrast-enhancement-over-time curve) higher than 30% per minute; 72% of benign tumors showed slopes lower than 30% per minute [1]. Both benign and malignant tumors showed some overlap resulting in an accuracy of approximately 80%. The slope values of the time intensity curve of postcontrast dynamic sequences and peak enhancement rates were calculated during the first minute after contrast administration on a pixel-by-pixel basis using a linear fitting algorithm. Tissues with high slopes were bright in the resultant image whereas slowly enhancing tissues with low slopes were dark. The first-pass slope value correlated well with tissue vascularization and perfusion. Highly vascularized or well-perfused benign lesions such as osteoid osteoma and giant cell tumor present with slope values similar to those of malignant tumors.

On conventional post-Gd-DTPA MRI, viable tumor and peritumorous edema exhibit marked contrast enhancement and cannot be differentiated [2]. Initial slope values of edematous muscle were lower than those of infil-trated muscle and viable tumor by 20% or more. Perineoplastic edema seen on MRI correlates with intratumoral prostaglandin concentration [3]. MRI after Gd-DTPA admin-istration is unique in that it may provide direct differentiation between viable and necrotic tumor. Viable tumor is characterized by marked contrast enhancement whereas necrotic tumor regions typically do not demonstrate contrast enhancement and remain low or intermediate in signal intensity on T_1-weighted postcontrast scans [4]. Sequential MRI with use of a fast gradient-echo MR sequence after bolus injection of Gd-DTPA may be used to assess tumor response to chemotherapy. In respon-ders, there was a reduction of the slope of the contrast enhancement–time curve by at least 60% on follow-up MRI after chemotherapy when compared with the prechemotherapy study; in nonresponders, the reduction was usually less than 60%. Following chemother-apy, residual viable tumor has been reported to show early and progressive enhancement at specific preferential sites [5]. In responders, a decrease in neovascularity and feeder vessels was observed on MR angiography. In nonresponders, there were persistent or increased neovascularity and feeder vessels (Figure 13.1) [6]. Differentiation between recurrent tumor and posttreatment tissue changes poses a difficult diagnostic problem. Tumors and posttreatment changes demon-strate contract enhancement and cannot be clearly differentiated on contrast-enhanced scans [7]. No or only slow increase in signal

FIGURE 13.1. Osteogenic sarcoma with high neovascularity and tumor encroachment onto popliteal artery. (A) T_1-postcontrast spin-echo MR coronal image shows intramedullary tumor with large enhancing soft tissue mass and perineoplastic edema (*arrows*). Note extensive cortical reaction with thickening and irregularity of the cortex. (B) 2-D time-of-flight MR coronal angiogram with maximum intensity projection shows medially displaced superficial femoral vessels (*long arrows*), multiple feeder vessels (*small arrows*), and marked neovascularity (*curved arrows*). (C) 3-D surface reconstruction provides simultaneous display of normal bone, extraosseous tumor, and vessels. The extraosseous tumor encroaches on the femoral vessels (*arrows*), but does not encase them. (From Lang et al. [6], with permission of *AJR*.)

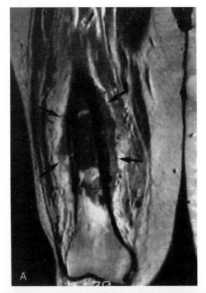

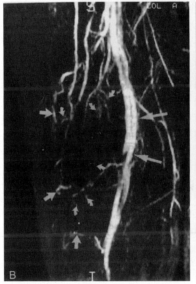
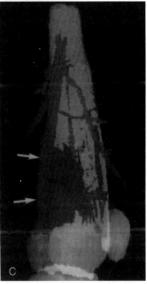

intensity observed with dynamic MRI is apparently indicative of a pseudomass, whereas an early and fast increase in signal intensity indicates recurrence.

MR Spectroscopy and Spectroscopic Imaging

MR spectroscopy exploits the chemical shift phenomenon, allowing different chemical substrates to be distinguished on the basis of their MR spectroscopic signature; this includes concentration, relaxation behavior, and interactions with other substrates. It provides direct access to biochemical components within living tissue, with concentration sensitivity down to the millimole per liter range. It can also be used to determine the rates of chemical reactions and thus provide further insights on metabolism and other in vivo biochemical processes. MR spectroscopy encompasses a wide range of techniques such as fat–water imaging, localized MR spectroscopy, and spectroscopic imaging [8].

Adrenal adenomas and nodular hyperplasia contain large amounts of intracellular fat, whereas most metastases and pheochromocytomas do not. Thus, chemical shift imaging with in-phase and opposed-phase gradient-echo images has been advocated to distinguish adenomas from nonadenomatous lesions. On a 1.5-tesla MR system (64 MHz), lipid and water spins have a frequency difference of about 224 Hz. The signal intensity of opposed phase images depends on the proportion of lipid and water content within the tissue. Compared to nonlipid-containing tissue, the signal from tissues containing fat and water cancels and yields low signal intensity on opposed-phase images [9].

MR spectroscopic imaging is more than just an additional imaging modality with a resolution of a few millimeters, and allows imaging-guided spectroscopic acquisition. The application of MR spectroscopy in the diagnostic clinic is driven by an increasing desire to obtain functional information that goes beyond diagnosis to prognosis and therapy planning or monitoring.

The proton MR spectra of intracranial tumors differ greatly from those of normal brain and reflect the metabolic alterations that accompany tumor growth. The elevation of choline signifies increased membrane turnover, and the presence of lactate marks for altered energy metabolism. N-Acetylaspartate present in normal brain is absent in tumors [9]. Thirty-four patients with cystic intracerebral mass lesions (28 tumors, 6 abscesses) were examined at ^{1}H-MR spectroscopy in vivo. Water-suppressed, double spin-echo sequences (TR1500/TE136 and 272) were used, and the acquisition time was 8 min for each sequence. The digital resolution of the spectroscopic imaging was 1 cm in the anteroposterior or left–right directions and 2 cm in the caudocranial direction. The diameter of the necrotic or cystic center was at least 2 cm. All lesions demonstrated Gd-DTPA enhancement in the regular or moderately irregular perilesional ring. Lactate (1.3 ppm) was present in 27 of 28 tumors, and peaks for alanine as well as lactate at 0.9 ppm, acetate at 1.9 ppm, and succinate at

2.4 ppm were identified in 6, 6, and 4 of the 6 abscesses, respectively [10]. The resonances of N-acetylaspartate, choline, and creatine were absent in all cases.

The addition of three-dimensional (3-D) MR spectroscopic imaging to MRI provides better detection and localization of prostate cancer in a sextant of the prostate than does use of MRI alone. At 3-D MR spectroscopic imaging, prostate cancer was diagnosed as possible if the ration of choline plus creatine to citrate exceeded 2 standard deviation (SD) above population norms or as definite if that ratio exceeded 3 SD above the norm. The spectroscopic volume was selected with the point-resolved spectroscopic (PRESS) technique, and the imaging data set was acquired with a spatial resolution of 0.24 to 0.70 cm^3 in 53 patients with biopsy-proved prostate cancer. The 3-D spectroscopic imaging diagnosis of definite cancer had higher specificity (75%) but lower sensitivity (63%). High specificity (to 91%) was obtained when combined MRI and 3-D MR spectroscopic imaging indicated cancer (Figure 13.2) [11]. Endorectal MRI and 3-D MR spectroscopic imaging were performed in 53 patients with prostate cancer. For the less experienced reader, the addition of 3-D MR spectroscopic imaging to MRI significantly improved accuracy [12]. Multisection proton MR spectroscopic imaging was feasible with a single spin-echo sequence for the acquisition of metabolic information in the human prostate [13].

Nonproton MR spectroscopic imaging has become clinically important. Phosphorus-13 MR spectroscopic imaging provides detailed information concerning bioenergics and lipid metabolism. ^{31}P-MR spectroscopy depicts metabolite changes in tumors after treatment [14] and is being investigated as a method to provide an early measure of response to cancer therapy. Carbon-13 MR spectroscopy depicts the flow of carbon metabolites through various biochemical pathways [15]. MR spectroscopy and spectroscopic imaging contribute most effectively to the achievement of basic physiological and pathological knowledge. These techniques are rapidly advancing as the result of new technical developments including high-

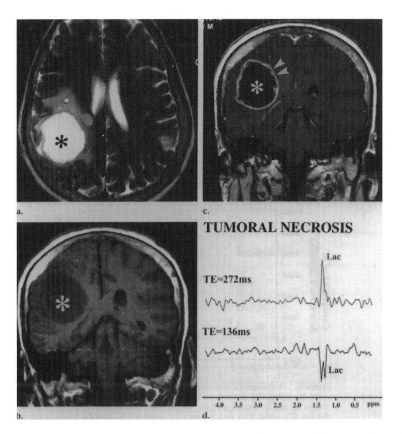

FIGURE 13.2. Transaxial T_2 (**a**) and coronal T_1-weighted images of the head without (**b**) and with (**c**) contrast enhancement show a cystic glioblastoma (*) with a Gd-DTPA enhanced ring (*arrowheads* in **c**) and surrounding edema (*dot* in **a**) in the right parietal lobe. Proton MR spectra (**d**) with the voxel in the necrotic center of the tumor show the absence of N-acetylaspartate, choline, and creatine peaks. Note relatively high lactate (Lac) peak, which is inverted with 136-ms TE. (From Grand et al. [11], with permission of *Radiology*.)

performance gradient systems, and will continue to expand as further advances are made, including more user-friendly software. Clinicians will increasingly use this new modality as they see diagnostic and therapeutic benefits for their patients [16].

Diffusion and Perfusion MRI

Diffusion is the externally induced behavior of molecules moving in a microscopic random pattern in a fluid, so-called Brownian movement. This motion can be quantified by means of a diffusion coefficient. Diffusion-weighted MRI is sensitive to microscopic motion that can be quantified by an apparent diffusion coefficient (ADC). The microscopic motions include molecular diffusion of water and microcirculation of blood in the capillary network (perfusion). The ADC is equal to the diffusion coefficient when diffusion is the only type of motion present, but ADCs in biological tissues are often higher than expected because they are affected by both diffusion and perfusion [17].

Diffusion-weighted imaging has been mostly limited to the brain because of many technical problems related to motion. Recently, an echo-planar imaging technique has been developed, and diffusion-weighted imaging of the abdomen has become possible because its fast imaging technique minimizes the effect of physiological motion [18]. Diffusion-weighted MRI images were acquired using the multisection spin-echo type single-shot echo-planar sequence in the transverse plane; 90° and 180° RF pulse series were applied, as well as two motion-probing gradients, one before and one after the 180° RF pulse. Motion-probing gradients were applied along all three directions, and the duration of the motion-probing gradient was 20 ms. Sequential sampling of the K-space was used with TE of 70 ms, bandwidth of 121 kHz, matrix of 92×128, field of view of 40 cm, section thickness of 10 mm, interscan gap of 5 mm, and one excitation. The ADC of the abdominal organs and hepatic lesions showed smaller values when calculated with the maxim b values ($846 \, s/mm^2$). Diffusion sensitivity is governed by the gradient factor b. The ADCs of the benign lesions calculated with b values of less than $850 \, s/mm^2$ were $2.49 \pm 1.39 \times 10^{-3} \, mm^2/s$ and significantly greater than those of the malignant lesions ($1.01 \pm 0.38 \times 10^{-3} \, mm^2/s$). Use of a threshold ADC of $1.6 \times 10^{-3} \, mm^2/s$ would result in 98% sensitivity and 80% specificity for differentiation of malignant from benign hepatic lesions when the maximum b value is used [18]. Signal intensity of hepatoma or hepatic metastasis decreased gradually in comparison with that of benign lesions as the b value became larger (Figure 13.3). Water-rich malignant lesions such as cystic ovarian cancer and mucinous adenocarcinoma may show large ADCs such as those produced by cyst or hemangioma. Fibrotic changes and thrombus in the hemangioma may reduce ADCs. Moderately heavy T_2-weighted MRI may help for the differentiation and reduce the necessity for Gd-enhanced MRI.

Diffusion-weighted MRI exploits the random motion of the molecules, which causes a phase dispersion of the spins with a resultant loss of signal. Tumor necrosis is characterized by increased membrane permeability and breakdown of the cell membrane and the intracellular membrane structures. These changes at the cellular level may result in less restricted, increased diffusion of water molecules in necrotic tumor than that in viable tumor with intact membrane. Necrotic tumor showed low signal intensity (mean normalized ADC, 0.46 ± 0.2) in 12 rats with osteogenic sarcoma, indicating rapid diffusion of water molecules as a

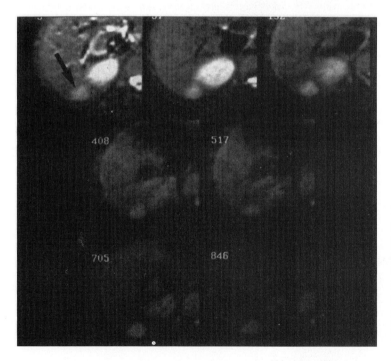

FIGURE 13.3. Diffusion-weighted transaxial single-shot echo-planar MR images of the liver show a metastatic adenocarcinoma (*arrow*) whose signal intensity decreases gradually as gradient factor b value (s/mm^2) numbers on each image become larger. (From Lang et al. [19], with permission of *Radiology*.)

result of loss of membrane integrity, whereas viable tumor showed high signal intensity (ADC, 0.16 ± 0.05) [19].

It is commonly accepted that tumors frequently induce angiogenesis and that highly vascular tumors are often more malignant than those that do not have increased vascularity. Benign lesions including posttreatment changes do not typically exhibit the same level of angiogenesis. Gd-DTPA bolus-infusion perfusion imaging has been proposed due to temporary decrease in T_2^*, resulting in a transient decrease in signal intensity on T_2 or T_2^*-weighted images. Time-of-flight (arterial spin labeling) techniques and echo-planar MRI and signal targeting with alternating radiofrequency (EPISTAR) use a variation of the inversion recover technique without injection of contrast

agents. They are under investigation for measuring tumor perfusion [20].

Magnetization Transfer Ratio

Magnetic resonance signal intensity is determined by three pools of protons: free water protons, water protons in proximity to macromolecules with restricted motion compared with that of free water protons, and immobile protons of macromolecules [21]. By using MR techniques that selectively address the contribution of magnetization transfer (MT) to signal intensity, one may be able to gain insight into the macromolecular basis of a session's appearance on MRI (Figure 13.4). MT has been used primarily to improve background

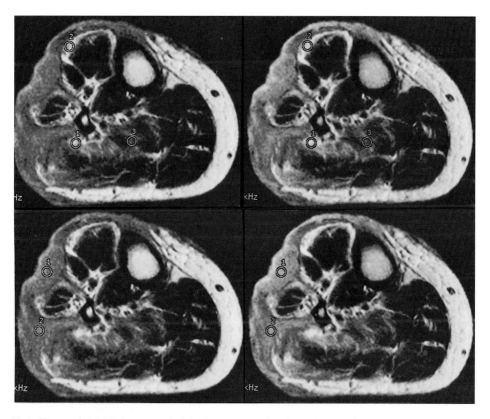

FIGURE 13.4. Transaxial MR images of right lower leg without (*left*) and with (*right*) MT pulse show necrotic masses in the anterior compartments with slight peripheral contrast enhancement. Diffuse mild contrast enhancement is also noted in the anterolat- eral subcutaneous flap muscles as well as soleus muscle. Regions of interest were placed in the enhanced areas, and MT ratios of 22% to 30% suggesting posttreatment changes were generated. No recurrent tumor was found by biopsy.

suppression for MR contrast-enhanced and angiographic sequences and T_2-weighting for gradient echo imaging. It has been suggested that hypercellular diseases such as tumors may produce a large amount of MT to free protons by cell wall protein interactions with free water [22].

Fifty-four patients with pathologically proved tumors underwent MT imaging using a 1.5-T scanner. Overall imaging time was 2min, 10s with and without application of MT pulse. The MT pulse had a duration of 19ms (offset from the resonance frequency of water by 2kHz) and utilized an area of waveform approximately 10 times greater than that of the 90° spin-echo pulse. The technique used a single-cycle sine pulse to induce broad homogeneous suppression. This suppression pulse was applied approximately 1ms before the imaging pulses. The regions of interest (4mm²) for signal intensity measurement were derived at the same site within the tumors. MT ratios, defined as 1 − intensity after suppression/intensity before suppression) were generated. Statistically significant differences were found between MRS of head and neck malignancies (0.381 ± 0.095) and benign lesions (0.255 ± 0.135). MTR of muscle (0.563 ± 0.097) were higher than those of benign or malignant head and neck lesions [23]. Fifteen patients with musculoskeletal tumors were also examined to assess the value of magnetization transfer contrast using spin-echo technique in tumor characterization. Multiplanar gradient-recalled (MPGR) echo sequences were used first without and then with magnetization transfer contrast (MTC) generated by a zero-degree binomial pulse (MTMPGR). The effect of magnetization transfer on individual tissues was determined as a ration of signal intensity (SI) on MTMPGR images (Ms) to signal intensity on MPGR images (Mo). Signal intensity ratios (SIR) and contrast-to-noise ratios (CNR) were calculated using these formulae:

$$SIR = SI_{tumor}/SI_{normal\ tissue}$$

and

$$CNR = (SI\ tumor - SI\ muscle)/standard\ deviation\ of\ background\ noise$$

All tissues had a Ms/Mo ratio less than 1. Tumors showed signal losses intermediate between marrow and muscle. Ms/Mo ratios for benign and malignant tumors did not differ significantly from each other. On MPGR scans without the saturation pulse, tumors showed signal intensities on average 30% greater than those of both muscle and fat and more than four times greater than those of marrow. Addition of MTC to the MPGR sequence increased the mean AIR between tumors and muscle by a factor of 1.2. Contrast between tumors and fat decreased on MTMPGR images by a factor of 0.7 [24]. As three-dimensional gradient-recalled echo imaging of musculoskeletal processes is used with increasing frequency, there may be a role for MTC that would greatly enhance otherwise poor tumor-to-muscle contrast.

References

1. Erlemann R, Reiser MF, Peters PE, et al. Musculoskeletal neoplasms: static and dynamic Gd-DTPA-enhanced MRI. Radiology 1989;171:767–773.
2. Hanna LS, Magill HL, Parham DM, et al. Childhood chondrosarcoma: MRI with Gd-DTPA. Magn Reson Imaging 1990;8:669–672.
3. Yamamura S, Sato K, Sugiura H, et al. Prostaglandin levels of primary bone tumor tissues correlated with peritumoral edema demonstrated by MRI. Cancer (Phila) 1997;79:255–261.
4. Erlemann R, Vassallo R, Bongartz G, et al. Musculoskeletal neoplasms: fast low-angle shot MRI with and without Gd-DTPA. Radiology 1990;17:494–495.
5. Van der Woude HJ, Bloem JL, Verstraete KL, et al. Osteosarcoma and Ewing sarcoma after neoadjuvant chemotherapy: value of dynamic MRI in detecting viable tumor before surgery. AJR 1995;165:593–598.
6. Lang P, Grampp S, Vahlensieck M, et al. Primary bone tumor value of MR angiography for preoperative planning and monitoring response to chemotherapy. AJR 1995;165:135–142.
7. Vanel D, Verstraete KL, Shapeero LG. Primary tumors of the musculoskeletal system. Radiol Clin North Am 1997;35:213–237.
8. Glover GH, Herfkens RJ. Research directions in MR imaging. Radiology 1998;207:289–295.
9. Tsushima Y, Ishizaka H, Matsumoto M. Adrenal masses: differentiation with chemical shift, fast

low-angle shot MRI. Radiology 1993;186:705–709.

10. Bruhn H, Frahm J, Gyngell ML, et al. Noninvasive differentiation of tumors with use of localized H-1 MR spectroscopy in vivo: initial experience in patients with cerebral tumors. Radiology 1989;172:541–548.

11. Grand S, Passaro G, Ziegler A, et al. Necrotic tumor versus brain abscess: importance of amino acids detected at ^{1}H MR spectroscopy—initial results. Radiology 1999;213:785–793.

12. Scheidler J, Hricak H, Vigneron DB, et al. Prostate cancer: localization with three-dimensional proton MR spectroscopic imaging—clinicopathologic study. Radiology 1999;213:473–480.

13. Yu KK, Scheidler J, Hricak H, et al. Prostate cancer: prediction of extracapsular extension with endorectal MRI and 3D proton MR spectroscopic imaging. Radiology 1999;213:481–488.

14. Van der Graaf M, van den Googert HJ. Human prostate: multisection proton MR spectroscopic imaging with a single spin-echo sequence—preliminary experience. Radiology 1999;213:919–925.

15. Negendank W. Studies of human tumors by MRS: a review. NMR Biomed 1992;5:303–324.

16. Cline GW, Magnusson I, Rothman DL, et al. Mechanism of impaired insulin-stimulated muscle glucose metabolism in subjects with insulin-dependent diabetes mellitus. J Clin Invest 1997;99:2219–2224.

17. LeBihan D. Molecular diffusion nuclear magnetic resonance imaging. Magn Reson Q 1991;7:1–30.

18. Kim T, Murakami T, Takahashi S, et al. Diffusion-weighted single-shot echoplanar MRI for liver disease. AJR 1999;173:393–399.

19. Lang P, Wendland MR, Saeed M, et al. Osteogenic sarcoma: noninvasive in vivo assessment of tumor necrosis with diffusion-weighted MRI. Radiology 1998;206:227–235.

20. Shames DM, Kuwatsura R, Vexler V, et al. Measurement of a capillary permeability to macromolecules by dynamic MRI: a quantitative noninvasive technique. Magn Reson Med 1993;29:616–622.

21. Eng J, Ceckler TL, Balaban RS. Quantitative H-1 magnetization transfer imaging in vivo. Magn Res Med 1991;17:304–314.

22. Yeung HN, Aisen AM. Magnetization transfer contrast with periodic pulsed saturation. Radiology 1992;183:209–214.

23. Yousem DM, Montone KT, Sheppard LM, et al. Head and neck neoplasms: magnetization transfer analysis. Radiology 1994;192:703–707.

24. Li KCP, Hopkins KL, Moore SG, et al. Magnetization transfer contrast MRI of musculoskeletal neoplasms. Skeletal Radiol 1995;24:21–25.

14
Targeted Imaging of Lymph Nodes

E. Edmund Kim

Lymphatic tissues are involved in many pathological processes, and the status of lymphatic tissue is especially important for cancer staging [1]. Clinical classification schedules have been developed that assess the local tumor, regional nodes, and metastatic (TNM) predilection sites. Such TNM schemes rely heavily upon imaging.

It is well known that lymphatic tissue is most prevalent in the peripheral layer of the skin, such that a subdermal injection will deliver the tracer to an area rich in lymph vessels. It is also well known that subcutaneous tissue has fewer lymphatic vessels and that direct injection of the diagnostic agent into a tumor will consequently entail the administration of the agent into a high-pressure system. Most lymph nodes are located deep inside fatty tissues and surrounded by a dense capsule that is impermeable to low molecular weight compounds. Therefore, diagnostic agents cannot be delivered to the intranodal compartments via diffusion from surrounding tissues. Mass transfer occurs exclusively through lymph node blood vasculature or lymphatic vessels. The liquid-phase transfer is accompanied by cell trafficking through both lymphatic and blood vessel walls. It has been known that large molecules may extravasate from the blood into the interstitium and thus reach lymph nodes [2]. Afferent lymphatic vessels penetrate the capsule and open into marginal sinuses, which in turn communicate with medullary sinuses and eventually converge into the efferent lymphatic vessel. The cortex of the lymphocytes constituting a lymph node is divided into lobules and contains follicles and germinal centers for B-cell proliferation. Nonlymphoid (accessory) cell types include interdigitating T cells (paracortex) and phagocytic macrophages. Blood vessels of lymph nodes contain specialized endothelial venules in the paracortical area where T- and B lymphocytes extravasate into the intranodal space. Circulating blood delivers fluids and substrates to all tissues, and most of the filtrate reenters the blood capillaries. Particles larger than about 10 nm in diameter cannot easily pass through this barrier [3]. External pathogens such as parasites and internal pathogens such as cancer cells can more easily enter the terminal lymphatics than the blood capillaries. Although endocytosis can transport small (<50 nm) particles into the lymphatic fluid, larger particles must enter through gaps between lymphatic endothelial cells and are more likely to be temporarily restrained within the gap upon partial closure.

Targeted Nuclear Imaging

Computed tomography (CT), magnetic resonance imaging (MRI), and nuclear imaging have been used for evaluating lymph nodes. All three techniques require administration of contrast agents or radiotracers to reliably detect metastases or to differentiate malignant from benign lymphadenopathy. Administration is performed either into the area drained by lymphatic vessel or into the lymphatic vessel itself. CT or MRI relies on the size and shape of the node for detecting cancer metastasis. Normal nodes are uniformly permeated with sinusoids, but pathological enlargement of germinal follicles or anatomical replacement of node by cancer or fat causes a distortion in sinusoidal pattern. Large nodes can be free of cancer whereas normal or small nodes may contain cancer. Lymphagiographic procedures using Ethiodol have become much less common with many adverse effects and limited opacification of certain nodal groups.

Sentinel lymph nodes (SNLs) are the first nodes draining a tumor, and the histological status of the sentinel nodes is predictive of the status of the regional nodes [4]. The sentinel nodes can be identified with blue dye, a radioisotope, or a combination. Technical parameters for sentinel lymph node biopsy are not standardized. Studies differ with respect to labeling agent, volume and site of injection, and interval between injection and surgery. For radioisotope methods, the particular size is important: the particles must be small (<20nm) enough to gain access to the lymphatic vessels but large enough to be trapped in the sentinel nodes. Krag et al. [5] reported that the highest technical success rate was achieved with unfiltered ^{99m}Tc sulfur colloid in breast cancer patients (Figure 14.1). Lymph nodes are not simply mechanical filters, and the filter function of a node is a complex physiological process of trapping, opsonization, and phagocytosis. The principal process ensuring that radiocolloids remain in the node is that of phagocytosis by the macrophages and histiocytes which line the subcapsular sinuses. Tracer in second-tier nodes is readily distinguished from tracer in SLNs because the lymph channels can be seen directly entering the SLNs. When using ^{99m}Tc antimony sulfide colloid, the lymph channels are almost always seen on dynamic imaging in melanoma patients after intradermal injection and are usually seen in breast cancer patients after peritumoral injection [6].

Intradermal or subdermal injections of the tracer over the surface of breast tumors may lead to a hot node in the axilla, but raise the possibility that lymph nodes that do not actually drain the primary tumor site will be removed as SLNs, perhaps leaving true SLNs.

In our 130 breast cancer patients with axillary drainage, 122 (94%) had one SLN, 7 (5%) had two SLNs, and 1 had four SLNs [6], suggesting that some of these hot SLNs were probably second-tier nodes. Drainage to exclusively the axillary node chain was found in 58% of 34 patients with breast cancer, to the axillary and internal mammary node chains in 19.4%, to the axillary, internal mammary, and subclavicular node chains in 13%, to the axillary and infraclavicular node chains in 3.2%, and to the internal mammary node chain in 6.4% [7]. Localized

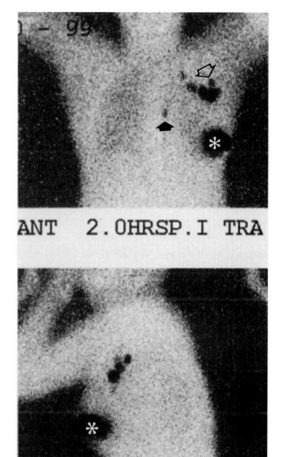

FIGURE 14.1. Anterior (*top*) and left lateral (*bottom*) static images of chest following injection of ^{99m}Tc sulfur colloid around palpable mass in left breast (*) superimposed on transmission images show drainage of radioactivity into the left internal mammary (*closed arrowhead*) and axillary (*open arrowhead*) lymphatic chains.

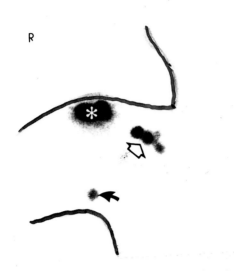
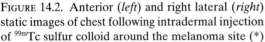
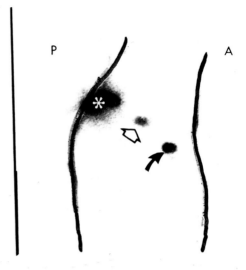

FIGURE 14.2. Anterior (*left*) and right lateral (*right*) static images of chest following intradermal injection of ^{99m}Tc sulfur colloid around the melanoma site (*) show drainage of radioactivity into the right para-clavicular (*open arrowhead*) and axillary (*closed arrow*) lymphatic chains.

breast cancer has a 5-year survival rate of 96%, dropping to 75% with regional spread and to 20% with distant spread. It has been known that axillary lymph node-positive patients are more likely to develop distant metastases and die earlier. Biopsy of the SLN was 98% accurate for the prediction of nodal metastases [8]. Skip metastases are only rarely encountered, and the probability of nonsentinel lymph node involvement is less than 0.1% [9]. Most (65%) melanomas are of the superficial spreading type. For melanomas less than 1.5 mm in thickness and without metastases, survival is greater than 90%; for melanomas greater than 4 mm in thickness, survival drops to 50%. The sentinel lymph node was positive in 30% of patients with a tumor thickness greater than 4 mm and 7% with a tumor thickness between 1.5 and 4 mm [10].

Lymphoscintigraphy (Figure 14.2) is probably the best way to identify basins draining a specific area of the skin, and SLNs could be mapped and identified individually. Nodal metastases from melanoma were orderly progressed, and no skip metastases were documented [11]. Carcino embryonic antigen (CEA)

antibodies labeled with ^{131}I could target and image primary and axillary breast cancers, the latter by lymphoscintigraphy after injection of antibodies into the webs of the fingers [12]. PET using ^{18}F-FDG was useful not only in the detection and staging of breast cancer [13] but also for monitoring preoperative chemotherapy effects with better sensitivity for primary cancer and better specificity for axillary nodal metastasis in comparison with ultrasonography [14]. Nuclear imaging after intravenous injection of ^{111}In poly-L-lysine (polyglucose macrocomplex, PGM) in rats showed brighter hyperplastic abdominopelvic lymph nodes than normal nodes. It is expected that lymphatic metastasis would decrease the uptake as the result of low PGM accumulation [15].

Targeted CT Imaging

Lymph nodes represent a difficult target for systemic drug delivery. Passive targeting of the lymphatic system can be obtained by injecting colloids or nanoparticulates into the interstitial space. The interstitial space is large, about 20%

of body weight, but individual distances between cells are tiny. The interstitial matrix may restrict movement of particles larger than 2 to 3 µm [16]. Small particles would experience a larger distribution space than larger particles, and surface charge as well as particle distensibility should be reflected in the movement of particles. Any potential lymphographic agent must achieve no detectable concentrations within the lymph node, and the detectable amounts depend on the imaging modality with the spatial resolution. Radiopaque emulsions and nanoparticles could target regional lymph nodes in the amounts sufficient for CT following the interstitial administration, and 1 mg of contrast medium per milliliter of node is required for visualization. The partially filled voxels at the edge of the node create an assignment or segmentation problem for quantitative CT. The parameters of mean content, total node content, and node volume are sensitive to the partial volume assignments at the node interface with unenhanced tissues. The maximum value is a good predictor of the contrast gradient that will exist relative to cancers growing within the node and containing no macrophages, but tends to overestimate actual contrast concentration due to the addition of quantum mottle [17]. Unenhanced lymph nodes average 50±3 Hounsfield unit (HU), and the agent that achieves enhancement with a measured mean attenuation of at least 80 HU or a maximum attenuation of at least 120 HU is potentially useful.

Targeted MRI

Magnetic compounds can be used as MRI contrast agents because of their ability to enhance proton relaxation. Colloidal iron oxide particles that generate high magnetic field gradients near their surface have been studied. Because colloids are usually stabilized by hydrophilic polymers, particularly dextran due to its low toxicity and biodegradability [18], one dextran-stabilized colloid was found in the lymph node at 3.6% of injected dose per gram of tissue [19]. Particle surface is the main factor that defines colloid biokinetics, and the accumulation of colloids in lymph nodes correlated with long blood clearance as well as lower amounts of surface-bound blood proteins [20]. It has been suggested that lymphotrophic particles are covered by a flexible dextran brush, which would be the factor responsible for colloid accumulation in lymph nodes (Figures 14.3, 14.4) [21]. Multilabeled graft copolymers of dextran such as polyglucose-associated macrocomplexes (PGM) have been synthesized, and the drug carriers were assembled by conjugation with modified poly-L-lysine, which is the backbone of graft copolymer and carries radioactive, paramagnetic, or fluorescent labels. Polymers were labeled with ^{111}In or gadolinium via transchelation from citrate complexes at pH 5.6 after polylysine amino groups were modified with DTPA and fluorescent dye such as fluorescein or rhodamin.

Biodistribution data in normal rates demonstrated high accumulation of PGM preparations in lymph nodes following intravenous administration. Lymphatic accumulation started in the peripheral nodes and continued to grow in all lymph node groups

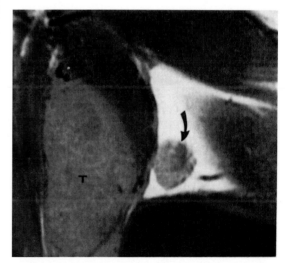

FIGURE 14.3. Sagittal T_1-weighted MR image after intravenous injection of MION (80 µmol Fe/kg) shows that VX2 tumor (T) implanted in the gastrocnemius muscle has metastasized to the regional lymph node, causing enlargement and lack of contrast agent uptake (*arrow*). (Reprinted from Weissleder et al. [21], with permission of *Radiology*.)

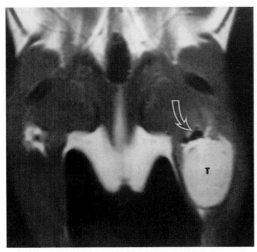 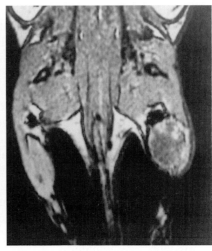

FIGURE 14.4. T_1-weighted spin-echo MR image (*left*) after intravenous injection of MION (80 μmol Fe/kg) shows decreased signal intensity of the left popliteal lymph node (*open arrow*), indicating absence of metastasis. R3230 tumor (T) was implanted in the left thigh of rats. Presence of intranodal iron oxide was confirmed on the coronal gradient-echo image (*right*). No tumor was found at histological study. (Reprinted from Weissleder et al. [21], with permission of *Radiology*.)

when PGM was practically eliminated from the blood. By 24h after injection of 12.7mg/kg, the accumulation was 23.8% ±4.1% of injected dose per gram of tissue in the mesenteric nodes, 12.3% ±3.6% in paraaortic nodes, and 5.9% ± 4.2% in the axillary nodes [15]. PGM recognition by phagocytes appears a complex and tissue-specific process, and the biokinetics of dextran copolymers is based on the macrokinetic balance of extravasation and phagocytosis process. Compared to lymphotropic superparamagnetic colloids, macromolecular paramagnetic agents have the advantage of lower and fewer imaging artifacts and also increased signal-to-noise ratio [22]. PGM labeled with 0.22mmol of gadolinium per gram through DTPA (diethylene triamininepentaacetic acid) moieties bound to the backbone increased Gd relaxivity from 4 to $5\,mM^{-1}s^{-1}$ to 22 to $24\,mM^{-1}s^{-1}$ due to restrictions in rotational reorientation; this allowed the relaxation enhancement in water at a polymer concentration as low as 1mg/l. The iron oxide-based superparamagnetic particles such as AMI-227 and USPIO may decrease the resolution power because of using T_2-weighted pulse sequences [22].

Liposomes as carriers of diagnostic agents have emerged as versatile tools possessing a variety of useful properties. They have been studied as delivery vehicles to the lymphatics. It has been shown that radioactively labeled, small, negatively charged liposomes are the most efficient in targeting rat regional lymph nodes after subcutaneous administration [23]. The optimal diameter of liposomes that localize in the lymph nodes after peritoneal administration in rats is approximately 200 nm [24]. Low molecular weight Gd-DTPA complexes were the first to be incorporated inside the liposomal internal aqueous compartment. They may leak from liposomes on contact with body fluids or components. Therefore, there was a creation of membranotropic chelating agents such as DTPA-stearylamine (SA) or phosphatidylethanolamine (PE), and amphiphilic acylated paramagnetic complexes of Mn and Gd [25]. Liposome surface modification with different polymers has been used to modify the in vivo properties of the vesicles. Modification with polyethylene glycol (PEG) is known to prolong the circulation times of the vesicles. PEG-coated Gd-containing vesicles produce the MR signal increase in both lymph nodes quickly and effectively (node-to-muscle ratio reaches 2.5 in 5–10 min). The main obstacles hindering the clinical use of liposome-based MR contrast agents are their toxicity and increased cost.

Conclusion

In nearly all cancer staging systems, the status of the lymph node strongly influences the clinical classification to assess prognosis and select therapy. Optimal localization of sentinel node requires lymphoscintigraphy and radiosensitive probes.

High-resolution CT or MRI has adequate spatial resolution to identify macroscopic disease in lymph nodes, and is able to detect particulate imaging agents that are directed into the terminal lymphatics. The size, shape, fluidity, charge, and coating of such colloids, emulsions, or nanoparticulate suspensions influence dose and temporal responses. Lymph nodes are a good target for visualization using particulate contrast agents because of the ability to concentrate the agent, thus enhancing the MR signal. Macromolecular drug carriers accumulate in lymph nodes after systemic administration and are able to deliver a variety of diagnostic agents to lymph nodes and allow lymph node nuclear and MR imaging. Liposomes possess certain unique features that make them good carriers of covalently attached chelated paramagnetic ions.

References

1. Berek JS, Hacker NF, Fu YS. Adenocarcinoma of the uterine cervix: histologic variables associated with lymph node metastasis and survival. Obstet Gynecol 1985;65:46–51.
2. Mayerson HS, Wolfram CG, Shirley HH, Wasserman K. Regional differences in capillary permeability. Am J Physiol 1960;198:155–160.
3. Seymour LW, Duncan R, Stahalm J, Kopecek J. Effect of molecular weight of N-(2-hydroxypropyl)methacrylamide copolymers on body distribution and rate of excretion after subcutaneous, intraperitoneal and intravenous administration to rats. J Biomed Mater Res 1987;21:1341–1346.
4. Krag DN, Weaver DL, Alex JC, Fairbank JT. Surgical resection and radiolocalization of the sentinel lymph node in breast cancer using a gamma probe. Surg Oncol 1993;2:335–340.
5. Krag DN, Ashikaga T, Harlow SP, Weaver DL. Development of sentinel node targeting technique in breast cancer patients. Breast J 1998;4:67–74.
6. Uren RF, Thompson JF, Howman-Giles R, Roberts JM. Sentinel lymph node detection and imaging. Eur J Nucl Med 1999;28:936–939.
7. Uren RF, Howman-Giles RB, Thompson JF, et al. Mammary lymphoscintigraphy in breast cancer. J Nucl Med 1995;36:1775–1780.
8. Borgstein PJ. SLN biopsy in breast cancer: guidelines and pitfalls of lymphoscintigraphy and gamma probe detection. J Am Coll Surg 1998;186:275–283.
9. Turner RR, Ollila DW, Krasne DL, Giuliano AE. Histopathological validation of the sentinel lymph node hypothesis for breast carcinoma. Ann Surg 1997;226:271–278.
10. Joseph E, Brobeil A, Glass F, et al. Results of complete lymph node dissection in 83 melanoma patients with positive SLN. Ann Surg Oncol 1998;5:119–125.
11. Reintgen D, Cruse CW, Wells K, et al. The orderly progression of melanoma nodal metastases. Ann Surg 1994;220:759–767.
12. DeLand F, Kim EE, Corgan R. Axillary lymphoscintigraphy in radioimmunodetection of carcinoembryonic antigen in breast cancer. J Nucl Med 1979;20:1243–1250.
13. Nieweg OE, Kim EE, Wong WH, Broussard WF. Positron emission tomography with F-18 deoxyglucose in the detection and staging of breast cancer. Cancer (Phila) 1993;71:3920–3925.
14. Bassa P, Kim EE, Inoue T, et al. Evauation of preoperative chemotherapy using PET with F-18 fluorodeoxyglucose in breast cancer. J Nucl Med 1996;37:931–938.
15. Papisov MI, Weissleder R, Bogdanor AA, Brady TJ. Intravenous lymph node-targeted carriers. In: Proceedings of International Symposium on Controlled Release of Bioactive Materials. Deerfield, IL: Controlled Release Society, 1994: 152–160.
16. Hirano K, Yamada H. Studies on the absorption of practically water-soluble drugs following injection. J Pharm Sci 1982;66:517–522.
17. Barnes JE. Characteristics and control of contrast in CT. Radiographics 1992;12:825–839.
18. Shen T, Weissleder R, Papisov MI, Bogdanov AA, Brady TJ. Monocrystalline iron oxide

nanocompounds (MION). J Magn Reson Imaging 1993;29:599–604.

19. Weissleder R, Stark DD, Engelstad BL, et al. Superparamagnetic iron oxide: pharmacokinetics and toxicity. Am J Radiol 1989;152:167–192.

20. Papisov MI, Savelyer VY, Sergienko VB, Torchilin VP. Magnetic drug targeting. In vivo kinetics of radiolabeled magnetic drug carriers. Int J Pharm 1987;40:201–205.

21. Weissleder R, Heautot JF, Schaeffer BK, Bogdanov A, Papisov M, Brady TJ. A high efficiency lymphotrophic agent for MR lymphography. Radiology 1994;191:225–230.

22. Tanoura T, Bernas M, Darkazanli A, et al. MR lymphography with iron oxide compound AMI-227. Am J Radiol 1992;159:875–881.

23. Patel H, Boodle C, Vaughan-Jones R. Assessment of the poteential uses of liposomes for lymphoscintigraphy and lymphatic drug delivery. Biochem Biophys Acta 1984;801:76–80.

24. Hirano K, Hunt A. Lymphatic transport of liposome-encapsulated agents. J Pharm Sci 1985;74:915–919.

25. Grant C, Karlik S, Florio E. A liposomal MRI contrast agent: phosphatidylethanolamine-DTPA. Magn Reson Med 1989;11:236–241.

15
Computed Tomography and Ultrasound Contrast Agents

E. Edmund Kim

Computed Tomography Contrast Agents

Contrast agent-assisted imaging of vasculature is widely employed during the diagnosis of many vascular and neoplastic diseases [1]. Conventional X-ray contrast media are ionic or neutral low molecular weight iodine-containing organic molecules and are able to delineate the vascular bed for a limited time following rapid extravasation into the interstitial space. Such a rapid disappearance of contrast material from the blood narrows the examination time window down to several minutes for the majority of diagnostic applications. Peak enhancement of the aorta takes place 10 to 20 s after the beginning of the injection. Within 2 min, the signal from the blood pool drops approximately fivefold [2].

Computed tomography (CT) has the best combination of spatial and temporal resolution of all tomographic modalities. There is a linear relationship between attenuation and electron density. CT is 10 times more sensitive to attenuation differences than film, and CT has good inherent contrast. CT is also a low-noise imaging modality. At the energies utilized for CT, attenuation is expected to depend on the number of electrons per unit mass (electrons/gram), which is approximately NZ/A density, where N is Avogadro's number, Z is the atomic number, and A is the atomic mass. The CT number is given as a Hounsfield unit (HU). As with air, fat, and bone, the imageability of X-ray contrast agents is attributable to their density. Barium sulfate used for gastrointestinal studies has a density greater than 4; water-soluble iodinated benzoic acid is greater than 1.4; and neat perflubron is greater than 1.8. This relative density must be retained or reestablished for imaging efficacy. Contrast enhancement refers to the administration of intravenous iodinated contrast medium to improve the detection of pathology or anatomical detail. Many pathological processes in the brain disrupt the blood–brain barrier and permit the leakage of iodinated contrast medium into the brain. This leakage appears on CT as a region of increased density. As intravenous iodinated contrast medium increases the density of circulating blood, the vascular structures increase in density (Figure 15.1).

Optimal rates of contrast medium administration for contrast enhancement depend on whether vessels or an abnormal blood–brain barrier is to be enhanced (Figure 15.2). High plasma iodine concentrations are achieved by injecting the intravenous iodine rapidly and then scanning as soon as the intravascular contrast medium equilibrates with the extravascular space (exclusive of the brain), within about 10 min. Once equilibrium has taken place, the contrast medium removed from the vascular circulation by renal filtration can be replaced by a slow intravenous infusion. About 30 to 40 g iodine is needed to enhance vascular structures, and one-half of a solution containing 42 g iodine is rapidly infused in a peripheral vein before scanning and the remainder during

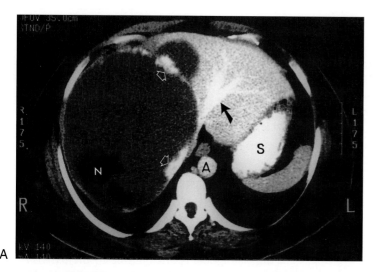

A

FIGURE 15.1. (**A**) Transaxial CT image of the liver following the oral and intravenous administration of iodine contrast agent shows a large lobulated hemangioma occupying the right hepatic lobe with a puddling (*open arrows*) of contrast agent in cavernous network along the anterior and medial margins. Note irregular nonenhanced necrosis (*N*) in the posterior portion of the hemangioma and also delineation of left hepatic veins (*arrow*). *S*, stomach; *A*, aorta. (**B**) Selected axial (SPECT) images of upper abdomen using 99^m Tc RBCs show a giant hemangioma taking labeled RBCs at 1.5h following the injection of radionuclide. Note a photon-deficient necrotic portion (*arrow*).

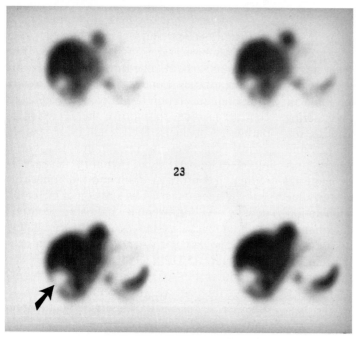

B

scanning. The additional dose of contrast medium, the so-called double dose technique, has a greater risk of renal damage than the conventional technique. Greater enhancement and more specific identification of arteries or veins may be achieved by dynamic scanning, which is a series of scans in rapid sequence after bolus injection of a contrast medium. It would be much more advantageous to diagnostic imaging to use a safe contrast medium that would stay in circulation longer but could be rapidly ex-

creted from the body after completion of the procedure. Organic iodine should be delivered to the target organ within a given time frame and excreted from the body after completion of a diagnostic procedure. Contrast medium has a small but predictable risk of mortality (1 in 40,000) and of serious morbidity (1 in 14,000). The risk is increased with renal failure and allergic conditions [3]. The major contraindication to contrast medium is a history of allergic reaction to iodine or contrast medium.

FIGURE 15.2. Transaxial CT image of the upper chest shows contrast-enhanced aortic arch (A) during the venous phase and also large malignant fibrous histiocytoma along the right chest wall with peripheral contrast enhancement and central necrosis (N).

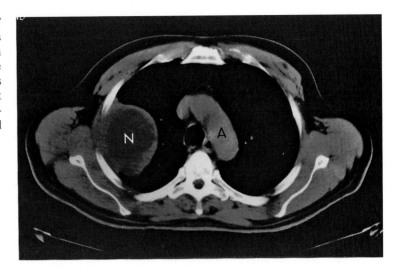

Rapid extravasation of CT contrast media negatively influences other areas of diagnostic imaging where precise delineation of the vascular bed is required. Some potential problems with enhanced extravasation appear during the measurement of abdominal organ perfusion. Potentially less leaky nonionic media are better for the determination of the functional parameters than highly diffusible ionic agents [4]. Macromolecular and particulate contrast media circulate for a long time and have been developed for nuclear and magnetic resonance imaging. To design water-soluble macromolecular blood-pool CT contrast agents, some iodine-containing polymers have been synthesized. Perfluoroctyl bromide (PFOB) and triiodobenzoyl carboxymethyldextran have been evaluated [5,6].

Ultrasound Contrast Agents

Ultrasonography is the most widely used imaging modality because of its low cost, availability, and safety. There are fundamental limitations in diagnosing diseases (Figure 15.3) that have acoustic properties similar to those of normal surrounding tissue as well as in the Doppler assessment of low-velocity blood flows and low-volume flow rates. Ultrasound technology continues to evolve, and new imaging algorithms are in development. Ultrasound

images are not as pictorial as CT or MRI and rely heavily on technical skills and mental integration of multiple images for accurate diagnosis. An excellent ultrasound contrast agent would benefit patient care and could be widely used. Ultrasound agents have been slow to

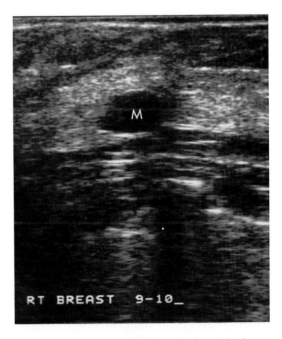

FIGURE 15.3. Ultrasonography of the right breast shows a fairly well-defined hypoechoic mass (M) measuring 1×1.5 cm, which was identified as an adenocarcinoma by biopsy.

develop, and the mechanisms of enhancement depend on the imaging algorithm, backscatter, attenuation, and sound speed [7]. The ideal ultrasound contrast agent should be safe, stable in the vascular system to survive capillary (about 5 μm) circulation, and be capable of modifying the acoustic properties of the interesting tissues.

Current contrast agents including microbubbles are well recognized to be the most effective backscatters. Microbubbles measure 2 to 8 μm in diameter and contain air or perfluorocarbon gas that has prolonged longevity because of its lower solubility. Stability of the microbubbles is provided in the shell made of denatured albumin, lipid or surfactant layers, or polybutylcyanoacrylate. Microbubbles have been shown to be highly effective in enhancing spectral/color/power Doppler signals, lasting up to 7 min following an intravenous bolus injection and up to 15 to 20 min after an infusion. Physiological embedding media such as albumin and galactose have very short blood persistence times of tens of seconds. This time is too brief for active targeting. Due to their large size, ultrasound contrast agents are mainly restricted to the blood pool, and are not too large for phagocytosis. Levovist (Schering AG), primarily designed as a blood-pool agent, has been shown to have a delayed liver-specific phase. SHU 563A (Schering AG) and NAI Investigational Drug (Nycomed Amersham) are selectively taken up by the Kupffer cells of the reticuloendothelial system after the vascular phase (5–10 min).

Numerous clinical studies have confirmed the usefulness of various blood-pool ultrasound contrast agents to improve diagnostic confidence. The contrast agents converted a previously suboptimal, nondiagnostic examination into a diagnostic one, thereby deferring referral to more costly or invasive procedures. The field of hepatic oncology is the model test platform where the application of these agents remains the most challenging and yet the most promising. Any success in this field could easily be extended to other systems.

Differential diagnosis of small hepatic tumors is important, but is not always possible, even with angiography. Sonographic angiography (sonography performed during intraarterial infusion of carbon dioxide microbubbles) was useful in the differential diagnosis of 222 hepatic tumors by depicting characteristic vascular features that reflect the vascular anatomy of specific types of hepatic tumors [8]. It detected a hypervascular pattern with peripheral blood supply in cases of hepatocellular carcinoma (90% sensitivity and 89% specificity). Typical vascular patterns of adenomatous hyperplasia, hemangioma, metastasis, and focal nodular hyperplasia were hypovascular (100% sensitivity and 91% specificity), spotty pooling (100% sensitivity and 100% specificity), peripherally hypervascular (64% sensitivity and 100% specificity), and centrally hypervascular (100% sensitivity and 100% specificity) on sonographic angiography, respectively. The detectability of hypervascularity was greater with sonographic angiography than with conventional angiography in hepatocellular carcinoma, metastasis, and hemangioma. The carbon dioxide microbubbles were prepared by vigorously mixing 10 ml of carbon dioxide, 10 ml of heparinized normal saline, and 5 ml of the patient's own blood. The results obtained by other studies made the diagnostic hypotheses for some of the ultrasound-angiographic patterns as follows [9]:

1. Hypervascular lesion with complete and centripetal filling in the early phase: hepatocellular carcinoma.
2. Hypervascular lesions with complete and centrifugal filling in the early phase: focal nodular hyperplasia (Figure 15.4).
3. Lesion vascularized only in the periphery (in early phase) with progressive and very persistent filling in the delayed phase: hemangioma.
4. Lesion vascularized in the periphery, with persistence of the contrast agent only in the periphery during the delayed phase: possible metastasis.
5. Iso- or hypovascular lesion whose direction of filling cannot clearly be defined as centripetal or centrifugal: regenerative nodule.

The early detection of hepatic metastases in patients with gastric carcinoma is important for

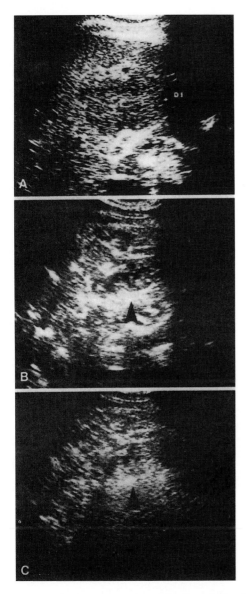

FIGURE 15.4. Ultrasonography of the liver following the injection of mixture of 10 ml CO_2, 10 ml saline, and 5 ml patient's own blood shows a typical central supply of CO_2 microbubbles that distributes them rapidly in a centrifugal direction to focal nodular hyperplasia (**A**). *Arrowheads* point to the center of lesion (**B,C**). (Reprinted from Veltri et al. [9], with permission of Springer-Verlag.)

determining the appropriate therapy. However, conventional imaging techniques are limited for detecting occult hepatic metastases. It has been known that the presence of even micro-

metastases is associated with changes in hepatic blood flow. Duplex/color Doppler ultrasonography has shown that measurement of the Doppler perfusion index (DPI), the ratio of hepatic arterial to total hepatic blood flow, can identify colorectal and gastric cancer patients with occult hepatic metastases [10]. Levovist-enhanced power Doppler imaging was developed to determine the same hepatic arterial contribution to total hepatic blood flow in an attempt to identify patients with hepatic metastases. The power Doppler signal intensity (PDSI) versus time curves for the hepatic artery and portal vein were obtained following quantification of the PDSI changes in each vessel, and the hepatic arterial contribution to total hepatic blood flow was calculated as the contrast-enhanced Doppler perfusion index (CEDPI). Significant increase of the CEDPI was found in patients with hepatic metastases. The transit time required for Levovist to arrive in the hepatic veins following the intravenous bolus injection was significantly reduced in patients with metastases when compared with controls.

References

1. Curtin JJ, Mewissen MW, Crain MR, Lipchik RJ. Postcontrast CT in the diagnosis and assessment of response to thrombolysis in massive pulmonary embolism. J Comput Assist Tomogr 1994;18:133–137.
2. Canty JM Jr, Judd RM, Brody AS, Klocke FJ. First-pass entry of nonionic contrast agent into the myocardial extravascular space: effects on radiographic estimates of transit time and blood volume. Circulation 1991;84:2071–2075.
3. Daniels DL, Haughton VM, Williams AL. Computed tomography of the jugular foramen. AJNR 1983;4:1227–1232.
4. Blomley MJK, Coulden R, Bufkin C, et al. Contrast bolus dynamic computed tomography for the measurement of solid organ perfusion. Invest Radiol 1993;28:S72.
5. Mattrey RF. Perfluorocytlbromide: a new contrast agent for CT, sonography and MRI. AJR 1989;152:247–251.
6. Doucet D, Meyer D, Chambon C, Bonnemain B. Blood-pool X-ray contrast agents: evalua-

tion of a new polymer. Invest Radiol 1991;26: S53.

7. Ophir J, Parker KJ. Contrast agents in diagnostic ultrasound. Ultrasound Med Biol 1989;15:319–327.

8. Kudo M, Tomita S, Tochio H, et al. Sonography with intra-arterial infusion of carbon dioxide microbubbles: value in differential diagnosis of hepatic tumors. AJR 1992;158:65–74.

9. Veltri A, Capello S, Faissola B, et al. Dynamic contrast-enhanced ultrasound with carbon dioxide microbubbles as adjunct to arteriography of liver tumors. Cardiovasc Intervent Radiol 1994;17:133–137.

10. Leen E, Anderson JR, Robertson J, et al. Perfusion in the detection of hepatic metastases secondary to gastric carcinoma. Am J Surg 1997;173:99–102.

16
Imaging of Anticancer Drugs for Therapeutic Response and Prognosis

David J. Yang, Chun Li, and E. Edmund Kim

To diagnose cancer, mammography is usually performed in patients with breast cancer; however, the detection rate is low among younger women because of their denser breast tissue. Computed tomography (CT), magnetic resonance imaging (MRI), and ultrasound provide anatomical information but not functional information about cancer. These imaging modalities also are not helpful in assessing or predicting therapeutic response. Thus, to develop an imaging technique to predict the responsiveness of tumors to chemotherapy for individual patients would be most helpful. Drug targeting through a receptor or enzymatic-mediated process is an effective way of cell-selective drug delivery because this process allows a satisfactory transport rate as well as ligand-dependent cell specificity.

Several reports have shown the possibility of using a labeled drug to select the patients who may benefit from such a drug therapy. For instance, ^{111}In-diethylene triaminepentraacetic acid (DTPA) octreotide, a somatostatin receptor antagonist, could provide useful information in the selection of patients who might benefit from treatment with octreotide [1–4]. The use of tumor hypoxia marker has been shown to be possible for predicting radiation resistance in individual tumors [5]. ^{99m}Tc-infecton, an antibiotic, is a useful marker in the differentiation of bacterial infection from inflammation. Consequently, the patients with bacterial infection respond well to infecton [6–8]. ^{111}In-Bleomycin targets head and neck cancer and identifies metastatic spread. It could

possibly be applied, using higher activities, for adjuvant Auger electron therapy of cancer [9–12]. In our laboratory, we developed DTPA–drug conjugates. Four ligands (adriamycin, methotrexate, paclitaxel, and tamoxifen) were selected for evaluation.

Imaging Adriamycin

Adriamycin (Doxorubicin, Rubex), a potent topoisomerase II inhibitor, has been widely used to treat breast, ovarian, leukemia, and lymphoma as well as other forms of cancer. The standard dose of adriamycin in cancer therapy is 60 to $75 \, mg/m^2$ every 21 days as a cycle [13,14]. The major side effect of adriamycin is cardiotoxicity. The patient with breast cancer undergoes four to six cycles of therapy. The treatment is expensive. If the binding of adriamycin to tumors can be detected with scintigraphy, then such a labeled adriamycin may predict the response of adriamycin therapy for breast cancer. Additionally, such a radiotracer may provide early diagnosis of cardiotoxicity induced by adriamycin.

Synthesis of ^{111}In-DTPA-Adriamycin (DTPA-ADR)

DTPA-ADR was synthesized by reacting the free base of adriamycin (100mg, 0.17mmol) with DTPA anhydride (62mg, 0.17mmol) in dimethylformaide (10ml) in the presence of dicyclohexyl carbodiimidazole (70mg, 0.34

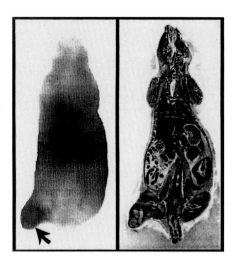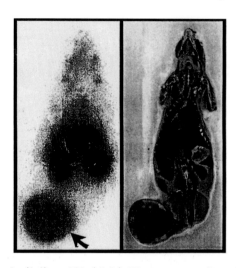

FIGURE 16.1. Autoradiographs of breast tumor-bearing rats with ^{111}In-DTPA-adriamycin (300 μCi/rat, i.v.) show the tumors (arrows) visualized from 30 min (*left*) to 48 h (*right*). The corresponding photos are next to the autoradiograms.

mmol). After dialysis (M.W. cutoff at 500), the product was lyophilized, yielded 70 mg (40%–50%). The structure was confirmed by mass spectrometry and proton NMR. The DTPA–ADR conjugate (5 mg), dissolved in 1 ml of water, was then added with [111]InCl$_3$ (0.7 mCi; NEN Dupont, Boston, MA, USA), sodium acetate (0.6 N, 20 μl) and sodium citrate (0.06 N, 20 μl). The mixture stood for 30 min. ^{111}In-DTPA-ADR reconstituted in saline was given to rats. Radiochemical purity was greater than 99% (10% ammonium formate in water/MeOH/0.2 M citric acid; 2:2:1, Rf=0.5; Bioscan, Washington, DC, USA).

Autoradiographic and Scintigraphic Studies

Female breast tumor-bearing rats (n=3) were killed at 30 min & 48 h after receiving ^{111}In-DTPA-ADR (300 μCi/rat, i.v.). Each body was fixed in carboxymethyl cellulose (4%). The frozen body was mounted onto a cryostat (LKB 2250 cryomicrotome) and cut into 40-μm coronal sections. Each section was thawed and mounted on a slide. The slide was then placed in contact with X-ray film (X-Omat AR; Kodak, Rochester, NY, USA) and exposed for 48 h.

Five breast tumor-bearing rats were administered 300 μCi of ^{111}In-DTPA-ADR, and whole-body planar images were obtained at 30 min to 48 h; 300,000 counts were acquired in a 128×128 matrix. In vivo autoradiographic (Figure 16.1) and planar imaging (Figure 16.2) studies in breast tumor-bearing rats indicated that the tumor could be visualized well at the time intervals studied. However, ^{111}In-DTPA showed little tumor uptake.

Imaging Methotrexate

Folic acid, an essential vitamin, enters into cells through a membrane-associated folate-binding protein (glycosylphosphatidylinositol-linked membrane folate-binding protein) in addition to classical high-affinity/low-capacity carrier system [15–17]. Folate-binding protein (FBP) is overexpressed by a number of neoplastic cell types (e.g., pulmonary, breast, ovarian, cervical, colorectal, nasopharyngeal, and renal adenocarcinomas, and ependymomas), but primarily expressed only in several normal differentiated tissues (e.g., choroid plexus, placenta, thyroid, and kidney) [16,18–23]. Low molecular weight folate–chelate conjugates, such as ^{67}Ga-deferoxamine-

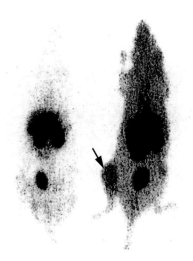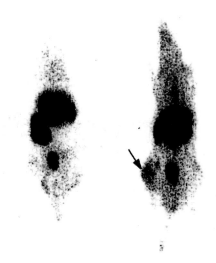

FIGURE 16.2. Whole-body images of breast tumor-bearing rats receiving ^{111}In-DTPA-adriamycin (300 µCi, i.v.) show the tumor uptake (*arrows*) at 30 min (*left*) and 48 h (*right*). Tumor has less uptake with ^{111}In-DTPA (rat at the *left* within the same panel).

folate and ^{111}In-DTPA-folate, have been used for diagnostic imaging of folate receptor-positive tumors [24–28]. Results of limited in vitro and in vivo studies with these agents suggest that folate receptors could be a potential target for tumor imaging.

It is known that membrane folic acid receptors are responsible for cellular accumulation of folate and folate analogs, such as methotrexate (MTX), and overexpressed on various tumor cells [29,30]. Cellular uptake of MTX has been shown to occur by an active process that is pH-, temperature-, and time-dependent. Evidence shows that MTX enters into cells by using both reduced folate carrier and FBP [15,22,31–35]. In vitro studies conducted with special cell lines that have only one type of folate receptor demonstrated that MTX influx by folate receptors shows different transport rates at different pH levels and that both receptors respond in a different way to the presence of folic acid [34–39]. Moreover, it has been suggested that there could be another MTX influx route distinct from the reduced folate carrier or the FBP [34].

MTX is an important chemotherapeutic agent for the treatment of variety of malignancies including breast cancer, non-Hodgkin lymphoma, osteogenic sarcoma, and choriocar-

cinoma [29,30]. It is known that MTX (4-amino, 4-deoxy, *N*-10-methyl pteroylglutamic acid) in vivo competes with folic acid for transport systems and target enzyme binding [15,22,31–35]. Hence, labeled MTX could be a potential tumor imaging agent for tumors overexpressing FBP.

Synthesis of DTPA-MTX

MTX-NH$_2$ (190 mg, 0.38 mmol) was dissolved in water (10 ml). The pH value was adjusted to 8 using NaOH (2 N). To this stirred solution, DTPA anhydride (700 mg, 1.96 mmol) was added slowly, and the pH value was maintained at 8 by adding NaOH (2 N). The mixture was completely dissolved and the color turned to a clear yellow. The mixture was stirred at room temperature for 48 h and dialyzed using a Spectra/POR molecularporous membrane with molecular cutoff at 500. After dialysis, the product was dried by lyophilizer. The product weighed 284 mg (85%); m.p., 152°–153°C (dec); ^{1}H-NMR (D$_2$O) δ 2.83–3.35 (m, 27H, -(CH$_2$)$_2$-DTPA and glutamate of MTX), 4.20–4.57 (m, 6H, -CH$_2$-pteridinyl, aromatic-NCH$_3$, NH-CH-COOH glutamate), 6.68–6.70 (d, 2H, aromatic-CO), 7.54–7.56 (d, 2H. aromatic-N), 8.40 (s, 1H, pteridinyl); FAB MS m/z calculated for

$C_{36}H_{45}N_{13}O_{13}$ $Na_4(M)^+$ 959.47, 871.9 (free), found 959.684, 870.575 (free).

A simple, fast, and high-yield aminoethyl-amido and DTPA analogues of MTX were developed. The structures of these analogues were confirmed by NMR and mass spectroscopic analysis. Radiosynthesis of DTPA-MTX with $^{111}InCl_3$ was achieved with 100% radiochemical purity. ^{111}In-DTPA-MTX was found to be stable at 0.5, 2, 24, and 48 h in dog serum samples. No degradation products were observed.

Radiolabeling of DTPA-MTX with $^{111}InCl_3$

DTPA-MTX (400–500 μg) was dissolved in water (0.1 ml). Sodium acetate (0.6 N, 20 μl) and sodium citrate (0.06 N, 20 μl) were added. Radiosynthesis of ^{111}In-DTPA-MTX was achieved by adding $^{111}InCl_3$ (37–128 MBq) into this vial. Radiochemical purity was determined by TLC (Fisher Scientific, Houston, Texas, USA) on ^{18}C-reversed-phase plates eluted with methanol. From radio-TLC (Bioscan, Washington, DC, USA) analysis, the radiochemical purity was 100%. The Rf values were 0.1 and 0.8 for $^{111}InCl_3$ and ^{111}In-DTPA-MTX, respectively.

Stability Assay of ^{111}In-DTPA-MTX

The stability of labeled ^{111}In-DTPA-MTX was tested in serum samples. Briefly, 740 KBq of 1 mg ^{111}In-DTPA-MTX was incubated in dog serum (200 μl) at 37°C for 48 h. The serum sample was diluted with 50% methanol in water, and radio-TLC was repeated at 0.5, 2, 24, and 48 h as described.

Tissue Distribution Studies

Female Fischer-344 rats (150±25 g) (Harlan Sprague-Dawley, Indianapolis, IN, USA) were inoculated subcutaneously with 0.1 ml of mammary tumor cells from the 13762 tumor cell line suspension (10^6 cells/rat, a tumor cell line specific to Fischer rats) into the hind legs using 25-gauge needles. Studies performed 14 to 17 days after implantation when tumors reached

approximately 1 to 2.5 cm in diameter. In tissue distribution studies, each animal was injected intravenously with 370 to 550 KBq of ^{111}In-DTPA-MTX or ^{111}In-DTPA (12 rats/group, 3 rats/time interval); the injected mass of ^{111}In-DTPA-MTX was 10 μg per rat. At 0.5, 2, 24, or 48 h following administration of the radiopharmaceuticals, the anesthetized animals were killed and the tumor and selected tissues excised, weighed, and counted for radioactivity by a gamma counter. The biodistribution of tracer in each sample was calculated as a percentage of the injected dose per gram of tissue wet weight (%ID/g). Student's t-test was used to assess the significance of differences between two groups.

In a separate experiment, blocking studies were performed to determine the receptor-mediated process. In blocking studies, ^{111}In-DTPA-MTX was coadministered (i.v.) with varying blocking doses of folic acid (0.0, 32, 320, or 500 μmol/kg) to tumor-bearing rats ($n=3$/group). Animals were killed 2 h post injection, and data were collected as previously described.

Biodistribution studies showed that tumor/blood count density ratios at 0.5 to 48 h gradually increased for ^{111}In-DTPA-MTX, whereas these values decreased for ^{111}In-DTPA in the same time period (Figure 16.3). In blocking studies, tumor/muscle and tumor/blood count density ratios were significantly decreased ($p < 0.05$) with high doses of folic acid coadministration (320 and 500 μmol/kg) (Figure 16.4).

Scintigraphic Studies

Preliminary clinical studies were performed in patients with bone metastasis and lung cancer. To each patient was administered ^{111}In-DTPA-MTX (2 mCi/patient, i.v.), and planar images were collected at 4 h post injection. Informed consent was obtained from each patient.

Scintigraphic ^{111}In-DTPA-MTX images showed that the bone metastasis lesion could be imaged (Figure 16.5). Bone scan confirmed the findings (Figure 16.6). In a patient with small-cell lung cancer, the tumor could be imaged by ^{111}In-DTPA-MTX (Figure 16.7).

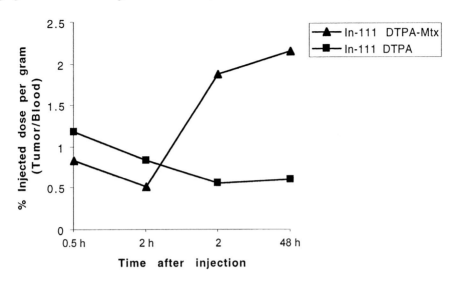

FIGURE 16.3. Time-dependent variation of tumor/blood activity ratios (%ID/g wet weight) with ^{111}In-DTPA-MTX versus ^{111}In-DTPA ($n=3$/time point).

Imaging Paclitaxel

Tubulin is the principal protein subunit of microtubules. Microtubules assemble when they are required by a cell for a particular function and depolymerize when they are no longer needed; therefore, it is the cellular target for antimitotic agents. The agents, such as vincristine, vinblastine, rhizoxin, maytansine, and podophyllotoxins, interact with tubulin on the colchicine-binding sites, inhibit tubulin polymerization, and cause cell arrest at metaphase. However, paclitaxel, another antitubulin agent, has a different mechanism, it promotes the

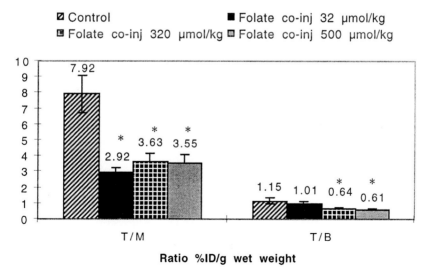

FIGURE 16.4. Tumor/muscle (T/M) and tumor/blood (T/B) activity ratios (%ID/g wet weight) with ^{111}In-DTPA-MTX significantly decreased ($*, p < 0.05$) with different doses of coinjected ($n=3$/group) cold folate.

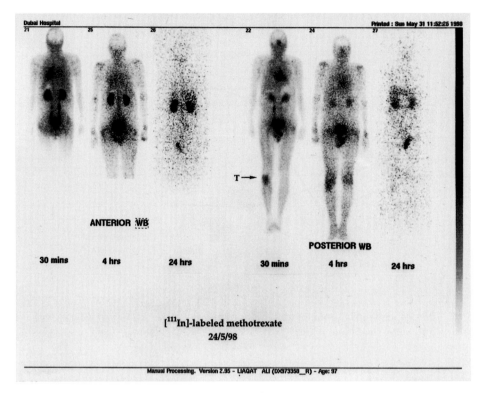

FIGURE 16.5. The tumor in the right proximal tibia (T) was well visualized with ^{111}In-DTPA-MTX in a patient at 0.5 to 4 h postinjection. Note also some focal increased activity in the left proximal femur.

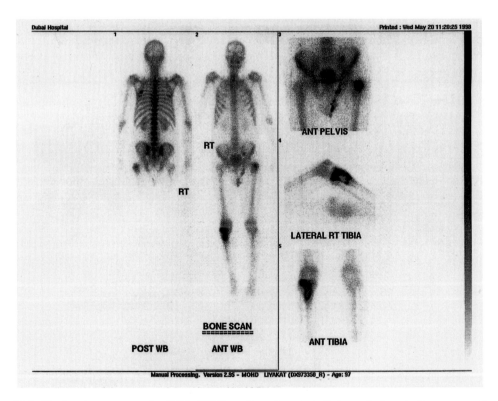

FIGURE 16.6. Nuclear bone scan using ^{99m}Tc-HDP confirmed metastatic bony lesions in the same patient.

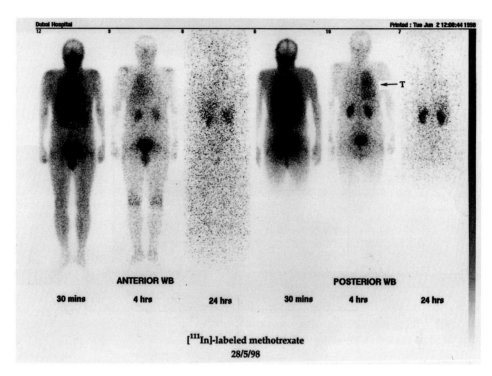

FIGURE 16.7. Small-cell lung carcinoma (T) tumor was well visualized with ^{111}In-DTPA-MTX in patient at 4 h post injection.

assembly of microtubules, resulting in highly stable, nonfunctional polymers that lead to mitotic arrest of proliferating cells [40–44]. The drug also induces apoptotic cell death in vitro and in vivo. [^{14}C]-Labeled and fluorescent-tagged paclitaxel derivatives were synthesized as new biological probes [45,46]; however, they are not suitable for human studies. Thus, ^{111}In-DTPA-paclitaxel was developed. To determine whether scintigraphy with ^{111}In-DTPA-paclitaxel could predict the response to chemotherapy with paclitaxel, four tumor models were selected for evaluation.

Ovarian carcinoma (OCA-1), mammary carcinoma (MCA-4), fibrosarcoma (FSA), and squamous cell carcinoma (SCC-VII) were inoculated into the thighs of female C3Hf/Kam mice. Mice bearing 8-mm tumors were treated with paclitaxel (40 mg/kg). The growth delay, which was defined as the time in days for tumors in the treated groups to grow from 8 to 12 mm in diameter minus the time in days for tumors in the untreated control group to reach

the same size, was measured to determine the effect of paclitaxel on the tumors. Sequential scintigraphy in mice bearing 10- to 14-mm tumors was conducted at 5, 30, 60, 120, 240 min, and 24 h post injection of ^{111}In-DTPA-paclitaxel (3.7 MBq) or ^{111}In-DTPA as a control tracer. The tumor uptakes (% injection dose/pixel) were determined.

^{111}In-DTPA-paclitaxel showed steady uptake from 0.5 to 24 h whereas ^{111}In-DTPA had less uptake (Figure 16.8). The growth delay of OCA-1, MCA-4, FSA, and SCC-VII tumors was 13.6, 4.0, −0.02, and −0.28 days, respectively. Both OCA-1 and MCA-4 were paclitaxel-sensitive tumors, whereas FSA and SCC-VII were paclitaxel-resistant tumors. The tumor uptakes at 24 h post injection of ^{111}In-DTPA-paclitaxel of OCA-1, MCA-4, FSA, and SCC-VII were 1.0×10^{-3}, 1.6×10^{-3}, 2.2×10^{-3}, and 9.0×10^{-3}% injection dose/pixel, respectively [42,43]. There was no correlation between the response to chemotherapy with paclitaxel and the tumor uptakes of ^{111}In-DTPA-paclitaxel. Scintigraphy

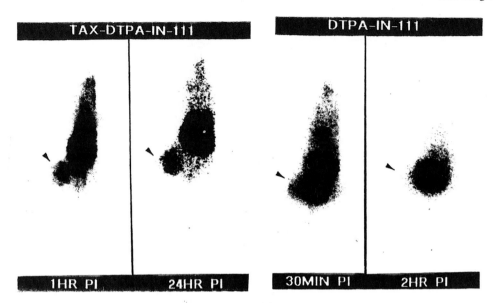

FIGURE 16.8. Whole-body images of breast tumor-bearing rats receiving ^{111}In-DTPA-paclitaxel (300 μCi, i.v.) show tumors (*arrowheads*) at 1 h (*left*) and 24 h (*right*) in the *left panel*. Tumor has much less uptake of ^{111}In-DTPA (*right panel*).

with ^{111}In-DTPA-paclitaxel could not predict the response to paclitaxel chemotherapy.

Imaging Tamoxifen

About one-third of all patients with advanced breast cancer respond to endocrine therapy, and the estrogen receptor (ER) assays of excised tumor tissue provide information about whether endocrine therapy is effective in each patient. However, only 60% of patients who have ER-positive breast cancer have an objective response to endocrine therapy [47,48]. Thus, the development of a supplemental technique to predict the responsiveness of breast cancer to adjuvant endocrine therapy for individual patients would be most helpful.

Radiolabeled estrogen and progesterone have been developed for use in positron emission tomography (PET) or single photon emission computed tomography (SPECT) to detect primary or metastatic breast cancer and to predict the responsiveness of breast cancer to endocrine therapy [49–55]. Tamoxifen, the trans isomer of a substituted triphenylethylene, is a nonsteroidal antiestrogenic drug that is widely used for endocrine therapy in patients with breast cancer. Tamoxifen binds to the cytoplasmic ER within the ER-positive breast tumor cell [56]. Both complexes cause a similar change in chromatin structure, but the antiestrogen–estrogen receptor DNA complexes are transcriptionally nonproductive [56,57]. In addition, tamoxifen reduces the amount of transforming growth factor-α (TGF-α), which stimulates tumor growth of ER-positive breast cancer. These mechanisms could explain the ER-mediated antitumor activity of tamoxifen. Recent reports have demonstrated that tamoxifen has several other antiproliferative effects, including inhibiting protein kinase C [58,59], binding to calmodulin [60], reducing sex hormone-binding globulin [61], and reducing insulin-like growth factor 1 [62]. Tamoxifen also stimulates tumor stromal cells (fibroblasts) and produces TGF-β, which can inhibit the growth of ER-negative breast cancer cells. Some patients with ER-negative breast cancer respond to tamoxifen, even if the objective responsive rate is less than 10% [63]. Considering these mechanisms of tamoxifen, radiolabeled tamoxifen should provide more accurate information about the effect of antiestrogen therapy than does radiolabeled estradiol.

PET Studies of Tamoxifen

Ten postmenopausal patients with ER-positive breast cancer, who were scheduled to receive tamoxifen therapy, were selected in this study. Informed consent was obtained from each patient. The age of the patients ranged from 52 to 68 years. ER concentration ranged from 19 to 1132 fmol/mg cytosol protein in nine primary and one metastatic lesions (Table 16.1). Pathological diagnoses of the primary tumor had been previously established for 9 of 10 patients. The primary tumor could not be confirmed pathologically in 1 patient (patient 6), but ER-positive axillary metastatic lesions were confirmed in the surgical specimen. Three of 10 patients (patients 1, 3, and 6 in Table 16.1) underwent diagnostic biopsies for primary lesions before PET studies, with lesions from the axillary lymph nodes of these patients being diagnosed pathologically after PET scanning. The other 7 patients were clinically suspected

TABLE 16.1. Summary of patients' Characteristics, PET imaging results, receptor assays and therapy response.

Patient	Age (yr)	Follow-up durationn (mo)	Lesion location	Number of lesions	Lesion size (cm)	Visual reading	SUV[a]	Receptor assay ER[b] (fmol/mg)	Response to therapy	Outcome	Comment
1	55	7	Left breast	1	3.0 × 3.0	−	1.6	125	Progression	Poor	Died 7 months later
			Spine	4	2.0 × 3.0	±	6.2			Poor	
					2.5 × 3.0	±	3.0			Poor	
					2.0 × 3.0	±	4.3			Poor	
					2.5 × 2.5	±	4.3			Poor	
			Sternum	1	2.5 × 6.0	±	4.2			Poor	
			Left axilla	1	ND	−	0.7			Poor	
2	58	5	Mediastinum	1	4.0 × 4.0	−	1.8	95[c]	Progression	Poor	Died 5 months later
3	52	24	Left breast	1	4.5 × 4.0	+	2.6	173	PR	Good	Improvement of
			Right axilla	1	1.5 × 1.5	+	2.2			Good	spine and liver
			Right breast	1	7.5 × 6.0	+	1.6			Good	lesions on CT scan
			Left axilla	1	2.0 × 1.0	+	2.6			Good	Improvement of
			Spine	4	3.5 × 2.5	+	3.0			Good	spine lesions on
					2.0 × 3.0	+	3.0			Good	bone scan
					2.5 × 2.5	+	3.0			Good	
					2.5 × 3.0	+	3.0			Good	
4	56	13	Right axilla	1	1.5 × 2.0	− (TN)	1.3	30[c]	NE	—	
5	66	14	Lung	1	1.5 × 1.5	±	3.3	185[c]	CR	Good	Improvement of lung lesion
6	65	26	Left axilla	1	3.0 × 3.0	+	2.9	19[d]	Not done	—	Surgical resection after PET study
7	54	8	Skull	1	3.0 × 4.0	−	0.9	54[c]	NC	Poor	
8	62	24	Neck	1	3.0 × 2.5	− (TN)	2.4	39[c]	Not done	—	Chemotherapy with 5-fluorouracil, doxorubicin and cyclophosphamide
9	63	24	Scapula	1	2.5 × 2.5	− (TN)	1.3	1132[c]	NE	—	No evidence of metastases in biopsy specimen
10	68	13	Spine	1	2.0 × 2.5	+	6.3	54[c]	PR	Good	Carcinoembryonic antigen down Improvement of pain and lesion on bone scan

ND, not defined; TN, true negative; PR, partial response; CR, complete response; NC, no change; NE, nonevaluable; +, positive; −, negative; ±, suspicious.

True positive ratio: paients: 5/7 (71.4%); lesion: 16/20 (80.0%).

[a] SUV, standardized uptake value.
[b] ER, estrogen receptor.
[c] ER concentration in the primary lesion removed before PET scan.
[d] ER concentration in the left axillar lesion.

to have metastatic lesions after their primary lesions had been resected.

The diagnoses of metastatic disease were based on radiological examinations that included mammograms, computerized tomographic (CT) and bone scans, magnetic resonance images, chest X-rays, or pathological findings. True-negative diagnoses were based on clinical follow-up for 13 months (patient 4), findings on CT scans and clinical follow-up for 24 months (patient 8), and results of a needle biopsy (patient 9).

Because each lesion in the axilla and the satellite lesion in the breast are difficult to identify simultaneously on PET images, a few small lesions in the same axilla and breast were estimated to be one lesion even if multiple metastatic lesions showed up on CT, MRI, or ultrasonography. Also, lesions in a spine are difficult to identify separately on PET images, and therefore a few lesions in one spine were estimated to be one lesion. Twenty-three lesions within the field of view (FOV) of PET images, which were clinically suspected to be primary or metastatic breast cancer, were subjects for the evaluation of diagnostic accuracy of PET with [18F]FTX. Tumor size of breast and axillary lesions was determined by direct measurement and that of the other metastatic lesions was measured by CT, MRI, or ultrasonography.

PET Technique

PET was performed with a Posicam 6.5 (Positron Corp., Houston, TX, USA) that provided an FOV of 42×11 cm for simultaneous acquisition of images in 21 sections [64]. Transmission scans were obtained with 185 MBq (5 mCi) of ^{68}Ga (approximately 300 million counts in 30 min) for attenuation correction. Patients had not eaten for at least 4 h before undergoing PET scanning. After the injection of 88.8 to 392.2 MBq (2.4–10.6 mCi) of [18F]FTX [65–67], four to six transaxial images (15 or 20 min each), centered on the suspected lesion, were obtained consecutively. The standardized uptake value, which is the ratio of the uptake of the radiotracer by tissue to the uptake of the radiotracer by the whole body (normalized for injected dose and body weight), was calculated pixel by pixel on each image.

Image Analysis

The venous blood samples were weighed and the radioactivity measured with a gamma counter to obtain percent injected dose per gram in blood. Regions of interest were drawn over the area corresponding to the lesion, lung, heart, liver, muscle, and normal breast on the color-coded images of the standardized uptake values. The maximum standardized uptake value in each region of interest was measured. Mean values of each maximum standardized uptake value from six regions of interest in the lung (upper, middle, and lower portions of each lung), three regions of interest in the heart (apex, septum, and lateral wall), three regions of interest in the liver (two in the right and one in the left hepatic lobes), two regions of interest in the muscle of the bilateral paraspinal region, and two regions of interest in the normal breast were calculated to analyze the biodistribution of [18F]FTX. Regions of interest were 1.0 cm in diameter for heart, muscle, and normal breast, and 2.6 cm in diameter for lung and liver. The size of the region of interest was changed to accommodate the tumor size. The maximum standardized uptake value (SUV) in the region of interest for each lesion was used for analysis.

For a biodistribution study, time activity (standardized uptake value) curves of each tissue or lesion were generated from four or five consecutive PET images obtained from 0 to 75 min or 80 min after the injection of [18F]FTX. Standardized uptake values of each tissue were compared between early image (0–15 min or 0–20 min after the injection of [18F]FTX) and delayed image (45–60 min or 40–60 min after the injection of [18F]FTX). The results are expressed as the mean ± SD. The differences in group means of standardized uptake values between early and delayed images were tested for significance by a paired Student's t-test. Differences were considered significant at $p < 0.05$.

Response to the tamoxifen therapy was evaluated for each patient, and judgment was based on the criteria of the recommendation of UICC [63]. The response of each lesion was judged as follows: good response, complete disappearance or decrease in tumor size on radiological examination or direct measurement, improvement of bone lesions on bone scan associated with decrease in tumor marker, and improvement of symptoms; and poor response, no change in tumor size or an increase in tumor size or the appearance of new lesions on radiological examination.

Visual interpretation of PET images with [18F]FTX and standardized uptake values of [18F]FTX in tumors were compared to the response to tamoxifen therapy and the concentration of ER in the tissue of primary lesions. The results of standardized uptake values were expressed with the mean and standard deviation. The differences in group means of standardized uptake values were tested for significance by an unpaired Student's t-test. Differences were considered significant at $p < 0.05$.

Higher uptake of [18F]FTX was observed in normal liver, lung, kidney, and heart regions on early and delayed images, whereas a lower accumulation of [18F]FTX was observed in normal breast and muscle regions. Mean standardized uptake values from early images of the lung and heart were higher than those on delayed images, but there were no significant statistical differences because of the small sample number (Table 16.2).

Patient characteristics, PET results, ER concentration of primary lesions (metastatic lesion in patient 6), and response to the tamoxifen

TABLE 16.2. Standardized uptake values of [18F]fluorotamoxifen in organs and tumors.

Organ	Results of PET images[a]		Significance
	Early	Delayed	
Lung ($n=4$)	4.5±1.8	2.9±0.8	None
Heart ($n=4$)	7.5±2.6	6.1±2.2	None
Liver ($n=4$)	19.2±9.8	21.5±8.4	None
Breast ($n=5$)	1.0±0.7	1.2±0.8	None
Muscle ($n=8$)	1.2±0.5	1.0±0.4	None
Tumor ($n=19$)	3.6±1.5	3.0±1.5	<0.01

[a] Mean±standard deviation.

therapy are summarized in Table 16.1. Three lesions in three patients (patients 4, 8, and 9) were considered to be truly negative for breast cancer on the basis of biopsy specimens or clinical course for more than 8 months. Five (71.4%) of 7 patients and 16 (80.0%) of 20 lesions were interpreted to be truly positive for breast cancer if the equivocal lesions were included in the positive results. As a whole, the mean standardized uptake values of [18F]FTX in tumors was 3.0 on the delayed images, which is significantly lower than that on early images (Table 16.2). Eight of 10 patients received tamoxifen therapy after the PET study. In 8 patients, 2 (patients 4 and 8) were excluded for the evaluation of response to tamoxifen therapy because there were no cancer lesions within the FOV of PET using [18F]FTX. Nineteen tumor lesions in 6 patients could be evaluated to compare the [18F]FTX uptake with response to tamoxifen therapy after the PET study. Three patients who had a good response to tamoxifen therapy showed positive lesions on PET images, whereas 2 of 3 patients who had a poor response to tamoxifen therapy showed a negative lesion and one showed mixed results. There was no significant difference of bone lesion uptake of [18F]FTX between good and poor responders. However, when bone lesions were excluded, [18F]FTX uptakes in tumors with good responses were significantly higher than those with poor responses (mean and SD of SUV: 2.46±0.62 versus 1.37±0.59; $p < 0.05$). Patient 3 in Table 16.1 showed an uptake of [18F]FTX in the primary tumor in the left breast, in metastatic lesions in the right breast, and in the bilateral axillary lymph node and the thoracic spine. This patient also had metastases in the liver and pelvic bone that were tremendously reduced in size (findings on CT scans) after tamoxifen therapy.

Conclusion

The distribution of 111In-DTPA-paclitaxel showed poor correlation with paclitaxel treatment response. Because DTPA-paclitaxel is more water soluble than paclitaxel, the distribution pattern may be different from paclitaxel.

After paclitaxel treatment, DTPA-paclitaxel may not have the same mechanism as paclitaxel. Using a smaller molecule, such as fluorine, results in less structural modification. Positron emission tomography (PET) imaging using [^{18}F]fluorotamoxifen as the radiotracer provides useful information in predicting the effect of tamoxifen therapy in patients with recurrent or metastatic ER-positive breast cancer. Those tumors that showed good uptake of the radiolabeled tamoxifen had positive responses to tamoxifen therapy.

The distribution of [^{18}F]fluorotamoxifen (FTX) showed low blood-pool activity but relatively high uptake in liver, lung, and heart. The distribution of tamoxifen in human tissue during tamoxifen treatment has been reported. Tamoxifen concentrations in various tissues are 10- to 60 fold higher than those in serum, with relatively high concentrations detected in liver and lung [68]. The apparent distribution volume for tamoxifen is about 50 to 60 l/kg [69], which suggests that extensive tissue binding is related to the lipophilic characteristics of this drug [68]. These pharmacokinetics may be responsible for the relatively low sensitivity of [^{18}F]FTX in detecting tumors because it is lipophilic.

Our preliminary patient data suggest that ^{111}In-DTPA-methotrexate may be a promising candidate to predict antifolate therapy. Further clinical studies should be performed to confirm the clinical utility of using ^{111}In-DTPA-methotrexate and ^{111}In-DTPA-adriamycin to predict treatment response.

References

1. Dorr U, Rath U, Sautter-Bihl ML, et al. Improved visualization of carcinoid liver metastases by ^{111}In-pentetreotide scintigraphy following treatment with cold somatostatin analogue. Eur J Nucl Med 1993;20:431–433.
2. Adrian HJ, Dorr U, Bach D, et al. Biodistribution of ^{111}In-pentetreotide and dosimetric considerations with respect to somatostatin receptor expressing tumor burden. Horm Metab Res (Suppl) 1993;27:18–23.
3. Breeman WA, de Jong M, Bernard BF, et al. Effects of ligand priming and multiple-dose injection on tissue uptake of ^{111}In-pentetreotide in rats. Nucl Med Biol 1997;24:749–753.
4. Dorr U, Frank-Raue K, Raue F, et al. The potential value of somatostatin receptor scintigraphy in medullary thyroid carcinoma. Nucl Med Commun 1993;14:439–445.
5. Cowan DS, Melo T, Park L, Ballinger JR, et al. BMS181321 accumulation in rodent and human cells: the role of P-glycoprotein. Br J Cancer (Suppl) 1996;27:S264–S266.
6. Hall AV, Solanki KK, Vinjamuri S, et al. Evaluation of the efficacy of ^{99m}Tc-Infecton, a novel agent for detecting sites of infection. J Clin Pathol 1998;51:215–219.
7. Vinjamuri S, Hall AV, Solanki KK, et al. Comparison of ^{99m}Tc infecton imaging with radiolabelled white-cell imaging in the evaluation of bacterial infection. Lancet 1996;347:233–235.
8. Britton KE, Vinjamuri S, Hall AV, et al. Clinical evaluation of ^{99m}Tc-infecton for the localization of bacterial infection. Eur J Nucl Med 1997;24:553–556.
9. Kairemo KJ, Ramsay HA, Paavonen T, et al. Imaging and staging of head and neck cancer using a low pH ^{111}In-bleomycin complex. Eur J Cancer B Oral Oncol 1996;32B:311–321.
10. Jekunen AP, Kairemo KJ, Ramsay HA, et al. Imaging of olfactory neuroblastoma by ^{111}In-bleomycin complex. Clin Nucl Med 1996;21(2):129–131.
11. Goodwin DA, Meares CF, DeRiemer LH, et al. Clinical studies with ^{111}In-BLEDTA, a tumor-imaging conjugate of bleomycin with a bifunctional chelating agent. J Nucl Med 1981;22:787–792.
12. Jaaskela-Saari HA, Kairemo KJ, Ramsay HA, et al. Labelling of bleomycin with Auger-emitter increases cytotoxicity in squamous-cell cancer cell lines. Int J Radiat Biol 1998;73:565–570.
13. Harrison K, Wagner NH Jr. Biodistribution of intravenously injected [^{14}C]doxorubicin and [^{14}C]daunorubicin in mice: concise communication. J Nucl Med 1978;19:84–86.
14. Fragu P, Klijanienko J, Gandia D, et al. Quantitative mapping of 4'-iododeoxyrubicin in metastatic squamous cell carcinoma by secondary ion mass spectrometry (SIMS) microscopy. Cancer Res 1992;52:974–977.
15. Westerhof GR, Jansen G, Emmerik NV, et al. Membrane transport of natural folates and antifolate compounds in murine L1210 leukemia cells: role of carrier- and receptor-mediated

transport systems. Cancer Res 1991;51:5507–5513.

16. Orr RB, Kreisler AR, Kamen BA. Similarity of folate receptor expression in UMSCC 38 cells to squamous cell carcinoma differentiation markers. J Natl Cancer Inst 1995;87:299–303.

17. Hsueh CT, Dolnick BJ. Altered folate-binding protein mRNA stability in KB cells grown in folate-deficient medium. Biochem Pharmacol 1993;45:2537–2545.

18. Weitman SD, Lark RH, Coney LR, et al. Distribution of folate GP38 in normal and malignant cell lines and tissues. Cancer Res 1992;52:3396–3400.

19. Campbell IG, Jones TA, Foulkes WD, Trowsdale J. Folate-binding protein is a marker for ovarian cancer. Cancer Res 1991;51:5329–5338.

20. Holm J, Hansen SI, Hoier-Madsen M, Sondergaard K, Bzorek M. Folate receptor of human mammary adenocarcinoma. APMIS 1994;102:413–419.

21. Ross JF, Chaudhuri PK, Ratnam M. Differential regulation of folate receptor isoforms in normal and malignant tissue in vivo and in established cell lines. Cancer (Phila) 1994;73:2432–2443.

22. Franklin WA, Waintrub M, Edwards D, et al. New anti-lung-cancer antibody cluster 12 reacts with human folate receptors present on adenocarcinoma. Int J Cancer (Suppl) 1994;8:89–95.

23. Weitman SD, Frazier KM, Kamen BA. The folate receptor in central nervous system malignancies of childhood. J Neuro-Oncol 1994;21:107–112.

24. Mathias CJ, Wang S, Lee RJ, et al. Tumor-selective radiopharmaceutical targeting via receptor-mediated endocytosis of ^{67}Ga-deferoxamine-folate. J Nucl Med 1996;37:1003–1008.

25. Wang S, Luo J, Lantrip DA, et al. Design and synthesis of [^{111}In]DTPA-folate for use as a tumor-targeted radiopharmaceutical. Bioconjugate Chem 1997;8:673–679.

26. Wang S, Lee RJ, Mathias CJ, et al. Synthesis, purification, and tumor cell uptake of ^{67}Ga-deferoxamine-folate, a potential radiopharmaceutical for tumor imaging. Bioconjugate Chem 1996;7:56–62.

27. Mathias CJ, Wang S, Waters DJ, et al. ^{111}In-DTPA-folate as a radiopharmaceutical for targeting tumor-associated folate binding protein. J Nucl Med (Suppl) 1997;38:133 (abstract).

28. Mathias CJ, Hubers D, Trump DP, et al. Synthesis of ^{99m}Tc-DTPA-folate and preliminary evaluation as a folate-receptor-targeted radiopharmaceutical. J Nucl Med (Suppl) 1997;38:87 (abstract).

29. Schilsky RL. Antimetabolites. In: Perry MC, ed. The Chemotherapy Source Book. Baltimore: Williams & Williams, 1992:301–306.

30. Chabner BA. Promising new drugs and combinations. Fulfilling our pledge. Oncologist 1999;4:VIII.

31. Deutsch JC, Elwood PC, Portillo RM, et al. Role of membrane-associated folate binding protein (folate receptor) in methotrexate transport by human KB cells. Arch Biochem Biophys 1989;274:327–337.

32. Kane MA, Portillo RM, Elwood PC, et al. The influence of extracellular folate concentration on methotrexate uptake by human KB cells. J Biol Chem 1986;261:44–49.

33. Wang X, Shen F, Freisheim JH, et al. Differential stereospecificities and affinities of folate receptor isoforms for folate compounds and antifolates. Biochem Pharmacol 1992;44:1898–1901.

34. Sierra EE, Brigle KE, Spinella MJ, et al. pH depedence of methotrexate transport by the reduced folate carrier and the folate receptor in L1210 leukemia cells. Further evidence for a third route mediated at low pH. Biochem Pharmacol 1997;53:223–231.

35. Westerhof GR, Schornagel JH, Kathmann I, et al. Carrier- and receptor-mediated transport of folate antagonists targeting folate-dependent enzymes: correlates of molecular-structure and biological activity. Mol Pharmacol 1995;48:459–471.

36. Chung KN, Saiwaka Y, Paik TH, et al. Stable transfectants of human MCF-7 breast cancer cells with increased levels of the human folate receptor exhibit an increased sensitivity to antifolates. J Clin Invest 1993;91:1289–1294.

37. Spinella MJ, Brigle KE, Freemantle SJ, et al. Comparison of methotrexate polyglutamation in L1210 leukemia cells when influx is mediated by reduced folate carrier or the folate receptor. Lack of evidence for influx route-specific effects. Biochem Pharmacol 1996;52:703–712.

38. Sierra EE, Brigle KE, Spinella MJ, et al. Comparison of transport properties of the reduced folate carrier and folate receptor in murine L1210 leukemia cells. Biochem Pharmacol 1995;50:1287–1294.

39. Spinella MJ, Brigle KE, Sierra EE, et al. Distinguishing between folate receptor-alpha-mediated transport and reduced folate carrier-

mediated transport in leukemia cells. J Biol Chem 1995;270:7842–7849.

40. Gehl J, Boesgaad M, Paaske T, et al. Paclitaxel and doxorubicin in metastatic breast cancer. Semin Oncol 1996;23(6 suppl 15):35–38.

41. Li C, Price JE, Milas L, et al. Antitumor activity of poly(L-glutamic acid)-paclitaxel on syngeneic and xenografted tumors. Clin Cancer Res 1999; 5:891–897.

42. Li C, Yu DF, Inoue T, et al. Synthesis, biodistribution and imaging properties of ^{111}In-DTPA-paclitaxel in mice bearing mammary tumors. J Nucl Med 1997;38(7):1042–1047.

43. Inoue T, Li C, Yang DJ, et al. Evaluation of ^{111}In-DTPA-paclitaxel scintigraphy to predict response on murine tumors to paclitaxel. Ann Nucl Med 1999;13:169–174.

44. Milross CG, Mason KA, Hunter NR, et al. Preclinical antitumor activity of water-soluble paclitaxel derivatives. Cancer Chemother Pharmacol 1997;39:486–492.

45. Rao CS, Chu JJ, Liu RS, et al. Synthesis and evaluation of [^{14}C]-labelled and fluorescent-tagged paclitaxel derivatives as new biological probes. Bioorg Med Chem 1998;6:2193–2204.

46. Evangelio JA, Abal M, Barasoain I, et al. Fluorescent taxoids as probes of the microtubule cytoskeleton. Cell Motil Cytoskeleton 1998;39:73–90.

47. Jordan VC. The role of tamoxifen in the treatment and prevention of breast cancer. Curr Probl Cancer 1992;16:129–176.

48. Wittliff JL. Steroid-hormone receptors in breast cancer. Cancer Res 1994;53:630–643.

49. Dehdashiti F, McGuire AH, Van Brocklin HF, et al. Assessment of 21-[^{18}F]fluoro-16α-ethyl-19-norprogesterone as a positron-emitting radiopharmaceutical for the detection of progestin receptors in human breast carcinomas. J Nucl Med 1991;32:1532–1537.

50. Mintun MA, Welch MJ, Siegel BA, et al. Breast cancer: PET imaging of estrogen receptors. Radiology 1988;169:45–48.

51. McGuire AH, Dehdashti F, Shiegel BA, et al. Positron tomographic assessment of 16α-[18F]fluoro-17β-estradiol uptake in metastatic breast carcinoma. J Nucl Med 1991;32:1526–1531.

52. Kiesewetter DO, Kilbourn MR, Landvatter SW, et al. Preparation of four fluorine-18-labeled estrogens and their selective uptake in target tissue of immature rats. J Nucl Med 1984;25:1212–1221.

53. Brodack JW, Kilbourn MR, Welch MJ, et al. Application of robotics to radiopharmaceutical preparation: controlled synthesis of fluorine-18-16α-fluoroestradiol-17β. J Nucl Med 1986;27:714–721.

54. Kenady DE, Pavlik EJ, Nelson K, et al. Images of estrogen-receptor-positive breast tumors produced by estradiol labeled with iodine ^{123}I at 16α. Arch Surg 1993;128:1373–1381.

55. Zielinski JE, Larner JM, Hoffer PB, et al. The synthesis of 11β-methoxy-[16α-^{123}I]iodoestradiol and its interaction with the estrogen receptor in vivo and in vitro. J Nucl Med 1989;30:209–215.

56. Yang DJ, Cherif A, Tansey W, et al. N,N-Diethylfluoro-methyltamoxifen: synthesis assignment of ^{1}H and ^{13}C spectra and receptor assay. Eur J Med Chem 1992;27:919–924.

57. Green S. Modulations of oestrogen receptor activity by oestrogens and antioestrogens. J Steroid Biochem Mol Biol 1990;37:747–751.

58. O'Brian CA, Liskamp RM, Solomon DH, et al. Inhibition of protein kinase C by tamoxifen. Cancer Res 1985;45:2462–2465.

59. Edashige K, Sato E, Akimaru K, et al. Nonsteroidal antiestrogen suppresses protein kinase C: its inhibitory effect on interaction of substrate protein with membrane. Cell Struct Funct 1991;16:273–281.

60. Lam HY. Tamoxifen is a calmodulin antagonist in the activation of cAMP phosphodiesterase. Biochem Biophys Res Commun 1984;118:27–32.

61. Pollak MN, Huynh HT, Lefevre SP. Tamoxifen reduces serum insulin-like growth factor 1 (IGF-1). Breast Cancer Res Treat 1992;22:91–95.

62. Rose DP, Chlebowski RT, Connolly JM, et al. Effects of tamoxifen adjuvant therapy and a low-fat diet or serum binding proteins and estradiol bioavailability in postmenopausal breast cancer patients. Cancer Res 1992;52:5386–5390.

63. Harris JR, Morrow M, Bonadonna G. Cancer of the breast. In: DeVita VT, Hellman S Jr, Rosenberg SA, eds. Cancer: Principles & Practice of Oncology. Philadelphia: Lippincott, 1993:1264–1332.

64. Mullani NA, Gould KL, Hartz RK, et al. Design and performance of Posicam 6.5 BGO positron camera. J Nucl Med 1990;31:610–616.

65. Yang DJ, Kuang L-R, Cherif A, et al. Synthesis of [^{18}F]fluoroalanine and [^{18}F]fluorotamoxifen

for imaging breast tumors. J Drug Targeting 1993;1:259–267.

66. Yang DJ, Li C, Kuang L-R, et al. Imaging, biodistribution and therapy potential of halogenated tamoxifen analogues. Life Sci 1994;55:53–67.

67. Yang DJ, Tewson T, Tansey W, et al. Halogenated analogues of tamoxifen: synthesis, receptor assay and inhibition of MCF7 cells. J Pharm Sci 1992; 81:622–625.

68. Lien EA, Solheim E, Ueland PM. Distribution of tamoxifen and its metabolites in rat and human tissues during steady-state treatment. Cancer Res 1991;51:4837–4844.

69. Lien EA, Solheim E, Lea O, et al. Distribution of 4-hydroxy-N-desmethyltamoxifen and other tamoxifen metabolites in human biological fluids during tamoxifen treatment. Cancer Res 1989; 49:2175–2183.

17
Imaging of Angiogenesis

Kenneth C. Wright and E. Edmund Kim

Angiogenesis is the process by which new vessels grow toward and into a tissue. It is required for several physiological processes including embryogenesis, corpus luteum formation, and wound healing. It is also a critical element in the pathogenesis of many disorders, most notably the rapid growth and metastasis of solid tumors.

Neovascularization is a fundamental prerequisite for expansive growth of solid tumors [1]. Initially, a tumor receives its sole supply of nutrients and oxygen by means of diffusion from preexisting host vasculature. In the absence of new vessel formation, cell proliferation equilibrates with the rate of cell death, and tumor size is limited to a few cubic millimeters [2,3]. This is termed the prevascular phase.

Once angiogenesis is upregulated, the tumor enters the vascular phase. Angiogenesis is a complex multistep process regulated by both stimulators and inhibitors in a system of checks and balances. Normally quiescent with slow rates of cell turnover, endothelial cells rapidly proliferate and form new blood vessels in response to a net positive balance of angiogenic factors secreted by tumor cells [4]. Stimulators are produced by neoplastic cells and tumor-associated inflammatory cells and act locally in a paracrine fashion to increase the production of endothelial cells and to prepare the local environment for the ingrowth of new vascular buds.

It is now generally assumed that microvessel formation around a tumor is stimulated by the tumor cells themselves. Hypoxia or factors associated with hypoxia such as decreased pH and increased lactate levels can induce tumor cells to secrete angiogenic factors, such as vascular endothelial growth factor (VEGF), which increases vascular permeability in addition to stimulating new vessel formation, basic fibroblast growth factor (bFGF), heparin-binding epidermal growth factor-like growth factor, pleiotrophin, and transforming growth factor-β (TGF-β). Tumors can also recruit macrophages and then activate them to secrete angiogenic activity such as bFGF [5]. Mast cells may be recruited by tumors as well, but mast cells alone do not cause angiogenesis. Instead, mast cells increase endothelial cell migration as the earliest event in the formation of a capillary sprout [6]. Inactivation of the p53 suppressor gene has also been shown to be capable of initiating angiogenesis because the p53 gene encodes the angiogenic suppressor thrombospondin 1 [7,8].

In addition to primary tumor growth, angiogenesis plays an essential role in tumor metastasis. For a tumor to disseminate hematogenously, malignant cells must enter the vasculature, survive, and implant and grow in the target organ [9,10]. Angiogenesis plays a key role in both the first and the last steps. The hyperpermeability of tumor vessels, which is tied to angiogenesis, may contribute to the transendothelial escape of tumor cells [11].

Angiogenesis is also necessary for a secondary tumor to grow following metastasis. On metastasizing to another organ, tumor cells are dependent on neovascularization to supply nutrients in much the same manner as the primary tumor. Often, tumor cells that metastasize are preselected for the angiogenic phenotype and thus grow rapidly after implantation because of neovascularization.

In 1972, Brem et al. [12] suggested that tumor aggressiveness could be correlated to neovascular intensity. The first report to confirm this hypothesis was in 1988, when Srivastava et al. [13] found that the degree of histological staining for vessels in patients with melanoma was associated with probability of metastasis. Since then, quantification of tumor neovascularity has been reported to provide prognostic information for more than a dozen different tumor types, including breast, lung, colon, and prostate [14]. Numerous studies have shown that increased microvessel density is correlated to poorer overall survival, poorer disease-free survival, and increased risk for metastasis.

Currently, there are two general methods of assessing the angiogenic capacity of a tumor. The first is done indirectly with a biochemical assay to detect angiogenic or antiangiogenic factors in the serum, urine, or cerebrospinal fluid of cancer patients. The second, more direct method is through the measurement of tumor vascularity in a biopsy specimen. The most widely used method of assessing tumor vascularity is the microvessel density technique first proposed by Weidner et al. [15] and summarized by Gasparini and Harris [16].

Although microscopic counting of capillaries on specially stained tumor specimens has been a useful surrogate of angiogenesis, microvessel density (MVD) is not a "gold standard" of angiogenesis, nor is it an ideal tool for clinical purposes. Being invasive, serial MVD assays to monitor progress of therapy are not practical. MVD is also subject to sampling errors because tumors are notoriously heterogeneous, the entire tumor cannot be examined, and MVD does not assess functional angiogenic activity.

Clearly, an imaging assay for angiogenic activity is needed, particularly if the method is quantitative, noninvasive, could sample the entire tumor, and could be repeated at frequent intervals. In actuality, radiologists have been imaging tumor angiogenesis for decades. It is called vascularity, and its relative density is noted on the capillary phase of angiograms.

Unlike other imaging methods, angiography permits excellent assessment of vessel morphology, showing caliber variations, coiling, or sinusoids. However, current efforts are mainly directed to extend vascularity-related diagnostics toward methods that are less invasive, and either cheaper, more widely available, and versatile (e.g., scintigraphy, power Doppler sonography, and perfusion CT), or more potent or flexible (e.g., MRI).

Radionuclide Imaging

The first reports on the use of radiotracers to define tumor perfusion demonstrated the utility of macroaggregated albumin to define arterial distribution and tumor volume [17,18] and quantitate response to therapy [19]. These studies suggested that the use of a large particle such as aggregated albumin, which results in transient small vessel occlusion, is most favorable for defining flow patterns.

With the development of technetium (Tc)-labeled particulates, ^{99m}Tc-sulfur colloid was suggested as the agent of choice. However, this radiopharmaceutical had a number of shortcomings. In the liver, perfusion information was limited to the initial first pass because of its rapid Kupffer cell sequestration. Additionally, normal splenic sequestration could lead to erroneous interpretation of extrahepatic perfusion.

The problems associated with ^{99m}Tc-sulfur colloid were overcome by the use of ^{99m}Tc-labeled macroaggregated albumin (MAA). The aggregated albumin particles produce capillary blockage, and the image represents the first-pass distribution of blood flow within a tumor (Figure 17.1). Additionally, an accurate assessment of the relative tumor vascularity can be obtained [20]. A dynamic, first-pass study using a high dose of ^{99m}Tc-DTPA can also be used to evaluate tumor blood flow and vascularity.

With the development of positron emission tomography (PET), spatial resolution and the ability to correct for attenuation were significantly improved. This imaging modality has allowed determination of tumor blood flow in absolute terms of milliliters per minute per

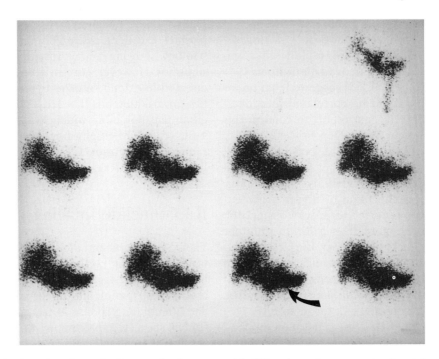

Figure 17.1. Anterior dynamic flow study (every 4s images) of the liver after infusion of ^{99m}Tc-MAA (macroaggregated albumin) particles through the hepatic arterial catheter show radioactivity accumulated in the right and left hepatic lobes in a patient with diffuse hepatic metastasis of rectal cancer, indicating good perfusion in the hepatic tumor bed. Note the radioactivity in the stomach (*arrow*) resulting from displacement of catheter tip.

gram of tissue [21]. In general, two means of quantitation of organ perfusion have been validated, but their application is somewhat organ- and tracer specific. One method is the normalization of tissue uptake to the amount of tracer injected. This approach is analogous to measuring perfusion with radiolabled particles such as MAA.

A second and more complicated method of quantitation is the application of parametric modeling to dynamic studies to determine organ perfusion. This approach was first applied to the diffusible tracer ^{15}O-water, but is has also been applied to the less highly extracted tracers ^{82}Rb and ^{13}N-NH$_3$ [21]. With this approach, distribution rate of the tracer in different cellular and extracellular compartments is estimated by fitting the dynamic data.

Although there has recently been a veritable explosion of ongoing research to develop unique functional tumor imaging agents, radiolabeled sestamibi (MIBI), initially developed for myocardial perfusion imaging, is frequently being used for tumor imaging. Sestamibi is a lipophilic cation that can accumulate in mitochondria driven by negative mitochondrial inner matrix and plasma membrane potentials. It is a suitable transport substrate for P-glycoprotein, and its efflux from tumor cells is related to P-glycoprotein expression [22].

It has been reported that ^{99m}Tc-labeled MIBI may be used to predict tumor angiogenesis and lymph node status. Scopinaro et al. [23] reported uptake of ^{99m}Tc-MIBI in breast cancer to be related to angiogenesis (Figure 17.2), one of the strong prognostic factors in this disease. In a study of 19 breast cancer patients, ^{99m}Tc-MIBI uptake in the primary tumor was used to classify tumors as positive or negative. These findings were then compared to microvessel density and surgically documented nodal status. In this relatively small study, results correlated extremely well to the microvessel density findings. In addition, ^{99m}Tc-MIBI

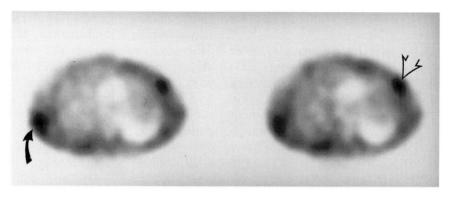

FIGURE 17.2. Selected axial SPECT images of the chest using ^{99m}Tc-sestamibi show focal areas of moderately increased activity in the biopsy-proven recurrent left breast carcinoma (*open arrow*) and also metastatic node (*closed arrow*) in the right axilla.

scanning had 100% specificity for prediction of nodal status.

In a more recent study, Yoon et al. [24] evaluated the relation of ^{99m}Tc-MIBI uptake and washout in untreated breast cancer patients with immunohistochemically determined angiogenesis and P-glycoprotein expression. A significant correlation was found between angiogenesis and the tumor-to-normal breast ratio (T:N) of the tracer in early and late scintigraphic images. Furthermore, the T:N ratios of early and late images and the washout index were not different according to tumor stage. However, no correlation was noted between tumor stage and angiogenesis or P-glycoprotein expression. Similar to the findings of Scopinaro et al. [23], an association between ^{99m}Tc-MIBI uptake and tumoral angiogenesis was found. This observation has also been reported by Omar et al. [25].

In addition to being a marker of breast cancer invasiveness and angiogenesis, tumoral uptake of ^{99m}Tc-MIBI can provide prognostic information. Bom et al. [26] found an association of low tumoral uptake of ^{99m}Tc-MIBI and poor response to chemotherapy in patients with small-cell lung cancer [26]. Mankoff et al. [27] and Ciarmiello et al. [28] reported that response to chemotherapy could be predicted by ^{99m}Tc-MIBI scintimammography in patients with breast cancer. They also related efflux rate to the outcome of chemotherapy. Recently, tumor angiogenesis or vascularity has been studied by using ^{99m}Tc-colchicine [29], heparin, and endostatin in animal tumor models.

As an indirect measure of tumor angiogenesis, radiolabeled ligands have been developed for imaging tumor hypoxia. Misonidazole (MISO), a hypoxic cell sensitizer, has been labeled with ^{18}F and used with PET [30]. However, because of the cost and availability of PET and PET isotopes, other radioligands are being developed for planar scintigraphic imaging of tumor hypoxia. MISO and erythronitroimidazol have been labeled with ^{131}I, but high thyroid uptake has been observed [31]. Recently, metronidazole has been labeled with ^{99m}Tc and experimentally shown to be as effective as MISO for imaging tumor hypoxia [32].

Ultrasound

The presence of blood flow and its velocity are registered with Doppler sonography if the related vessels are large enough. Doppler also permits estimation of the intratumoral flow resistance, which may reflect interstitial pressure. However, Doppler sonography has limited sensitivity for recognition of slow flow. Flow velocities less than 1 cm/s are difficult to detect because of artifacts caused by tissue movement, which only to some degree are suppressed by motion discrimination algorithms. Therefore, capillary blood flow thus far remains undetectable with available conventional Doppler methods.

In contrast to conventional Doppler Ultrasonography (US), color Doppler (CD) mapping allows the demonstration of even very slow blood flow velocities, which are found in newly formed microvessels of malignant tumors. Use of CD in contemporary examinations is mainly directed at detecting vessels and determining their spatial orientation. The CD approach allows mapping of flow signals for the entire tumor volume in a real-time ultrasonographic imaging method and thus offers a noninvasive, easily applicable method for direct measurement of actual blood flow in intratumoral blood vessels. However, it does not permit measurement of the volume of blood flow.

CD is based on the mean Doppler frequency shift and therefore is a measure of a directional component of the velocity of blood moving through the sample volume. As such, it suffers from inherent limitations [33,34]. In the mean frequency mode, noise can look like blood flow in any direction. Hence, if the color gain is too high or the Doppler display threshold is too low, noise will dominate the image and make the identification of true blood flow impossible. By turning down the color gain, artifacts will be eliminated, but sensitivity will also be greatly reduced. Moreover, CD imaging is angle dependent, and therefore it loses sensitivity to blood flow that is perpendicular to the sound field. Finally, because it is a frequency-detection technique, color CD has the potential to alias. Low-flow settings in CD typically use very low pulse repetition frequencies, often resulting in aliasing artifact, which obscures directional information.

Power Doppler US is a technique that was developed in an attempt to overcome some of the drawbacks of color Doppler imaging [33]. Power Doppler (PD) displays the integrated power of the Doppler signal instead of its mean Doppler frequency shift and extends the dynamic range of the Doppler scale [35]. PD encodes the power of the Doppler signal in color [33]. The hue and brightness of the color signal represent the power in the Doppler signal, which is related to the number of red blood cells producing the Doppler shift [36,37]. This parameter is fundamentally different from the mean frequency shift. The relationship can be very complex and can depend in nonlinear ways on such variables as shear rates, blood flow velocity, and hematocrit [38]. This hematocrit dependence tends to decrease the pulsatility in the vessels imaged. PD has been employed previously in cardiological examinations mainly to better characterize stenotic and regurgitant jets [39–41]. The hypothesis behind these measurements was that power was presumed to be more sensitive to low-flow states [41].

PD has several advantages over CD. Probably the most important advantage is that in PD, noise may be assigned to a homogeneous background (e.g., blue) even when the gain is increased greatly over the level at which noise begins to obscure the CD image. This contrasts with the appearance of noise on a CD image, which appears as random color, totally obscuring any information-containing signal. Doppler noise, like noise in general, is a random process (often referred to as Gaussian white noise), and therefore has a random phase angle. Because the frequency shift recorded in CD is dependent on the rate of change of the phase angle, noise at any point can appear as any frequency shift, including very high or low values, and can also appear as flow from any direction. Therefore, as CD is based on the mean frequency shift, CD noise can look like flow of any velocity. Additionally, because of the random fluctuation of noise, the noise signal appears as rapidly changing velocities. Thus, if the Doppler gain is too high or the threshold too low, any vascular signal is quickly buried in a noisy background with CD. In contrast, noise has a much different appearance in the power mode. Noise has a very low power compared with information-containing signal. Therefore, if the Doppler gain is increased or if the threshold is lowered to the noise floor in the power mode, the resulting image noise assumes a nearly uniform appearance, corresponding to low-power background. Any information-containing signal, displayed as a signal of higher power, appears as a different color relative to the noise floor. PD uses more of the available dynamic range when producing flow images, thus increasing flow sensitivity.

Other advantages that PD has over CD ultrasound are that it is essentially angle independent and that it is not subject to aliasing, so it elicits more precise, angiogram-like pictures without the salt-and-pepper appearance of conventional CD imaging. The mean-frequency representation of CD varies with the degree of aliasing. The PD image is unaffected by aliasing because the integral of the power spectrum is the same whether or not the signal wraps around.

CD also has advantages over PD, the most significant being that PD is more sensitive to tissue motion. However, development of more sophisticated motion-suppressing techniques should expand the applicability of the PD method. Furthermore, CD displays directional and velocity information.

Although color Doppler signals are detected in most malignant tumors studied, no significant correlation has been found between MVD and intratumoral blood flow velocity assessed by color-coded Doppler. Using color Doppler US, Lee et al. [42] observed a relative increase in blood flow within malignant breast tumors compared with benign breast lesions, especially at the tumor periphery. However, neither color signal intensity nor flow velocity correlated to extent of angiogenesis as measured with histological microvessel density techniques, which suggests that the vessels assessed at color Doppler US are larger than those measured with microvessel counts. These findings are similar to those previously reported for breast cancer [42] and uterine myomas [43]. Instead, a high Doppler tumor blood flow was associated with a greater extent of disease [44].

Furthermore, not only malignant but also some benign tumors show detectable Doppler signals [45,46]. As a rule, up to 10% of malignant breast tumors show no or only weak Doppler signals. Consequently, methods of quantification using computer-assisted image analysis have been applied to both color and spectral Doppler information [47–49]. Although quantitative color Doppler enables assessment of vascularity (i.e., flow velocities and vessel density) for an entire tumor cross

section, it is subject to potential flaws because of the Doppler angle, aliasing, and interpolation algorithms as well as spatial and temporal irregularities of tumor blood flow. In comparison, spectral Doppler quantification is physically more precise but is limited to a few intratumoral vessels.

With the advantage of relative angle and velocity independence, extended dynamic range, and higher sensitivity, power Doppler ultrasound has been shown to be a more useful tumor flow mapping technique [50]. Using power Doppler ultrasonography, contours of vessels are shown clearly, somewhat mimicking angiography. In cervical carcinoma, assessment of intratumoral vascular index, the in vivo indicator of angiogenic activity, by power Doppler ultrasound and a quantitative image processing system showed high correlation with MVD, the conventional indicator of tumor angiogenic activity.

Recently, microbubble contrast agents have become available for clinical use with ultrasonography. The increased echogenicity of these agents enables improved detection of parenchymal organ blood flow when compared with routine color Doppler and power Doppler US. As a result, differences in vascularity between benign and malignant lesions may be detected. Contrast-enhanced US can depict residual tumor after radiofrequency ablation, thereby enabling additional directed therapy [51].

In summary, it is not possible to identify the vascular architecture and detect vascular pathology with spectral and conventional color Doppler techniques. Power Doppler US is superior to conventional color Doppler imaging in the depiction of tumor vascularity. The findings of power Doppler US correlate well with the findings at angiography. However, although Doppler sonography may indeed increase diagnostic confidence, at the present time it does not obviate biopsy.

Computed Tomography

New tumor vessels are too small to be resolved using current structural diagnostic imaging methods. However, high tumor microvessel

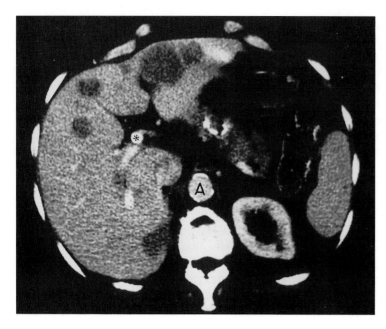

FIGURE 17.3. Axial CT image of the upper abdomen following the injection of iodine contrast agent shows multiple metastatic lesions with slight contrast enhancement in the right and left hepatic lobes in a patient with neuroendocrine tumor. Note enhanced aorta (A) and portal vein (*).

density is associated with an increase in perfusion (i.e., blood flow per unit volume of tissue). New tumor vessels also demonstrate increased fenestration of the basement membrane, resulting in an increase in the permeability of these vessels. These physiological changes alter contrast enhancement during computed tomography (CT). Functional CT techniques that quantify these physiological changes can provide greater insight into how angiogenesis alters contrast enhancement. By providing a marker for tumor angiogenesis, quantitative contrast-enhanced CT can improve the diagnostic assessment of patients with cancer. The functional information obtained can aid with tissue characterization, such as type or grade of tumor, improve detection of metastases, produce clearer delineation of tumors with benefits for radiotherapy planning and biopsy, and provide prognostic information.

A conventional unenhanced CT image displays a map of X-ray attenuation values within a cross section of the body. Following intravenous injection of iodinated contrast media, structures within the image demonstrate an increase in attenuation that is proportional to the concentration of iodine within them (Figure

17.3). There is minimal intracellular uptake of contrast agents, and excretion is via glomerular filtration. For the initial period following injection, enhancement is largely due to the contrast medium within the intravascular space. The delivery of contrast medium to the tissues during the first pass is determined primarily by blood flow. With time, the contrast medium passes from the intravascular space into the extravascular space. In the later phases, tissue enhancement is partly the result of intra- and extravascular contrast medium. The intravascular component depends on the volume of the blood space within the tissue concerned whereas the extravascular component depends on the permeability of the capillaries to contrast medium.

Recently developed CT scanners utilizing slip-ring technology permit very high spatial resolution (<0.05 µl) images to be obtained at rapid intervals (<100 ms) because the X-ray tube can rotate continuously around an object, making uninterrupted data acquisition possible. The combination of the high spatial and temporal resolutions makes this tool an ideal method for the investigation of tissue vascular physiology, allowing the measurement of contrast agent pharmacokinetics and biodistribution in vivo [52].

The introduction of continually rotating (spiral) CT systems has resulted in a wider ability to image organs within the first pass of contrast medium during which the relationship between physiology and contrast enhancement is simpler. It has also enabled the development of functional CT techniques that can provide insight into the relationship between contrast enhancement and pathophysiology.

There are two basic functional CT paradigms, perfusion measurements and permeability studies. Both techniques employ a series of images acquired at the same location over a period of time from which it is possible to generate a time-attenuation curve displaying the temporal changes in iodine concentration resulting from injection of the contrast medium. CT perfusion measurements are derived from a study performed within the first pass of contrast medium during which the agent can be assumed to be intravascular. Permeability measurements employ a slower dynamic study during which a proportion of the injected contrast medium passes out of the vascular system into the extracellular space. With appropriate mathematical modeling of data from the tissue of interest and from the vascular system, quantitative functional information can be derived.

Tumor angiogenesis is associated with increased perfusion, blood volume, and permeability resulting in increased contrast enhancement to a magnitude determined by the intensity of neovascularization. Perfusion CT combines functional information with high spatial resolution, enabling direct visualization and quantification of variations in perfusion [53,54]. CT-derived perfusion images of tumors demonstrate high perfusion within the peripheral portions of tumors where new vessel density is known to be greatest [53,54]. This change may be seen as "ring enhancement" on conventional contrast-enhanced CT or as high peripheral perfusion, blood volume, or permeability on functional CT techniques with parametric imaging.

Distinguishing cancerous tissue from a benign lesion using structural criteria is frequently difficult. However, functional CT techniques that quantify perfusion, blood volume, and permeability are useful in tissue characterization, tumor detection, tumor delineation, and prognostic information. Using a spiral CT system, Swenson et al. [55] measured peak enhancement in solitary pulmonary nodules and found that malignant nodules showed greater enhancement than benign lesions. Furthermore, the degree of enhancement correlated with the intensity of angiogenesis as determined by histopathological assessment of MVD. Malignant and inflammatory nodules showed higher values of all parameters than benign nodules, with the clearest separation provided by perfusion measurements.

A similar diagnostic problem occurs with determination of the malignant status of lymph nodes. When relying on structural imaging, lymph nodes are often classified as benign or malignant depending on whether they exceed a predetermined size. Clearly, this approach will fail to diagnose small nodes that contain tumor. However, it has been shown for gastric cancer that malignant nodes enhance more avidly than benign nodes, a finding that can be attributed to tumor-associated angiogenesis [56].

The grade of a specific tumor can be inferred from quantitative analysis of contrast enhancement. Angiogenesis within high-grade gliomas is not only more intense, but also more heterogeneous than that seen in low-grade tumors of the same type. This difference is not usually appreciable on conventional contrast-enhanced CT images or simple enhancement measurements. However, separate evaluation of the intra- and extravascular components of contrast enhancement using Patlak analysis with parametric imaging enables visualization of the heterogeneity in blood volume within high-grade gliomas [57].

Use of angiogenesis as a marker for the presence of tumor can improve the delineation of tumor from adjacent normal tissues or from peritumoral edema. Accurate definition of tumor borders is essential for radiotherapy planning. CT permeability images derived using Patlak analysis can markedly improve the visualization of tumor [57].

The high spatial resolution of functional CT makes the technique ideally suited to visualize and quantify physiological changes within areas of angiogenesis. By highlighting the area of most intense angiogenesis, high-resolution CT perfusion and permeability imaging can be used to guide percutaneous biopsy to the site of the most active tumor, reducing the chance of sampling error.

Magnetic Resonance Imaging

Magnetic resonance imaging (MRI) is potentially useful in estimating tumor angiogenesis and may prove superior to histological methods because it is noninvasive, can sample the entire tumor, can be repeated frequently, and reflects both the anatomy (vascular volume) and the physiology (permeability) of the tumor. In addition, MRI is capable of providing morphological information important in evaluating features such as parenchymal distortion, tumor border, pattern of enhancement, and homogeneity of enhancement [58] (Figure 17.4). Potentially, a combination of these morphological criteria and kinetic information could lead to improved cancer diagnosis and follow-up.

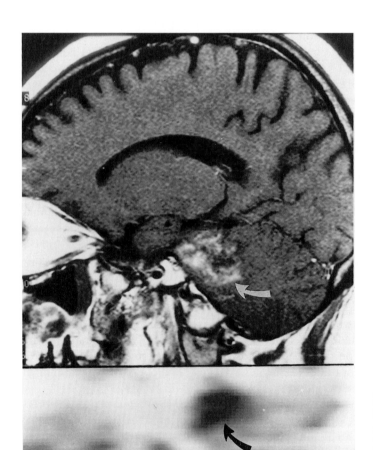

FIGURE 17.4. Sagittal T_1-weighted MR image (*top*) of the head near the midline following the injection of Gd-DTPA shows a heterogeneous contrast enhancement in the pons (*arrow*). Selected sagittal PET image (*bottom*) at the comparable level shows a moderately increased uptake of ^{18}F-FDG (*arrow*), indicating active malignant tumor. Biopsy confirmed a glioma.

MR Angiography

MR angiography (MRA) is a truly noninvasive imaging technique that requires no contrast agent. This technique has exploited the flow sensitivity of the MR signal and rapid scanning methods to obtain the images. However, its clinical application has been hampered by long acquisition times, sensitivity to motion artifacts, and limited spatial resolution. The introduction of contrast-enhanced rapid MRA has made this technique applicable for the macroscopic assessment of the vascular system supplying a tumor. Vessel diameters as small as 4 mm can be reliably imaged. Furthermore, multiphasic angiography allows a sequential imaging of the arterial and venous system [59].

In addition to morphological features, functional flow parameters can be determined by phase-contrast angiography [60]. Although this method is highly accurate, its clinical application is currently limited to vessels of 3 mm or larger.

Dynamic Contrast-Enhanced MRI

In addition to nonenhanced MRA, a variety of contrast-enhanced MRI and analytical techniques have been used for detection and characterization of tumors [58,61–64]. Microvascular density and permeability are the major factors that influence the detectable contrast enhancement pattern for a given tissue. Correlative MRI studies and histopathological analysis have shown this to be true for tumors [61–64] as well as normal tissues. Dynamic contrast-enhanced MRI can be used to estimate both vascularity and microvascular permeability.

Tumors with active angiogenesis enhance rapidly, with an early peak followed by subsequent contrast washout. A correlation exists between the rate of contrast enhancement and tumor MVD, indicating that tumor neovascularity plays an important role in the rapid early contrast enhancement of tumors and suggesting that the rate of contrast enhancement may

depend more on the density of tumor neovascularity than the inherent degree of malignancy of the tumor [58,65].

Although vascular density in malignant tumors is higher than in normal parenchyma, there is a great overlap with benign lesions. Vascular density is the major factor contributing to the overall intensity of enhancement, but the latter does not help for differential diagnosis. Therefore, the main diagnostic potential of MRI relies on its ability to detect differences in vascular permeability.

However, small molecular contrast media, either iodinated compounds or gadolinium chelates, are not well designed to measure the hyperpermeability of microvessels. The characteristic of hyperpermeability in malignant tissues has been shown repeatedly using macromolecular probes [66,67], but has not been shown for molecules smaller than 1000 daltons. Gadopentetate and similar small molecular contrast media quickly equilibrate between the intravascular and interstitial spaces. Due to this high vascular extraction rate, even in normal microvessels, small molecules have inherent disadvantages for estimating blood volume and abnormal capillary permeability, exclusive of central nervous system tissues [68–70]. This rapid and variable transcapillary exchange in normal tissues limits the potential to detect or measure hyperpermeability associated with neoplasms. Thus, only a modest dynamic range in permeability measures is possible using small molecular contrast media.

Because of the limitations of small molecular contrast agents, macromolecular contrast materials (MMCM) are being developed for both MRI and CT. These MMCM have molecular sizes that approximate those of serum proteins and are well suited to define the increased vascularity and permeability inherent to tumor microvasculature [71–73]. These large molecules diffuse very slowly, if at all, through normal endothelial barriers. Therefore, MMCMs recirculate in the blood for an hour or longer and can yield quantitative measurements of blood volume and permeability, expressed as the permeability-surface area product [68,74]. Recent studies in nude rats implanted with a human breast cancer line demonstrated that MMCM-enhanced MRI can be applied in living subjects to quantitatively document an acute reduction, within 24h, in tumor microvascular permeability in response to anti-VEGF antibody therapy [75].

In conclusion, dynamic contrast-enhanced MRI is proving to be a powerful tool to assess the spatial and temporal variations of tumor microcirculation [58,76,77]. Contrast-enhanced dynamic MRI uniquely enables the mapping of areas with high microcirculation in the entire tumor. Furthermore, contrast-enhanced MRI reflects the functionally active tumor parts that may better mirror angiogenic activity in terms of disease outcome.

Functional MRI

Presently, there is no single validated method that can sufficiently describe the functional status of tumor angiogenesis. Studies have shown that differences in tumor angiogenesis are correlated with different patterns of contrast enhancement observed by MRI [58,76–80]. The regenerated signal–time curves depend on the local microvessel density, regional blood flow, microvessel permeability for the contrast agent, and on the size and physiochemical nature of the extracellular space accessible for gadolinium-based contrast agents [78,79].

Intratumoral MVD is a characteristic of malignant tumors that also contains clinically relevant prognostic information that may guide treatment of the patient. Hawighorst et al. [81] examined the relationship between functional MRI-based parameters and established histomorphological markers of tumor angiogenesis (MVD and VEGF expression) in patients with cervical carcinoma. Results showed that areas with a high contrast enhancement coincided significantly with focal "hot spots" of MVD, especially in tumors with a rimlike pattern of enhancement. Although findings also showed that areas of high MVD and high microvessel permeability did not necessarily colocalize, MR imaging of microvascular permeability has been shown to correlate with histological tumor grade [82].

In conclusion, information about the tumor microvasculature can be obtained by functional MR imaging techniques [83]. Quantitative MRI methods developed in conjunction with suitable pharmacokinetic models allow detailed parameterization of contrast enhancement with respect to tumor microcirculation [78,79].

Pulsed Arterial Spin Labeling MRI

Pulsed arterial spin labeling MRI may be applicable to tumor perfusion imaging. Arterial spin tagging has been applied previously for the study of a number of organs, and particularly to the noninvasive mapping of brain, heart, and kidney perfusion [84–90]. Detailed analysis of this method has indicated a number of parameters that should be considered for accurate determination of perfusion, including T_1 relaxation of water within the artery between the position of labeling and the imaging slice, the degree of arterial labeling and off-resonance magnetization transfer due to the exchange of free water with water associated with macromolecules, and the extraction fraction of blood water [85,88,90].

Application of this approach for determination of cerebral perfusion by arterial spin labeling has been validated by correlation with the results of radioactive microsphere infusion [91]. It has also been shown that the technique can be used to follow vascular remodeling and angiogenesis during the ovarian cycle in the rat [92]. However, no studies have been reported for tumor perfusion.

Targeted MRI

MRI cannot always differentiate benign from malignant lesions. In an effort to overcome this problem, techniques are being developed to target contrast agents to specific tumor markers.

The expression of a particular angiogenesis marker, the endothelial integrin $\alpha_v\beta_3$, has been shown to correlate with tumor grade [93–95]. Because the degree of angiogenesis and $\alpha_v\beta_3$

expression may be predictive of malignant potential, MR imaging of $\alpha_v\beta_3$ may aid in distinguishing benign from aggressive lesions [15,95].

Recently, a novel approach to detecting angiogenesis in vivo using MRI and a paramagnetic contrast agent targeted to endothelial $\alpha_v\beta_3$ via the LM609 monoclonal antibody has been described [96]. This approach provided enhanced and detailed imaging of rabbit squamous cell carcinomas (V2) by directly targeting paramagnetic agents to the angiogenic vasculature. In addition, angiogenic "hot spots" not seen by standard MRI were detected. This strategy represents a noninvasive means to assess the growth and malignant phenotype of tumors.

MR Spectroscopy

MR spectroscopy can be used to assess indirectly tumor vasculature through the evaluation of tumor bioenergetics, pH status, and lactate levels with use of both phosphorus-31 and hydrogen-1 MR spectroscopic techniques [97,98].

References

1. Folkman J. Intratumoral microvascular density as a prognostic factor in cancer. Am J Pathol 1995;147:9–19.
2. Folkman J. The role of angiogenesis in tumor growth. Semin Cancer Biol 1992;3:65–71.
3. Folkman J. Clinical applications of research on angiogenesis. N Engl J Med 1995;333:1757–1763.
4. Folkman J. Introduction: angiogenesis and cancer. Semin Cancer Biol 1992;3:47–48.
5. Polverini PJ, Leibovich JS. Induction of neovascularization in vivo and endothelial proliferation in vitro by tumor-associated macrophages. Lab Invest 1984;51:635–642.
6. Azizkhan RG, Azizkhan JC, Zitter BR, et al. Mast cell heparin stimulates migration of capillary endothelial cells in vitro. J Exp Med 1980;152:931–944.
7. Ziche M, Morbidelli L, Donnini S. Angiogenesis. Exp Nephrol 1996;4:1–14.
8. Dameron K, Volpert O, Tainsky M, Bouck N. Control of angiogenesis in fibroblasts by p53 reg-

ulation of thrombospondin 1. Science 1994;265:1582–1584.
9. Weidner N. Tumor angiogenesis: review of current applications in tumor prognostication. Semin Diagn Pathol 1993;10:302–313.
10. Weinstat-Saslaw D, Steeg P. Angiogenesis and colonization in the tumor metastatic process: basic and applied advances. Fed Am Soc Exp Biol J 1994;8:401–407.
11. Jain R, Gerlowski L. Extravascular transport in normal and tumor tissues. Crit Rev Oncol Hematol 1984;5:115–170.
12. Brem S, Cotran R, Folkman J. Tumor angiogenesis: a quantitative method of histologic grading. J Natl Cancer Inst 1972;48:347–356.
13. Srivastava A, Laidler P, Davies R, et al. The prognostic significance of tumor vascularity in intermediate thickness (0.76–4.0 mm thick) skin melanoma: a quantitative histologic study. Am J Pathol 1988;133:419–423.
14. Weidner N. Intratumor microvessel density as a prognostic factor in cancer (comment). Am J Pathol 1995;147:9–19.
15. Weidner N, Semple JP, Welch WR, et al. Tumor angiogenesis and metastasis—correlation in invasive breast carcinoma. N Engl J Med 1991;324:1–8.
16. Gasparini G, Harris A. Clinical importance of the determination of tumor angiogenesis in breast carcinoma: much more than a new prognostic tool: review. J Clin Oncol 1995;13:765–782.
17. Kirkham BC, Tyson IB, Wirtanen GW. Comparison of ^{131}I-macroaggregated liver scanning in selective hepatic arteriography. J Nucl Med 1970;11:196–202.
18. Kaneko M, Sasaki T, Kido C. Positive scintigraphy of tumor by means of intra-arterial injection of radioiodinated macroaggregated albumin. AJR (Am J Roentgenol) 1968;102:81–87.
19. Blank RJ, Tyson IB. Intra-arterial ^{131}I-macroaggregated albumin to define intrahepatic tumors: a possible method of quantitating tumor response to therapy. J Nucl Med 1969;10:514–516.
20. Gyves JW, Ziessman HA, Ensminger WD, et al. Definition of hepatic tumor microcirculation by single photon emission computed tomography (SPECT). J Nucl Med 1984;25:972–977.
21. Perlman SB, Stone CK. Clinical positron emission tomography. In: Wilson MA, ed. Textbook of Nuclear Medicine. Philadelphia: Lippincott-Raven, 1998:331–351.
22. Piwnica-Worms D, Chiu ML, Budding M, et al. Functional imaging of multidrug-resistant P-

glycoprotein with an organotechnetium complex. Cancer Res 1993;53:977–984.

23. Scopinaro F, Schillaci O, Scarpina M, et al. Technetium-99m sestamibi: an indicator of breast cancer invasiveness. Eur J Nucl Med 1994;21:984–987.

24. Yoon JH, Bom HS, Song HC, et al. Double-phase Tc-99m sestamibi scintimammography to assess angiogenesis and p-glycoprotein expression in patients with untreated breast cancer. Clin Nucl Med 1999;5:314–318.

25. Omar WS, Eissa S, Moustafa H, et al. Role of thallium-201 chloride and Tc-99m methoxy-isobutyl-isonitrile (sestaMIBI) in evaluation of breast masses: correlation with the immuno-histochemical characteristic parmeters (Ki-67, PCNA, Bcl, and angiogenesis) in malignant lesions. Anticancer Res 1997;17:1639–1644.

26. Bom HS, Kim YC, Min JJ, et al. Tc-99m sestamibi uptake in small cell lung cancer. J Nucl Med 1998;39:91–94.

27. Mankoff DA, Dunnwald LK, Gralow JR, et al. Monitoring and predicting the response of breast cancer to neo-adjuvant chemotherapy using [Tc-99m] MIBI scintimammography. J Nucl Med 1997;38:46 (abstract).

28. Ciarmiello A, Del Vecchio S, Carriero MV, et al. Efflux rate of Tc-99m MIBI as a predictor of the outcome of therapy in patients with advanced breast carcinoma. J Nucl Med 1997;38:241 (abstract).

29. Zareneyrizi F, Yang DJ, Oh C-S, et al. Synthesis of Tc-99m ethylenedicysteine-colchicine for evaluation of antiangiogenic effect. Anti cancer Drugs (1999);10:685–692.

30. Yang DJ, Wallace S, Cherif A, et al. Development of F-18-labeled fluoroerythronitromidazole as a PET agent for imaging tumor hypoxia. Radiology 1995;194:795–800.

31. Cherif A, Wallace S, Yang DJ, et al. Development of new markers for hypoxic cells: [131I]iodomisonidazole and [131I]iodoerythroni-tromidazole. J Drug Targeting 1996;4:31–39.

32. Yang DJ, Ilgan S, Higuchi T, et al. Noninvasive assessment of tumor hypoxia with 99mTc labeled metronidazole. Pharm Res 1999;16:743–750.

33. Rubin JM, Bude RO, Carson PL, et al. Power Doppler US: a potentially useful alternative to mean-frequency-based color Doppler US. Radiology 1994;190:853–856.

34. Bude RO, Rubin JM, Adler RS. Power versus conventional color Doppler sonography: comparison in the depiction of normal intrarenal vasculature. Radiology 1995;192:777–780.

35. Newman JS, Adler RS, Bude RO, et al. Detection of soft-tissue hyperemia: value of power Doppler sonography. AJR (Am J Roentgenol) 1994;163: 385–389.

36. Dymling SO, Persson HW, Hertz CH. Measurement of blood perfusion in tissue using Doppler ultrasound. Ultrasound Med Biol 1991;17: 433–444.

37. Shung KK. Scattering of ultrasound by blood. IEEE Trans Biomed Eng 1976;23:460–467.

38. Shung KK. In vitro experimental results on ultrasonic scattering in biological tissues. In: Shung KK, Thieme GA, eds. Ultrasonic Scattering in Biological Tissues. Boca Raton: CRC Press, 1993:291–312.

39. Sahn DJ. Instrumentation and physical factors related to visualization of stenotic regurgitant jets by Doppler color flow mapping. Am Coll Cardiol 1988;12:1354–1365.

40. Simpson IA, Valdes-Cruz LM, Sonn DJ, et al. Doppler color flow mapping of simulated in vitro regurgitant jets: evaluation of the effects of orifice size and hemodynamic variables. Am Coll Cardiol 1989;13:1195–1207.

41. Jain SP, Fan PH, Philpot EF, et al. Influence of various instrument settings on the flow information derived from the power mode. Ultrasound Med Biol 1991;17:49–54.

42. Lee WJ, Chu JS, Hong SJ, et al. Breast cancer angiogenesis: a quantitative morphologic and Doppler imaging study. Ann Surg Oncol 1995;2: 246–251.

43. Huang SC, Yu CH, Huang RT, et al. Intratumoral blood flow in uterine myoma correlated with a lower tumor size and volume, but not correlated with cell proliferation or angiogenesis. Obstet Gynecol 1996;87:1019–1024.

44. Peters-Engl C, Medl M, Mirau M, et al. Color-coded and spectral Doppler flow in breast carcinomas—relationship with the tumor microvasculature. Breast Cancer Res Treat 1998;47:83–99.

45. Raza S, Baum JK. Solid breast lesions: evaluation with power Doppler US. Radiology 1997; 203:164–168.

46. Sahin Akyar G, Sumer H. Color Doppler ultrasound and spectral analysis of tumor vessels in the differential diagnosis of solid breast masses. Invest Radiol 1996;31:72–79.

47. Delorme S, Weisser G, Zuna I, et al. Quantitative characterization of color Doppler images: reproducibility, accuracy and limitations. J Clin Ultrasound 1995;23:537–550.

48. Fein M, Delorme S, Weisser G, et al. Quantification of color Doppler for the evaluation of tissue vascularization. Ultrasound Med Biol 1995;21: 1013–1019.

49. Bell DS, Bamber JC, Eckersley RJ. Segmentation and analysis of colour Doppler images of tumour vasculature. Ultrasound Med Biol 1995; 21:635–647.

50. Bude RO, Rubin JM. Power Doppler sonography. Radiology 1996;200:21–23.

51. Solbiati L, Goldberg SN, Ierace T, et al. Radio-frequency ablation of hepatic metastases: post-procedural assessment with a US microbubble contrast agent—early experience. Radiology 1999;211:643–649.

52. Hamberg LM, Hoop B, Hunter GJ, et al. Functional imaging with slip-ring CT and echo planar MRI: a preliminary report. Med Rev 1994;49: 10–19.

53. Miles KA, Hayball MP, Dixon AK. Functional imaging of changes in human intrarenal perfusion using quantitative dynamic computed tomography. Invest Radiol 1994;29:911–914.

54. Miles KA, Hayball MP, Dixon AK. Measurement of human pancreatic perfusion using dynamic computed tomography with perfusion imaging. Br J Radiol 1995;68:471–475.

55. Swensen SJ, Brown LR, Colby TV, et al. Lung nodule enhancement at CT: prospective findings. Radiology 1996;201:447–455.

56. Fukuya T, Honda H, Hayahi T, et al. Lymph-node metastases: efficacy of detection with helical CT in patients with gastric cancer. Radiology 1995; 197:705–711.

57. Leggett DAC, Miles KA, Kelley BB. Blood-brain barrier and blood volume imaging of cerebral glioma using functional CT: a pictorial review. Eur J Radiol 1999;30:185–190.

58. Buadu L, Murakami J, Murayama S, et al. Breast lesions: correlation of contrast medium enhancement patterns on MR images with histopathologic findings and tumor angiogenesis. Radiology 1996;200:639–649.

59. Goldfarb JW, Prasad PV, Li W, et al. Dynamic contrast-enhanced breath-hold 3D magnetic resonance abdominal angiography and renal perfusion. Proc ISMRM 1997;1:200 (abstract).

60. Schoenberg SO, Knopp MV, Bock M, et al. Renal artery stenosis: grading of hemodynamic changes with cine phase-contrast MR blood flow measurements. Radiology 1997;203:45–53.

61. Stomper P, Herman S, Kippenstein D, et al. Suspect lesions: findings at dynamic gadolinium-enhanced MRI correlated with mammographic and pathologic features. Radiology 1995;197: 387–395.

62. Griebel J, Mayr NA, de Vries A, et al. Assessment of tumor microcirculation: a new role of dynamic contrast MR imaging. J Magn Reson Imaging 1997;7:111–119.

63. Hawighorst H, Engenhart R, Knopp MV, et al. Intracranial meningiomas: time- and dose-dependent effects of irradiation on tumor microcirculation by dynamic MR imaging. Magn Reson Med 1997;15:423–432.

64. Hawighorst H, Knapstein PG, Schaeffer U, et al. Pelvic lesions in patients with treated cervical carcinoma; efficacy of pharmacokinetic analysis of dynamic MR images in distinguishing recurrent tumors from benign conditions. AJR (Am J Roentgenol) 1996;166:401–408.

65. Frouge C, Guinebretiere J, Contesso G, et al. Correlation between contrast enhancement in dynamic magnetic resonance imaging of the breast and tumor angiogenesis. Invest Radiol 1994;29:1043–1049.

66. Jain RK. Transport of molecules across tumor vasculature. Cancer Metasis Rev 1987;6:559–593.

67. Gerlowski LE, Jain RK. Microvascular permeability of normal and neoplastic tissues. Microvasc Res 1986;31:288–305.

68. Schwickert H, Stiskal M, van Dijke C, et al. Tumor angiography using high resolution 3D MRI: comparison of Gd-DTPA and a macromolecular blood pool contrast agent. Acad Radiol 1995;2:851–858.

69. Weinmann H, Laniado M, Mutzel W. Pharmacokinetics of DTPA/dimeglumine after intravenous injection into healthy volunteers. Physiol Chem Phys Med NMR 1984;16:167–172.

70. Schmiedl U, Moseley ME, Ogan MD, et al. Comparison of initial biodistribution patterns of Gd-DTPA and albumin-Gd-DTPA using rapid spin echo imaging. J Comp Assist Tomogr 1987;11: 306–313.

71. van Dijke C, Brasch R, Roberts T, et al. Mammary carcinoma model: correlation of macromolecular contrast enhanced MR imaging characterizations of tumor microvasculature and histologic capillary density. Radiology 1996;198: 813–818.

72. Schwickert H, Stiskal M, Roberts T, et al. Contrast-enhanced MRI assessment of tumor capillary permeability: the effect of pre-irradiation on the tumor delivery of chemotherapy. Radiology 1996;198:893–898.

73. Cohen F, Kuwatsuru R, Shames D, et al. Contrast enhanced MRI estimation of altered capillary

permeability in experimental mammary carcinomas following x-radiation. Invest Radiol 1995; 29:970–977.

74. Kuwatsuru R, Shames D, Mühler A, et al. Quantification of tissue plasma volume in the rat by contrast-enhanced magnetic resonance imaging. Magn Reson Med 1993;30:76–81.

75. Brasch R, Pham C, Shames D, et al. Assessing tumor angiogenesis using macromolecular MR imaging contrast media. J Magn Reson Imaging 1997;7:68–74.

76. Verstraete KL, De-Deene YD, Roels H, et al. Benign and malignant musculoskeletal lesions: dynamic contrast-enhanced MR imaging: parametric first-pass images depict tissue vascularization and perfusion. Radiology 1994;192: 835–843.

77. Degani H, Gussi V, Weinstein D, et al. Mapping pathophysiological features of breast tumors by MRI at high spatial resolution. Nat Med 1997;3: 780–782.

78. Hoffmann U, Brix G, Knopp MV, et al. Pharmacokinetic mapping of the breast: a new method for dynamic MR-mammography. Magn Reson Med 1995;33:506–514.

79. Brix G, Semmler W, Port R, et al. Pharmacokinetic parameters in CNS Gd-DTPA enhanced MR imaging. J Comput Assist Tomogr 1991;15: 621–627.

80. Takashima S, Noguchi Y, Okumara T, et al. Dynamic MR imaging in the head and neck. Radiology 1993;189:813–821.

81. Hawighorst H, Weikel W, Knapstein PG, et al. Angiogenic activity of cervical carcinoma: assessment by functional magnetic resonance imaging-based parameters and a histomorphological approach in correlation with disease outcome. Clin Cancer Res 1998;4:2305–2312.

82. Brasch RC, Daldrup H, Shames D, et al. Macromolecular contrast media-enhanced MRI estimates of microvascular permeability correlate with histopathologic tumor grade. Acad Radiol 1998;5(suppl 1):S2–S5.

83. Passe TJ, Bluemke DA, Siegelman SS. Tumor angiogenesis: tutorial on implications for imaging. Radiology 1997;203:593–600.

84. Roberts DA, Detre JA, Bolinger L, et al. Renal perfusion in humans: MR imaging with spin tagging of arterial water. Radiology 1995;196: 281–286.

85. Silva AC, Zhang W, Williams DS, et al. Estimation of water extraction fractions in rat brain using magnetic resonance measurement of perfusion with arterial spin labeling. Magn Reson Med 1997;35:58–68.

86. Roberts DA, Rizi R, Lenkinski RE, et al. Magnetic resonance imaging of the brain: blood partition coefficient for water: application to spin-tagging measurement of perfusion. J Magn Reson Imaging 1996;6:363–366.

87. Pekar J, Jezzard P, Roberts DA, et al. Perfusion imaging with compensation for asymmetric magnetization transfer effects. Magn Reson Med 1996;35:70–79.

88. Zhang W, Silva AC, Williams DS, et al. NMR measurement of perfusion using arterial spin labeling without saturation of macromolecular spins. Magn Reson Med 1995;33:370–376.

89. McLaughlin AC, Ye FQ, Pekar JJ, et al. Effects of magnetization transfer on the measurement of cerebral blood flow using steady-state arterial spin tagging approaches; a theoretical investigation. Magn Reson Med 1997;37:501–510.

90. Williams DS, Grandis DJ, Zhang W, et al. Magnetic resonance imaging of perfusion in the isolated rat heart using spin inversion of arterial water. Magn Reson Med 1993;30:361–365.

91. Walsh EG, Minematsu K, Leppo J, et al. Radioactive microsphere validation of a volume localized continuous saturation perfusion measurement. Magn Reson Med 1994;31:147–153.

92. Tempel C, Neeman M. Perfusion of the rat ovary: application of pulsed arterial spin labeling MRI. Magn Reson Med 1999;41:113–123.

93. Brooks PC, Clark RAF, Cheresh DA. Requirement of vascular integrin $\alpha_v\beta_3$ for angiogenesis. Science 1994;264:569–571.

94. Brooks PC, Stromblad S, Klemke R, et al. Antiintegrin alpha v beta 3 blocks human breast cancer growth and angiogenesis in human skin. J Clin Invest 1995;96:1815–1822.

95. Gladson CL. Expression of integrin $\alpha_v\beta_3$ in small blood vessels of glioblastoma tumors. J Neuropathol Exp Neurol 1996;55:1143–1149.

96. Sipkins DA, Cheresh DA, Kazemi MR, et al. Detection of tumor angiogenesis in vivo by $\alpha_v\beta_3$-targeted magnetic resonance imaging. Nat Med 1998;4:623–626.

97. Castillo M, Kwock L, Mukherji S. Clinical applications of proton MR spectroscopy. Am J Neuro-Radiol 1996;17:1–15.

98. Kaplan O, Cohen J. Metabolism of breast cancer cells as revealed by non-invasive magnetic resonance spectroscopy studies. Breast Cancer Res Treat 1994;31:285–299.

18
Imaging of Apoptosis and Hypoxia

David J. Yang and E. Edmund Kim

Tumor cells are more sensitive to conventional irradiation in the presence of oxygen than in its absence; even a small percentage of hypoxic cells within a tumor could limit the response to radiation [1–4]. Hypoxic radioresistance has been demonstrated in many animal tumors but only in a few tumor types in humans [5–9]. The occurrence of hypoxia in human tumors has, in most cases, been inferred from histological findings and from animal tumor studies. In vivo demonstration of hypoxia has required tissue measurements with oxygen electrodes, and the invasiveness of these techniques has limited their clinical application. Additionally, this technique can only be used on accessible tumors such as head and neck tumor. Many attempts to increase the radiosensitivity of tumors by administration of chemical radiosensitizers have not been successful [10–14].

Misonidazole (MISO) is a hypoxic cell sensitizer, and labeling MISO with different halogenated radioisotopes (e.g., ^{18}F, ^{123}I, ^{99m}Tc) may be useful for differentiating a hypoxic but metabolically active tumor from a well-oxygenated active tumor by positron emission tomography (PET) or planar scintigraphy. Moreover, the assessment of tumor hypoxia with labeled MISO would provide a rational means of selecting patients for treatment with radiosensitizing or bioreducing drugs (e.g., mitomycin C). Such selection would permit more accurate evaluation of patients for cost-effective management.

[^{18}F]fluoromisonidazole (FMISO) has been used with PET to evaluate tumor hypoxia. Recent studies have shown that PET, with its ability to monitor cell oxygen content through [^{18}F]FMISO, has a high potential to predict tumor response to radiation [15–20]. PET gets a higher resolution without collimation; however, the cost of using PET isotopes in a clinical setting is prohibitive. Although labeling MISO with iodine was the choice because of chemical similarity to [^{18}F]FMISO, high uptake in thyroid tissue was observed [21]. Therefore, it is desirable to develop compounds for planar scintigraphy such that the isotope costs are less expensive than PET and can be used clinically in most medical facilities. Because of its favorable physical characteristics as well as its extremely low price, ^{99m}Tc has been preferred to label radiopharmaceuticals. Several nitroimidazole analogues have been labeled with ^{99m}Tc using nitrogen and sulfur chelates [22–25]; however, the synthetic route involves several steps. Metronidazole (MN), a known hypoxic marker, has been used to treat trichomoniasis [26] and was chosen for its structural similarity to nitroimidazole. To demonstrate its diagnostic potential in hypoxic tissue detection, we have imaged patients with stroke.

Apoptosis, programmed cell death, is a natural, orderly, energy-dependent process that causes cells to die without inducing an inflammatory response. Apoptosis is triggered either by a decrease in factors required to maintain the cell in good health or by an increase in factors that cause damage to the cell. When these factors tilt in the direction of death and the cell has sufficient time to respond, a common proteolytic cascade involving cysteine aspartic acid-specific proteases (caspases) is activated to initiate apoptosis. As caspase members have been identified as effectors of apoptosis, the role of CPP32/caspase-3 in hypoxia was explored. The findings emphasize the critical role of caspase-3 in tissue injury consecutive to hypoxia [27–29]. Recent studies have shown that hypoxia induces cell apoptosis in various diseases [30–32]. The mechanisms of hypoxia-induced endothelial cell death and role of p53 and bcl-2 in apoptosis have been well documented [30–33].

Cells that die by apoptosis autodigest their DNA and nuclear proteins, change the phospholipid composition on the outer surface of their cell membrane, and form lipid-enclosed vesicles, which contain noxious intracellular contents, organelles, autodigested cytoplasm, and DNA. The compositional cell membrane phospholipid change that occurs with the onset of apoptosis is marked by the sudden expression of phosphatidylserine (PS), a phospholipid that ordinarily appears on the inner leaflet of the membrane, on the external leaflet of the membrane. The constant exposure of PS during apoptosis makes it an attractive target for radiopharmaceutical imaging [34]. Imaging apoptosis was achieved by ultrasound [35], confocal laser scanning microscopy [36], and a fluorescent probe [37]. There is a need to use a radiolabeled technique to image in vivo real time apoptosis because of the sensitivity, specificity, accessibility, and the cost compared to these techniques.

Assessment of apoptosis would be useful to evaluate the efficacy of therapy such as disease progression or regression. Annexin V, an endogenous human protein, has a high affinity (kd = 7nmol/l) for phosphotidylserine (PS) bound to the cell membrane [38,39]. Fluorescence-labeled annexin V is used for histological and cell-sorting studies to identify apoptotic cells. In vivo detection of apoptosis using ^{99m}Tc-HYNIC annexin V has been reported [40]. However, this labeling process requires two additional chemicals (tricine and triphenylphosphine), which is inconvenient. ^{99m}Tc-L,L-ethylenedicysteine (^{99m}Tc-EC) is the most recent and successful example of N_2S_2 chelates [40–43]. EC, a new renal imaging agent,

can be labeled with ^{99m}Tc easily and efficiently with high radiochemical purity and stability and is excreted through the kidney by active tubular transport [40–48]. We have developed an ethylenedicysteine (EC)-annexin V conjugate, which is stable and easy to label with ^{99m}Tc.

Synthesis of L,L-Ethylenedicysteine

The mass spectral analysis was conducted at the University of Texas Health Science Center (Houston, TX, USA). Nuclear magnetic resonance (NMR) spectra were recorded on a Bruker-300 spectrometer. The mass data were obtained by fast atom bombardment on a Kratos MS 50 instrument (England). N-Hydroxysulfosuccinimide (sulfo-NHS) and 1-ethyl-3-(3-dimethylaminopropyl) carbodiimide-HCl (EDC) were purchased from Pierce Chemical (Radford, IL, USA). All other chemicals were purchased from Aldrich Chemical (Milwaukee, WI, USA). Silica gel coated thin-layer chromatography (TLC) plates were purchased from Whatman (Clifton, NJ, USA). ^{99m}Tc-pertechnetate was obtained from a commercial ^{99}Mo/^{99m}Tc generator (Ultratechnekow FM™; Mallinckrodt Diagnostica, Holland).

EC was prepared in a two-step synthesis according to the previously described methods [49,50]. The precursor, L-thiazolidine-4-carboxylic acid, was synthesized (m.p. 195°, reported 196°–197°). EC was then prepared (m.p. 243°C, reported 251°C).

Radiolabeling of EC-MN and EC with ^{99m}Tc

The amino analogue of metronidazole (MN) was synthesized in a three-step manner according to the previously described methods [51]. The structure was confirmed by ^{1}H-NMR and fast-atom bombardment mass spectroscopy (FAB-MS). Synthesis of ethylenedicysteine-metronidazole (EC-MN) and radiosynthesis of ^{99m}Tc-EC-MN were achieved according to our previously reported method [52]. Radiochemical purity was determined by TLC (ITLC SG; Gelman Sciences, Ann Arbor, MI, USA) eluted with, respectively, acetone (system A) and ammonium acetate (1M in water):methanol (4:1) (system B). From radio-TLC (Bioscan, Washington, DC, USA) analysis, the radio-chemical purity was greater than 95%. Stability assay was tested in serum samples. Briefly, 740 KBq of 1mg ^{99m}Tc-EC-MN was incubated in dog serum (200μl) at 37°C for 4h. The serum samples were diluted with 50% methanol in water and radio-TLC repeated at 0.5 to 4h.

Oxygen Microelectrode pO$_2$ Measurements in Tumor-Bearing Rats

To confirm tumor hypoxia detected by imaging, intratumoral pO$_2$ measurements were performed using the Eppendorf computerized histographic system. Twenty to 25 pO$_2$ measurements along each of two to three linear tracks were performed at 0.4-mm intervals on each tumor (40–75 measurements in total). Tumor pO$_2$ measurements were made on three tumor-bearing rats. Using an online computer system, the pO$_2$ measurements of each track were expressed as absolute values relate to the location of the measuring point along the track, and as the relate frequencies within a pO$_2$ histogram between 0 and 100mmHg with a class width of 2.5mm.

Intratumoral pO$_2$ measurements of tumors indicated the tumor oxygen tension range was 4.6±1.4mmHg as compared to normal muscle, 35±10mmHg. The data indicate that the tumors are hypoxic.

Imaging Apoptosis and Hypoxia

Imaging Apoptosis

Synthesis of EC-annexin V (EC-ANNEX)

Sodium bicarbonate (1N, 1ml) was added to a stirred solution of EC (5mg, 0.019mmol). To this colorless solution, sulfo-NHS (4mg, 0.019mmol) and EDC (4mg, 0.019mmol) were added. Annexin V (M.W. 33kDa, human; Sigma)

(0.3mg) was then added. The mixture was stirred at room temperature for 24h. The mixture was dialyzed for 48h with cutoff at M.W.10,000. After dialysis, the product was frozen dried; the product in salt form weighed 12mg.

Radiolabeling of EC-ANNEX with ^{99m}Tc

Radiosynthesis of ^{99m}Tc-EC-ANNEX was achieved by adding the required amount of ^{99m}Tc-pertechnetate into EC-ANNEX (3mg) and SnCl$_2$ (100μg). The mixture was loaded on a Sephadex gel column (PD-10, G-25; Pharmacia Biotech, Switzerland) and eluted with phosphate-buffered saline (pH 7.4); 1ml of each fraction was collected. The product was collected at fraction 3 as evidenced by radio-TLC using the same solvent as described in ^{99m}Tc-EC-MN. After column purification, the product yield was 65%.

Imaging Tumor Apoptotic Cells

To demonstrate the different uptake in various tumors, three animal models were selected: breast, ovarian, and sarcoma tumor-bearing rodents. Both breast and ovarian tumor-bearing rodents are considered to be highly apoptotic animal models whereas sarcoma tumor-bearing rodents are a low apoptotic animal model [53–59]. Scintigraphic images were obtained 0.5 to 4h after i.v. injection of 100 to 300mCi of ^{99m}Tc-EC-annexin V to tumor-bearing rodents.

^{99m}Tc-EC-ANNEX was found to be stable at 0.5 to 4h in dog serum samples. There were no degradation products observed. Scintigraphic images obtained at different time points showed visualization of tumor in ^{99m}Tc-EC-ANNEX group (Figures 18.1–18.3). The images indicated that highly apoptotic tumor-bearing animal models have more uptake of ^{99m}Tc-EC-ANNEX compared to sarcoma tumor-bearing rodents (a low apoptotic animal model).

Imaging Tumor Hypoxia and Hypoxic Tissue

Scintigraphic images, using a gamma camera (Siemens Medical Systems, Hoffman Estates, IL, USA) equipped with a low-energy, parallel-hole collimator, were obtained 0.5 to 4h after i.v. injection of 100mCi of ^{99m}Tc-EC-MN to

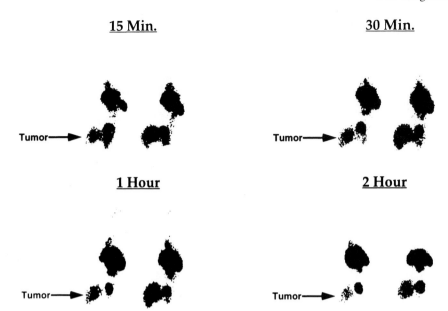

FIGURE 18.1. Planar images of breast tumor-bearing rats following administration of ^{99m}Tc-EC-annexin V (300mCi/rat, i.v.) show that tumor uptake could be visualized after 15min to 2h.

tumor-bearing rats. Whole-body autoradiogram was obtained by a quantitative image analyzer (Cyclone Storage Phosphor System; Packard, Meridian, CT, USA). Following i.v. injection of 100mCi of ^{99m}Tc-EC-MN, each animal was killed at 1h and the body was fixed in carboxymethyl cellulose (4%). The frozen body was mounted onto a cryostat (LKB 2250 cry-

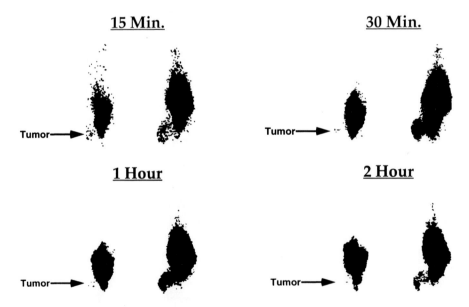

FIGURE 18.2. Planar images of ovarian (OCA-1) tumor-bearing mice after administration of ^{99m}Tc-EC (*left*) and ^{99m}Tc-EC-annexin V (*right*) (100mCi/ mouse, i.v.) demonstrate that the tumor could be visualized 15min post injection with ^{99m}Tc-EC-annexin V.

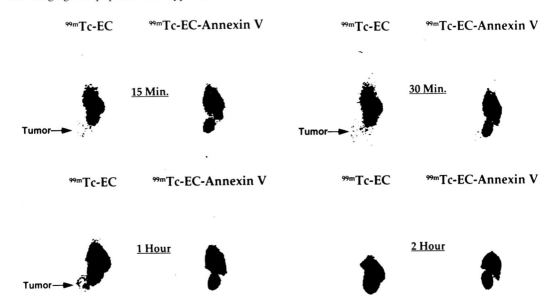

FIGURE 18.3. Planar images of sarcoma-bearing mice (low apoptosis) after administration of ^{99m}Tc-EC and ^{99m}Tc-EC-annexin V (100 mCi/mouse, i.v.) indicate that tumor uptake was low with both tracers.

omicrotome) and cut into 100-μm coronal sections. Each section was thawed and mounted on a slide. The slide was then placed in contact with a multipurpose phosphor storage screen and exposed for 15 h.

Scintigraphic and autoradiographic images of tumor-bearing rodents obtained at 1 h showed visualization of tumor in ^{99m}Tc-EC-MN (Figures 18.4, 18.5) whereas EC (control) had less uptake in the tumor (Figure 18.4).

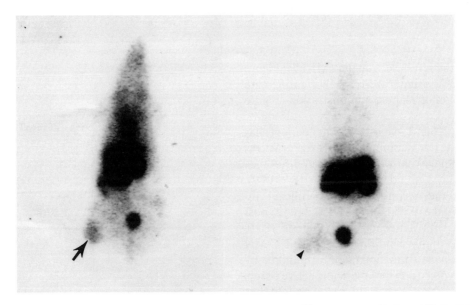

FIGURE 18.4. Selected scintigraphic images (*ventral view*) of a rat with a subcutaneous breast tumor in the right hind leg at 1 h following intravenous admin- istration of ^{99m}Tc-EC-MN (*left*) and ^{99m}Tc-EC (*right*) show very minimal radiotracer uptake (*arrowheads*) in the tumor area with ^{99m}Tc-EC.

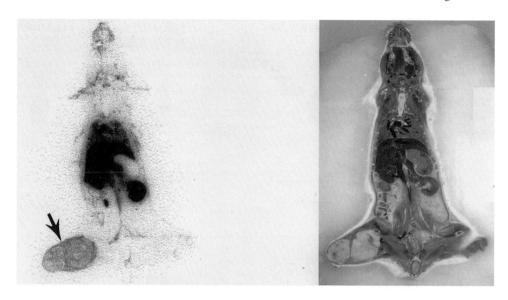

FIGURE 18.5. Whole-body autoradiogram (coronal section) obtained 1 h after intravenous injection of ^{99m}Tc-EC-MN demonstrated tumor (*arrow*) activity. A corresponding photo image is on the *right*.

To image hypoxic tissue, in clinical studies, we decide to image patients with stroke because the tissue at stroke area is hypoxic. Each patient with brain infarction was administered ^{99m}Tc-EC-MN (i.v., 30–40 mCi), and planar and SPECT images were acquired at 1 to 3 h post administration. The images were compared to CT and MRI findings.

Four selected cases are presented.

Case 1. This 59-year-old male patient has stroke in the left basal ganglia (MRI T_1; Figure 18.6). SPECT using ^{99m}Tc-EC-MN identified the stroke lesion at 1 h post administration (Figure 18.7).

Case 2. This 73-year-old male patient has stroke in the left medium cerebral artery (MCA) area. CT images showed no marked difference between day 1 and day 12 (Figures 18.8, 18.9). However, the lesions showed significant increased uptake of ^{99m}Tc-EC-MN at day 12 (post treatment with anticoagulant) (Figures 18.10, 18.11). The findings indicate that ^{99m}Tc-EC-MN could provide functional information by imaging hypoxic and metabolically active tissue.

Case 3. This 72-year-old male patient has stroke in the right MCA and PCA area. CT images exaggerate the lesion size (Figure 18.12) when compared to SPECT ^{99m}Tc-EC-MN (1 h post administration) (Figure 18.13).

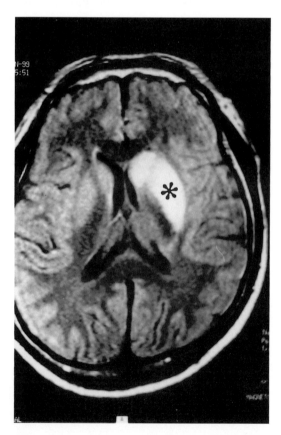

FIGURE 18.6. Case 1. This 59-year-old male patient had a stroke in the left basal ganglia with high signal intensity on T_1-weighted image, indicating hemorrhage(*).

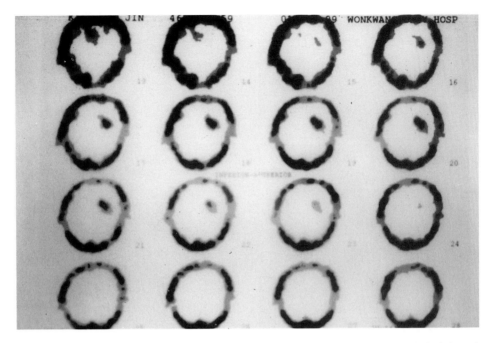

FIGURE 18.7. SPECT ^{99m}Tc-EC-MN of case 1 identified the stroke lesion at 1 h post administration.

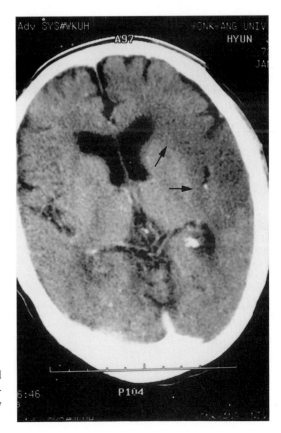

FIGURE 18.8. Case 2. This 73-year-old male patient had a stroke in the left middle cerebral artery (MCA) distribution. This figure shows CT image of low-density lesion (*arrows*) between day 1 and day 12.

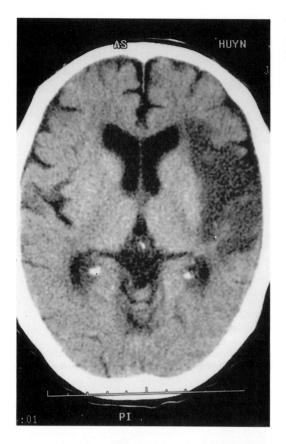

FIGURES 18.9. CT image of low-density lesion of patient shown in Figure 18.8 on day 12. Note that there is no marked difference.

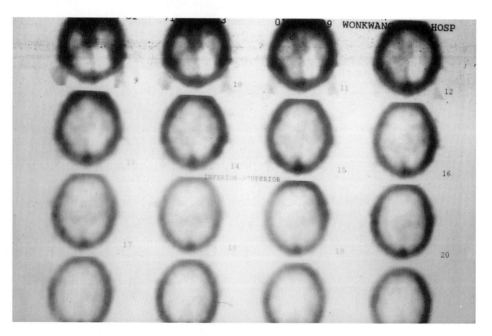

FIGURES 18.10. Figure shows significantly increasing uptake of ^{99m}Tc-EC-MN on day 1, for the lesions shown in Case 2, to day 12.

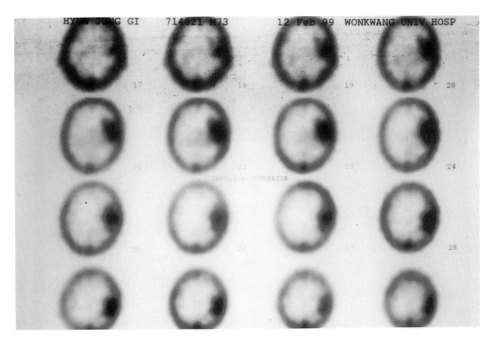

FIGURES 18.11. The same patient as in Figure 18.10 on day 12. Note significant increasing uptake of ^{99m}Tc-EC-NN (post-treatment with anticoagulant). The findings suggest that ^{99m}Tc-EC-MN could provide functional information by imaging hypoxic and metabolically active tissue.

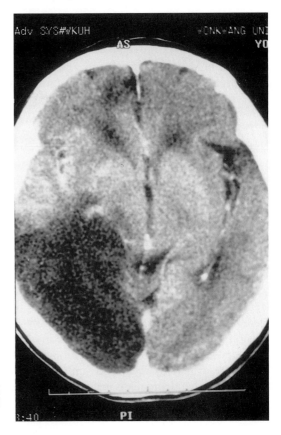

FIGURE 18.12. Case 3. This 72-year-old male patient had a stroke in the right middle and posterior cerebral artery distribution with a low density on CT.

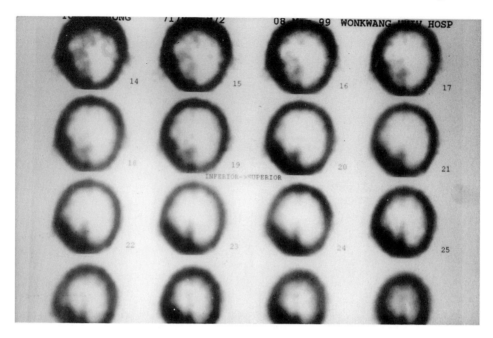

FIGURE 18.13. Compared to SPECT, a small area of ^{99m}Tc-EC-MN (1 h post administration) uptake on CT images exaggerates the lesion size (see Figure 18.12).

Case 4. A 59-year-old male patient with brain infarction (left). Planar whole-body image of ^{99m}Tc-EC-MN were obtained at 1 h post administration. Less uptake in thyroid and stomach was observed, suggesting the in vivo stability of ^{99m}Tc-EC-MN (Figure 18.14).

The development of new tumor hypoxia agents is clinically desirable for detecting primary and metastatic lesions as well as for predicting radioresponsiveness and time to recurrence. None of the contemporary imaging modalities accurately measures hypoxia because the diagnosis of tumor hypoxia requires pathological examination. It is often difficult to predict the outcome of a therapy for hypoxic tumor without knowing at least the baseline of hypoxia in each tumor treated. Although the Eppendorf polarographic oxygen microelectrode can measure the oxygen tension in a tumor, this technique is invasive and needs a skillful operator. Additionally, this technique can only be used on accessible tumors (e.g., head and neck, cervical), and multiple readings are needed. Therefore, an accurate and easy method of measuring tumor

hypoxia will be useful for patient selection. However, tumor to normal tissue uptake ratios varies depend upon the radiopharmaceuticals used. Therefore, it would be rational to correlate tumor to normal tissue uptake ratio with the gold standard Eppendorf electrode measures of hypoxia when new radiopharmaceuticals are introduced to clinical practice.

[^{18}F]FMISO has been used to diagnose head and neck tumors, myocardial infarction, inflammation, and brain ischemia. Tumor to normal tissue uptake ratio was used as a baseline to assess tumor hypoxia. Although tumor hypoxia using [^{18}F]FMISO was clearly demonstrated, introducing new imaging agents into clinical practice depends on other factors such as easy availability and cost. For reasons of better imaging characteristics and lower price, attempts are made to replace the ^{123}I-, ^{131}I-, ^{67}Ga-, and ^{111}In-labeled compounds with corresponding ^{99m}Tc-labeled compounds when possible. EC can be labeled with ^{99m}Tc very easily and efficiently at room temperature with high radiochemical purity and the preparation remains stable. Because of reported labeling capacity and rapid renal

FIGURE 18.14.   Case 4. A 59-year-old male patient had a left cerebral infarction. Planar whole-body images of ^{99m}Tc-EC-MN (*left*) and spot views of head (*right*) obtained at 1h post administration show abnormally increased activity in the left brain. Less uptake in thyroid and stomach was observed, suggesting the in vivo stability of ^{99m}Tc-EC-MN.

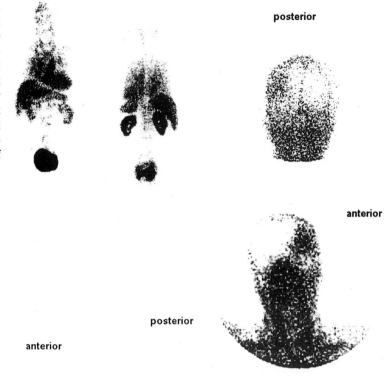

clearance, EC was selected to synthesize a new ^{99m}Tc-labeled metronidazole. EC-MN was prepared using a relatively simple and fast chemistry.

Scintigraphic images obtained at different time points showed visualization of tumor in the ^{99m}Tc-EC-MN-injected group. In the same animal model, ^{99m}Tc-EC-ANNEX also showed visualization of tumor, suggesting the area of tumor hypoxia and apoptosis may be overlapped. Further studies using microautoradiographic technique to demonstrate the distribution difference between hypoxic marker and apoptotic marker would be necessary. An animal model with high apoptotic tumor cells has more ^{99m}Tc-EC-ANNEX uptake than a low apoptotic tumor model. The findings support further studies on therapeutic efficiency evaluation using this marker. The apoptotic process could occur in the early stage (4–24h) after chemotherapy and radiation therapy [53,58]; therefore, proper timing is necessary to image apoptosis.

To image stroke patients, ^{99m}Tc-EC-MN seems to map the lesion area more accurately than CT and MRI. Because ^{99m}Tc-EC-MN could detect hypoxic tissue, it may be useful for follow-up of treatment response.

Conclusion

^{99m}Tc-EC-ANNEX and ^{99m}Tc-EC-MN were developed to assess tumor hypoxia and apoptosis. Due to easier chemistry, cost-effectiveness of the isotope, reasonable tumor-to-tissue uptake ratios, and SPECT imaging potential, ^{99m}Tc-EC-ANNEX and ^{99m}Tc-EC-MN could possibly be used to evaluate tumor response to radiotherapy, chemotherapy, and time of tumor recurrence.

References

1. Hall EJ. The oxygen effect and reoxygenation. In: Hall EJ, ed. Radiobiology for the Radiobiologist. Philadelphia: Lippincott, 1988:137–160.

2. Bush RS, Jenkins RDT, Allt WEC, et al. Definite evidence for hypoxic cells influencing cure in cancer therapy. Br J Cancer 1978;37:302–306.

3. Hohman WF, Palcic B, Skarsgard LD. The effect of nitroimidazole and nitroxyl radiosensitizers on the post-irradiation synthesis of DNA. Int J Radiat Biol Relat Stud Phys Chem Med 1976; 30:247–261.

4. Gray LH, Conger AD, Elbert M. The concentration of oxygen dissolved in tissues at the time of irradiation as a factor in radiotherapy. Br J Radiol 1953;26:638–648.

5. Dische S. A review of hypoxic-cell radiosensitization. Int J Radiat Oncol Biol Phys 1991; 20:147–152.

6. Gray LH, Conger AD, Ebert M, et al. The concentration of oxygen dissolved in tissue at the time of irradiation as a factor in radiotherapy. Br J Cancer 1953;26:638–642.

7. Dische S, Gray AJ, Zanelli GD. Clinical testing of the radiosensitizer Ro-07-0582. II. Radiosensitization of normal and hypoxic skin. Clin Radiol 1976;27:159–166.

8. Gatenby RA, Kessler HB, Rosenblum JS, et al. Oxygen distribution in squamous cell carcinoma metastases and its relationship to outcome of radiation therapy. Int J Radiat Oncol Biol Phys 1988;14:831–838.

9. Nordsmark M, Overgaard M, Overgaard J. Pretreatment oxygenation predicts radiation response in advanced squamous cell carcinoma of the head and neck. Radiother Oncol 1996; 41:31–39.

10. Martin FD, Porter EA, Fischer JJ, et al. Effect of a perfluorochemical emulsion on the radiation response of BA1112 rhabdomyosarcomas. Radiat Res 1987;112:45–53.

11. Martin DF, Porter EA, Rockwell S, et al. Enhancement of tumor radiation response by the combination of a perfluorochemical emulsion and hyperbaric oxygen. Int J Radiat Oncol Biol Phys 1987;13:747–751.

12. Peters LJ, Withers HR, Thames HD, et al. Keynote address—The problem: tumor radioresistance in clinical radiotherapy. Int J Radiat Oncol Biol Phys 1982;8:101–108.

13. Phillips TL. Chemical modification of radiation effects. Cancer (Phila) 1977;39:987–998.

14. Mohindra JK, Rauth AM. Increased cell killing by metronidazole and nitrofurazone of hypoxic compared to aerobic mammalian cells. Cancer Res 1976;36:930–936.

15. Koh W-J, Rasey JS, Evans ML, et al. Imaging of hypoxia in human tumors with [18F]fluoromisonidazole. Int J Radiat Oncol Biol Phys 1992;22:199–212.

16. Valk PET, Mathis CA, Prados MD, et al. Hypoxia in human gliomas: demonstration by PET with [18F]fluoromisonidazole. J Nucl Med 1992;33: 2133–2137.

17. Martin GV, Caldwell JH, Rasey JS, et al. Enhanced binding of the hypoxic cell marker [18F]fluoromisonidazole in ischemic myocardium. J Nucl Med 1989;30:194–201.

18. Rasey JS, Koh WJ, Grieson JR, et al. Radiolabeled fluoromisonidazole as an imaging agent for tumor hypoxia. Int J Radiat Oncol Biol Phys 1989;17:985–991.

19. Rasey JS, Nelson NJ, Chin L, et al. Characterization of the binding of labeled fluoromisonidazole in cells in vitro. Radiat Res 1990;122:301–308.

20. Yang DJ, Wallace S, Cherif A, et al. Development of F-18-labeled fluoroerythronitroimidazole as a PET agent for imaging tumor hypoxia. Radiology 1995;194:795–800.

21. Cherif A, Wallace S, Yang DJ, et al. Development of new markers for hypoxic cells: [131I]iodomisonidazole and [131I]iodoerythronitroimidazole. J Drug Targeting 1996;4:31–39.

22. Johnson G, Nguyen KN, Lui Z, et al. HL91 Technetium-99m: a potential new marker of myocardial viability assessed by nuclear imaging early after reperfusion. J Nucl Cardiol 1998; 5:285–294.

23. Fukuchi K, Kusuoka H, Yutani K, et al. Assessment of reperfused myocardium using new hypoxia avid imaging agent 99mTc-HL91. J Nucl Med 1996;37:94P.

24. Melo T, Duncan J, Ballinger JR, et al. BMS 194796, a second generation 99mTc labeled 2-nitroimidazole for imaging hypoxia in tumors. J Nucl Med 1998;39:219P.

25. Zhang X, Melo T, Ballinger JR, et al. Evaluation of 99mTc-butyleneamino oxime (BnAO), a non-nitroaromatic agent for imaging hypoxia in tumors. J Nucl Med 1998;39:216P.

26. Foster JL, Conroy PJ, Searle AJ, et al. Metronidazole (Flagyl): characterization as a cytotoxic drug specific for hypoxic tumour cells. Br J Cancer 1976;33(5):485–490.

27. Bossenmeyer-Pourie C, Koziel V, Daval J. CPP32/CASPASE-3-like proteases in hypoxia-induced apoptosis in developing brain neurons. Brain Res Mol Brain Res 1999;71:225–237.

28. Banasiak KJ, Cronin T, Haddad GG. bcl-2 prolongs neuronal survival during hypoxia-induced apoptosis. Brain Res Mol Brain Res 1999;72: 214–225.

29. Chen EY, Fujinaga M, Giaccia AJ. Hypoxic microenvironment within an embryo induces apoptosis and is essential for proper morphological development. Teratology 1999;60:215–225.

30. Suzuki H, Tomida A, Tsuruo T. A novel mutant from apoptosis-resistant colon cancer HT-29 cells showing hyper-apoptotic response to hypoxia, low glucose and cisplatin. Jpn J Cancer Res 1998;89:1169–1178.

31. Gee MS, Koch CJ, Evans SM, et al. Hypoxia-mediated apoptosis from angiogenesis inhibition underlies tumor control by recombinant interleukin 12. Cancer Res 1999;59:4882–4889.

32. Khan S, Cleveland RP, Koch CJ, et al. Hypoxia induces renal tubular epithelial cell apoptosis in chronic renal disease. Lab Invest 1999;79:1089–1099.

33. Stempien-Otero A, Karsan A, Cornejo CJ, et al. Mechanisms of hypoxia-induced endothelial cell death. Role of p53 in apoptosis. Biol Chem 1999;274:8039–8045.

34. Blankenberg F, Narula J, Strauss HW. In vivo detection of apoptotic cell death: a necessary measurement for evaluating therapy for myocarditis, ischemia, and heart failure. J Nucl Cardiol 1999;6:531–539.

35. Czarnota GJ, Kolios MC, Abraham J, et al. Ultrasound imaging of apoptosis: high-resolution non-invasive monitoring of programmed cell death in vitro, in situ and in vivo. Br J Cancer 1999;81:520–527.

36. Zucker RM, Hunter ES III, Rogers JM. Apoptosis and morphology in mouse embryos by confocal laser scanning microscopy. Methods 1999;18:473–480.

37. Mizukami S, Kikuchi K, Higuchi T, et al. Imaging of caspase-3 activation in HeLa cells stimulated with etoposide using a novel fluorescent probe. FEBS Lett 1999;453:356–360.

38. Blankenberg FG, Katsikis PD, Tait JF, et al. Imaging of apoptosis (programmed cell death) with ^{99m}Tc-annexin. J Nucl Med 1999;40:184–191.

39. Tait JF, Smith C. Site-specific mutagenesis of annexin V: role of residues from Arg-200 to Lys-207 in phospholipid binding. Arch Biochem Biophys 1991;288:141–144.

40. Vriens PW, Blankenberg FG, Stoot JH, et al. The use of technetium ^{99m}Tc annexin V for in vivo imaging of apoptosis during cardiac allograft rejection. J Thorac Cardiovasc Surg 1998;116:844–853.

41. Davison A, Jones AG, Orvig C, Sohn M. A new class of oxotechnetium(+5) chelate complexes containing a $TcON_2S_2$ Core. Inorg Chem 1980;20:1629–1632.

42. Verbruggen AM, Nosco DL, Van Nerom CG, et al. ^{99m}Tc-L,L-Ethylenedicysteine: a renal imaging agent. Labelling and evaluation in animals. J Nucl Med 1992;33:551–557.

43. Van Nerom CG, Bormans GM, De Roo MJ, et al. First experience in healthy volunteers with ^{99m}Tc-L,L-ethylenedicysteine, a new renal imaging agent. Eur J Nucl Med 1993;20:738–746.

44. Surma MJ, Wiewiora J, Liniecki J. Usefulness of ^{99m}Tc-N,N'-ethylene-1-dicysteine complex for dynamic kidney investigations. Nucl Med Commun 1994;15:628–635.

45. Verbruggen A, Nosco D, Van Nerom C, et al. Evaluation of ^{99m}Tc-L,L-ethylenedicysteine as a potential alternate to ^{99m}Tc-MAG3. Eur J Nucl Med 1990;16:429.

46. Van Nerom C, Bormans G, Bauwens J, et al. Comparative evaluation of ^{99m}Tc-L,L-ethylenedicysteine and ^{99m}Tc-MAG3 in volunteers. Eur J Nucl Med 1990;16:417.

47. Jamar F, Stoffel M, Van Nerom C, et al. Clinical evaluation of ^{99m}Tc-L,L-ethylenedicysteine, a new renal tracer, in transplanted patients. J Nucl Med 1993;34:129P.

48. Jamar F, Van Nerom C, Verbruggen A, et al. Clearance of the new tubular agent ^{99m}Tc-L,L-ethylenedicysteine: estimation by a simplified method. J Nucl Med 1993;34:129P.

49. Ratner S, Clarke HT. The action of formaldehyde upon cysteine. J Am Chem Soc 1937;59:200–206.

50. Blondeau P, Berse C, Gravel D. Dimerization of an intermediate during the sodium in liquid ammonia reduction of L-thiazolidine-4-carboxylic acid. Can J Chem 1967;45:49–52.

51. Hay MP, Wilson WR, Moselen JW, et al. Hypoxia-selected antitumor agents. Bis(nitroimidazolyl)alkanecarboxamides: a new class of hypoxia-selected cytotoxins and hypoxic cell radiosensitizers. J Med Chem 1994;37:381–391.

52. Yang DJ, Ilgan S, Higuchi T, et al. Noninvasive assessment of tumor hypoxia with ^{99m}Tc-labeled metronidazole. Pharm Res 1999;16:743–750.

53. Meyn RE, Milas L, Stephens LC. Apoptosis in tumor biology and therapy. Adv Exp Med Biol 1997;400B:657–667.

54. Meyn RE, Stephens LC, Milas L. Programmed cell death and radioresistance. Cancer Metastas Rev 1996;15(1):119–131.

55. Meyn RE, Stephens LC, Hunter NR, Milas L. Apoptosis in murine tumors treated with chemotherapy agents. Anticancer Drugs 1995;6: 443–450.

56. Meyn RE, Stephens LC, Hunter NR, Milas L. Induction of apoptosis in murine tumors by cyclophosphamide. Cancer Chemother Pharmacol 1994;33:410–414.

57. Meyn RE, Stephens LC, Ang KK, et al. Heterogeneity in the development of apoptosis in irradiated murine tumours of different histologies. Int J Radiat Biol 1993;64:583–591.

58. Stephens LC, Hunter NR, Ang KK, et al. Development of apoptosis in irradiated murine tumors as a function of time and dose. Radiat Res 1993;135:75–80.

59. Stephens LC, Ang KK, Schultheiss TE, et al. Apoptosis in irradiated murine tumors. Radiat Res 1991;127:308–316.

19
Imaging of Signal Transduction and Antisense Imaging

David J. Yang and E. Edmund Kim

Imaging of Signal Transduction in Cancer

An estimated 600,000 human deaths result from cancer, and 1.5 million new cases of cancer are diagnosed each year. Approximately 5% of cancers are hereditary. The survival rate of patients diagnosed with early-stage cancer is higher than those with advanced-stage disease [1–3]. The diagnosis of cancer is made by pathological evaluation of tissue. Due to rapid developments in molecular biology, more and more biomarkers and gene markers are being developed for early detection of tumors. Trends in molecular biology research have focused from drug administration followed by angiogenesis to drugs in the micromolecular pathway. Molecular pathways that mediate signal transduction, cell-cycle traversal, apoptosis, hypoxia, and necrosis provide better understanding of molecular-targeted therapy. Although several molecular biomarkers have proven to be useful serum tumor markers for cancer early detection, these markers could not provide localization, staging, and characterization of tumor tissue.

Positron emission tomography/single photon emission computed tomography (PET/SPECT) are unique forms of computed tomography that produce images of biochemical and physiological processes in tissues, compared to anatomically based imaging methods such as X-ray computed tomography (CT) and magnetic resonance imaging (MRI). Use of PET/SPECT radiotracers can monitor the effectiveness or ineffectiveness of therapies [4]. With a quantitative biochemical imaging tool, the oncologist can maximize the proper therapeutic regimen by quantifying and predicting a tumor-specific biological response to a chemotherapeutic agent in each patient. In addition, quantitative PET/SPECT imaging may allow the rapid development of new chemotherapeutic drugs.

Due to the favorable physical characteristics of ^{99m}Tc and its extremely low price, ligands that can be labeled with ^{99m}Tc have been preferred. ^{99m}Tc can be obtained from a ^{99}Mo generator. ^{99m}Tc-ethylenedicysteine (^{99m}Tc-EC) is a successful example of N_2S_2 chelates [5–7]. This study is aimed to develop molecular targets for cancer imaging using ^{99m}Tc-EC or ^{111}In-DTPA conjugated with signal transduction ligands. If the uptake of radiolabeled ligands can be measured by planar scintigraphy, these tracers may be used to redirect early cancer diagnosis and therapeutics. In addition, they may predict the effectiveness of chemotherapy. These ligands fall into the following several categories.

Receptor-Targeting Ligands

Imaging Folate Receptors

The human folate receptor (FR) is a plasma membrane protein that is anchored to the membrane via a glycosylphosphatidylinositol (GPI) tail in some cell types. A carboxyl-terminal hydrophobic domain is an essential component of the processed signal for attachment of the GPI membrane anchor to proteins, and it is linked to the site (omega) of GPI modification by a spacer domain [8–10]. A carboxyl-terminal peptide in folate receptors is efficiently proteolyzed intracellularly by a pathway that is independent of GPI signal recognition, resulting in proper protein folding and secretion. Such carboxyl-terminal sequences could represent a simple adaptation for proteins whose physiological functions reside both at the cell surface and in extracellular fluids, allowing their selective and tissue-specific release.

Folic acid uptake is initiated by binding to an external folate receptor that cycles to an internal, but membrane-bound, compartment. When assayed in confluent nonmitotic cells, two-thirds of the FR pool is located in an internal (acid-resistant) compartment, but phorbol 12-myristate 13-acetate (PMA) causes a shift such that 65% to 75% of the receptor pool resides on the surface of the plasma membrane. PMA is the first reported positive modulator of receptor-mediated folate uptake. PMA may be activating more than one protein kinase C-independent signal transduction pathway [11–14]. Folate-binding protein is overexpressed by a number of neoplastic cell types (e.g., pulmonary, breast, ovarian, cervical, colorectal, nasopharyngeal, renal adenocarcinomas, and ependymomas), but primarily expressed in only several normal differentiated tissues (e.g., choroid plexus, placenta, thyroid, and kidney) [15–22]. To target tumor FR, we developed ^{99m}Tc-EC-folate.

Imaging Estrogen Receptors

The presence of sex hormone receptors in a receptor-mediated disease is an important factor for both prognosis and choice of therapy in breast and certain types of endometrial cancer [23–28]. Currently, estrogen receptors are identified by in vitro analysis of biopsy specimens and the use of antiestrogens. Tamoxifen is the therapy of choice for estrogen receptor-positive (ER+) disease. Tamoxifen therapy is effective in 30% of unselected patients with breast cancer. A response rate of 50% to 60% was obtained in patients with estrogen receptor-positive tumors [29,30]. Patients with metastatic cancer who do respond to the treatment have a response duration of 10 to 18 months and prolonged survival [31,32]. Although tamoxifen has been reported to induce endometrial cancer, the risk of endometrial cancer in tamoxifen-treated patients is 2 per 1000 women [33–35]. Therefore, the detection and measurement of estrogen receptors by the use of a radiolabeled tamoxifen should provide a useful tool for the detection of ER+ diseases as it may assist in selecting and following the most favorable choice of therapy, as well as predict its outcome. In addition, radiolabeled tamoxifen would also be useful in investigating tamoxifen's mechanisms of action because it would provide more accurate information about the effectiveness of antiestrogen (tamoxifen) therapy. In this report, we evaluated the imaging potential of $[^{123}I]/[^{131}I]$iodotamoxifen and $[^{111}In]$DTPA-tamoxifen in animal models with endometriosis.

Tyrosine Kinases

The relationship between intracellular signal transduction, cell cycles, and cell growth is likely to detect specific mechanisms to induce normal cell cycling and apoptosis in tumor cells without damaging normal cells. Tyrosine kinase-specific and Ras farnesyltransferase inhibitors for signal transduction in cancer cells are the major focuses on drug development. For instance, increased tyrosine kinase activity is known to be associated with overexpression of oncogenes (e.g., HER-2/neu proto-oncogene in breast cancer). There are two classes of protein tyrosine kinases: receptor (RTK) and non-receptor (non-RTK). For RTK, ligand binds to epidermal growth factor (EGFR) and triggers phosphorylate tyrosine residues that provide binding sites for the adaptor protein Grb2. A signaling pathway is then initiated, for instance, GDP-bound Ras in inactive form is converted to GTP-bound Ras active form. Activation of Ras can also be induced by non-RTKs. Ras activation has been coupled to mitogen-activated protein kinases (MAPK), which leads to cell proliferation and differentiation [36].

Farnesyl protein transferase (FPTase) catalyzes the first of a series of posttranslational modifications of Ras required for full biological activity. Farnesylation is required for the membrane partition and function of several proteins, including Ras. Specific farnesyl transferase inhibitors (FTIs) have been developed that selectively inhibit the processing of these proteins [37–39]. FTIs have been shown to be potent inhibitors of tumor cell growth in cell culture and in murine models and at doses that cause little toxicity to the animal. The mechanism of FTI action may involve in regulating p53 function [40].

We labeled genistein, a tyrosine kinase inhibitor, with ^{99m}Tc, and evaluated tissue distribution in tumor-bearing rodents.

Hypoxia and Apoptosis Signaling

Malignant tumors contain a significant fraction of microregions that are chronically or transiently hypoxic. Experimental evidence shows that hypoxia may have a profound impact on malignant progression and on responsiveness to therapy. Hypoxia was found to induce apoptosis in cells expressing wild-type p53 [41]. Hypoxic cells activate target genes such as p21/waf-1, which interact with cell-cycle machinery or participate in apoptosis. Apoptosis is a genetically encoded program of cell death that can be activated under physiological conditions like hypoxia, and it may be an important safeguard against tumor development. During the apoptotic process, the disruption of mitochondrial membrane function and the release of protease activators is involved. The disruption of mitochondrial membrane function in response to different oxygen content leads to the inhibition of gluconeogenesis and apoptosis in hypoxic cells [42,43].

During the hypoxic-induced apoptosis process, it is known that tumor tissue has a high level of nitroreductase in the cytoplasm. Agents with a nitroimidazole (NIM) moiety could be reduced by nitroreductase and subsequently bound to macromolecules [44–46]. In this report, tissue distribution of ^{99m}Tc-EC-NIM in tumor-bearing rodents was evaluated before and after chemotherapy.

Scintigraphic Studies of ^{99m}Tc-Ethylenedicysteine-Folate (EC-Folate)

Radiosynthesis of ^{99m}Tc-EC-folate was achieved using a previously described method [47,48]. In a 59-year-old patient with recurrent glioblastoma, SPECT images, using a gamma camera equipped with a low-energy, parallel-hole collimator, were obtained 2 h after i.v. injection of 30 mCi of ^{99m}Tc-EC-folate. The images were compared to MRI findings. Although MRI T_1-weighted images showed the lesions (Figure 19.1), the viability of tumor tissue was unclear. SPECT ^{99m}Tc-EC-folate demonstrated the feasibility of using a folate receptor-targeting tracer to image tumors (Figure 19.2).

Synthesis of [^{123}I]/[^{131}I]Iodotamoxifen

Tosyl analogue [49,50] of tamoxifen (10 mg) was dissolved in acetone (1 ml). Na^{123}I or Na^{131}I (3.15 mCi in 0.2 ml borate buffer, pH 8.5) was added. The reaction mixture was heated at 100°C for 2 h. Acetone was then evaporated under N_2. The unreacted tosyl analogue was hydrolyzed with 2 N HCl (1 ml) at 110°C for 15 min. The mixture was basified with 2 N NaOH (1.5 ml). The product was extracted from CH_2Cl_2 (2 ml) and purified from a silica gel-packed column (SPE 500 mg; Waters, Cliffton, NJ, USA). The column was eluted with 10% triethylamine in ether:petroleum ether (1:1). The solvent was evaporated and the final product was reconstituted in 0.05 M citric acid (10 ml). The isolated product was 690 μCi. The specific activity was 0.5 Ci/μmol.

Radiosynthesis of ^{111}In-DTPA-Tamoxifen (TX) Conjugate

A stirred solution of aminoethylanilide-DTPA (100 mg, 0.195 mmol) [51] and aldotamoxifen (83.3 mg, 1 equivalent, 0.195 mmol) [52,53] in CH_3CN-H_2O (1:1) (8 ml) was treated with a solution of NaCNBH$_3$ (1 M in THF) (0.13 ml, 0.67 equivalent, 0.13 mmol). The mixture was stirred under nitrogen atmosphere at room

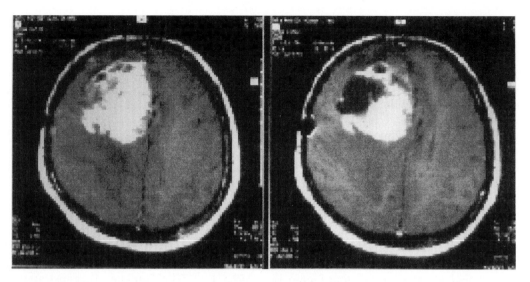

FIGURE 19.1. Patient with recurrent glioblastoma in the right brain. Selected MRI images show the lesion with marked contrast enhancement.

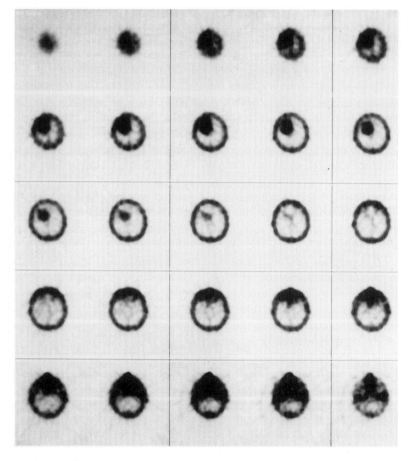

FIGURE 19.2. SPECT using ^{99m}Tc-EC-folate of patient with recurrent glioblastoma identified the lesion at 2 h post administration.

temperature for 2h; the solvent was then evaporated. The unreacted aldotamoxifen was removed by excessive washing with CH_2Cl_2 (3×5ml). The DTPA-TX product was used without further purification. The DTPA-TX conjugate (5mg) was dissolved in 1ml of ethanol/water (2:1) mixture. An aliquot containing 0.1mg DTPA-TX was added with [111]InCl_3 (0.7mCi, in 20µl, 0.04N HCl; NEN Dupont, Boston, MA, USA). Sodium acetate (0.6N, 20µl) and sodium citrate (0.06N, 20µl) were then added. The mixture stood for 30min. The final solution was then formulated in 5% ethanol/saline solution. Radiochemical purity was determined to be greater than 99% (using $CHCl_3/MeOH;1:1$, Rf=0.2; Bioscan, Washington, DC, USA).

Scintigraphic Study of Endometriosis in Animal Models

Endometriosis was produced in four monkeys. After orotracheal intubation, general anesthesia was maintained by administration of 0.5% to 2.5% isoflurane mixed with 100% oxygen. To produce monkeys with endometriosis, four monkeys underwent hysterectomy. The uterus was sectioned into 4-cm squares. The animal uterine tissues were sutured onto the peritoneum of the anterior abdominal wall. The serosal side of the uterine tissue faced the peritoneum and the endometrium faced the peritoneal cavity. Six weeks after recovering from surgery, the animals were administered [123I]/[131I]iodotamoxifen and 111In-DTPA-TX (0.1 mCi/kg, i.v.). Whole-body planar images were obtained at 30min, 2h, 24h, and 48h; 300,000 counts were acquired in a 256×256 matrix.

At the end of the experiments, the multiple peritoneal implants were removed. After the preparation, a midline laparotomy was performed, exposing the four grafted areas. Adequate biopsy samples were surgically resected under direct vision and fixed in 10% buffered formalin. After complete examination of the abdominal cavity, the muscle and subcutaneous layers were closed with 3/0 vicryl. The skin was sutured with 3/0 monofilament stainless steel.

Gamma scintigraphy of 111In-DTPA-tamoxifen in monkeys indicates that the hydrophilic tamoxifen analogue has greater uterine-to-muscle ratio counts than do halogenated tamoxifen analogues (Figure 19.3).

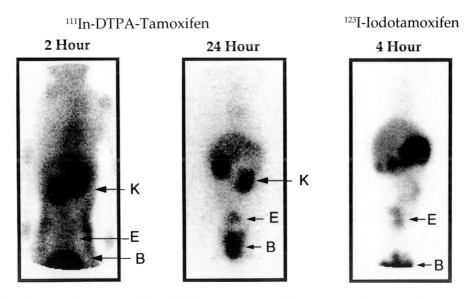

FIGURE 19.3. Planar scintigraphy of 111In-DTPA-tamoxifen and 123I-iodotamoxifen (0.1mCi/kg, 10µg, i.v.) in monkeys simulated with endometriosis. K, kidney; E, endometrium graft; B, bladder.

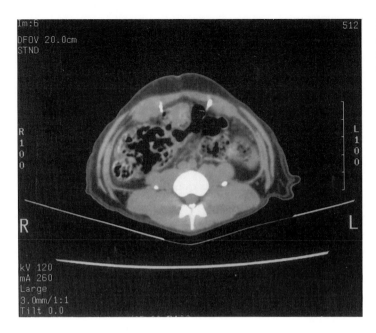

FIGURE 19.4. CT abdominal image of the section with a lesion in the anterior lower abdomen that corresponds to the planar scinitigraphy.

The selected planar images correspond to CT findings (Figure 19.4). Histopathological examinations (data not shown) revealed that sections through each of the peritoneal implants at multiple levels consisted of a well-defined layer of skeletal muscle (abdominal wall) with a layer of dense mature fibrous connective tissue partially covered by mesothelial cells (peritoneum) along one border. Each section contained a variably sized mass of implanted endometrial tissue intimately attached to a segment of the peritoneal surface of the abdominal wall. In some areas the serosal surface of the implant blended imperceptibly with the peritoneal surface of the abdominal wall; however, in some areas there existed a narrow cleft between the deep border of the implant and the peritoneal surface of the abdominal wall. Immediately adjacent to the peritoneal and serosal interface were two broad layers of smooth muscle cells (myometrium). Within the myometrium there was extensive atrophy of the smooth muscle cells. The remaining portion of the implant consisted of streaming intertwining bundles of fibrous connective tissue with extensive neovascularization. Along portions of the surface of the implant were irregular glands partially lined by a tall columnar epithelium (endometrium). Most of the glands, however, were lined by markedly attenuated to necrotic epithelial cells with pyknotic nuclei and shrunken eosinophilic cytoplasm. Large portions of the endometrial surface of the implants were denuded of epithelium. In areas primarily at the border of the implants there were fragments of suture material surrounded by granulation tissue. Numerous scattered individual smooth muscle cells in the myometrium had pyknotic nuclei.

Tyrosine Kinase Imaging

Female Fischer-344 rats (150 ± 25 g) (Harlan Sprague-Dawley, Indianapolis, IN, USA) were inoculated subcutaneously with 0.1 ml of mammary tumor cells from the 13762 tumor cell line suspension (10^6 cells/rat, a tumor cell line specific to Fischer rats) into the hind legs using 25-gauge needles. Studies were performed 14 to 17 days after implantation when tumors reached approximately 1 cm in diameter. Tissue distribution of ^{99m}Tc-EC-genistein was evaluated in breast tumor-bearing rats at 30 min, 2 h, or 4 h ($n = 3$/time interval, 10μCi/rat, i.v.).

In animal studies, the count density ratios at 30 min to 4 h were from 0.73 ± 0.03 to 0.75 ± 0.14 for tumor/blood and from 3.45 ± 1.82 to 7.63 ± 0.96 for tumor/muscle (Table 19.1). Both

TABLE 19.1. Biodistribution of ^{99m}Tc-EC-genistein in breast tumor-bearing rats.

| Tissue/organ | Percent of injected ^{99m}Tc-EC-genistein dose per organ or tissue: | | |
	30 min	2 h	4 h
Blood	0.635±0.167	0.367±0.109	0.335±0.086
Lung	0.454±0.082	0.256±0.068	0.216±0.043
Liver	0.723±0.066	0.602±0.022	0.449±0.124
Stomach	1.022±0.137	1.544±0.920	2.696±0.835
Kidney	5.222±0.880	7.689±1.058	6.499±0.351
Thyroid	8.809±2.184	7.613±1.688	6.040±2.225
Muscle	0.159±0.072	0.050±0.021	0.033±0.010
Spleen	0.392±0.045	0.431±0.013	0.444±0.117
Uterus	0.355±0.141	0.209±0.016	0.172±0.113
Tumor	0.460±0.056	0.271±0.070	0.244±0.061
Tumor/blood	0.747±0.137	0.748±0.065	0.729±0.032
Tumor/muscle	3.450±1.820	5.651±1.011	7.633±0.963

Values shown represent the mean±SD of data from three animals.

tumor/lung and tumor/uterus are greater than 1. ^{99m}Tc-EC-genisten may be useful as a marker for imaging the activity of tyrosine kinase and to assess therapeutic responses.

Hypoxia and Apoptosis Signaling Imaging

Using the same animal protocol previously described, tissue distribution studies were conducted at 0.5 to 4h. To ascertain whether ^{99m}Tc-EC-NIM (nitroimidazole) could monitor tumor response to chemotherapy, a group of rats with tumor volume of 1.5 cm were treated with paclitaxel (40 mg/kg, i.v.) at one single dose. Each animal was injected intravenously with 10 µCi of ^{99m}Tc-EC-NIM (biodistribution dose) and with 300 µCi of ^{99m}Tc-EC-NIM (imaging dose) both before- and after treatment (on day 4). The injected mass of ^{99m}Tc-EC-NIM was 10 µg per rat.

Gradually increased tumor/blood and tumor/muscle count density ratios were observed (Table 19.2). High tumor/intestine ratios (>6) were seen. ^{99m}Tc-EC-NIM may be a useful agent to assess tumor hypoxia at the abdomen region. After chemotherapy at a single dose on day 4, there was no marked difference between tumor/blood and tumor/muscle ratios (Table 19.2). Similar results were observed in scinti-

graphic images (Figure 19.5). The findings indicated that there was an improvement in cancer treatment due to no changes in count density ratios.

Clinical Imaging of Cancer Signal Transduction

The development of new tumor-seeking agents is clinically desirable for detecting primary and metastatic lesions as well as monitoring tumor response to therapy. Adequately high tumor specificity could also provide a favorable tumor-selective radiation therapy by using appropriate α- or β-emitting nuclides, and also proper selection of patients for chemotherapy.

The potential use of folate receptor imaging could be for prediction of the therapeutic effectiveness of antifolates. In a in vitro study, Chung et al. reported that increased expression of FRs by human mammary carcinoma and Chinese hamster ovary cells resulted in increased folic acid binding and increased methotrexate uptake and cytotoxicity [54]. If the uptake of folate is directly related to the effectiveness of antifolate therapy, EC-folate imaging could possibly be used to predict the therapeutic effectiveness of antifolates in cancer patients who will be treated with antifolates.

TABLE 19.2. Biodistribution of ^{99m}Tc-EC-NIM in breast tumor-bearing rats.

Organ/tissue	Percent of injected ^{99m}Tc-EC-NIM dose per organ or tissue:			
	30 min	2 h	4 h	2 h[a]
Blood	0.544±0.020	0.291±0.037	0.201±0.018	0.381±0.023
Lung	0.325±0.005	0.189±0.036	0.125±0.005	0.503±0.075
Liver	2.197±0.110	1.940±0.221	1.679±0.176	1.157±0.066
Stomach	0.110±0.004	0.790±0.015	0.054±0.002	0.148±0.061
Kidney	1.770±0.097	2.393±0.354	2.539±0.110	3.379±0.166
Thyroid	2.276±0.427	1.155±0.543	0.968±0.497	1.548±0.657
Muscle	0.035±0.001	0.021±0.002	0.022±0.009	0.029±0.003
Intestine	0.092±0.007	0.087±0.022	0.064±0.012	0.194±0.146
Urine	5.605±2.925	3.381±1.756	0.644±0.113	8.301±1.047
Tumor	0.172±0.012	0.151±0.018	0.139±0.003	0.179±0.014
Tumor/blood	0.316±0.022	0.521±0.018	0.677±0.079	0.471±0.055
Tumor/muscle	4.890±0.448	7.317±1.000	8.356±0.749	6.819±1.278

Values shown represent the mean±SD of data from three animals.
[a] Values are from 5 days post treatment with paclitaxel (40 mg/kg, i.v., single dose).

Tamoxifen binds to the cytoplasmic ER within the ER (+) breast tumor cells [55]. The complexes cause a similar change in chromatin structure, but the antiestrogen–estrogen receptor DNA complexes are transcriptionally nonproductive [55,56]. In addition, tamoxifen reduces the amount of transforming growth factor (TGF-α), which stimulates tumor growth of ER (+) breast cancer. These mechanisms could explain the ER-mediated antitumor

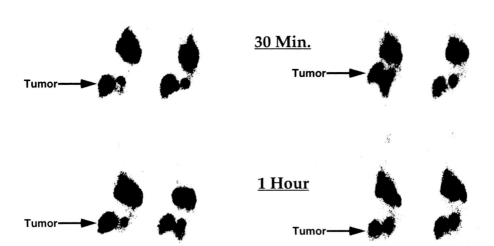

FIGURE 19.5. Planar images of breast tumor-bearing rats without (*left*) and with (*right*) paclitaxel treatment (40 mg/kg, i.v., single injection on day 14) following the administration of ^{99m}Tc-EC-NIM (300 µCi/rat, i.v.) on day 18 indicated that tumor volume and tumor uptake decreased after paclitaxel treatment.

activity of tamoxifen. Recent reports have demonstrated that tamoxifen has several other antiproliferative effects, including inhibiting the binding of protein kinase C [57,58] to calmodulin [59], reducing sex hormone-binding globulin [60], and reducing insulin-like growth factor [61]. Tamoxifen also stimulates tumor stromal cells (fibroblasts) and produces TGF-β, which can inhibit the growth of ER-negative breast cancer cells, and this is important because more than 10% of patients with ER-negative breast cancer respond to tamoxifen [62]. The adverse reactions to tamoxifen include hot flashes, nausea, and vomiting. There is increasing concern about the potential of tamoxifen for causing endometrial cancer [55]. Considering these mechanisms of tamoxifen, radiolabeled tamoxifen should provide more accurate information about the effect of anti-estrogen therapy.

In identifying the optimal tamoxifen treatment for each patient, lymph node status is not a useful predictive marker of response to tamoxifen therapy. Numerous genetic biomarkers and apoptosis regulators have been evaluated. For instance, high levels of progesterone receptors (>100 fmol/mg protein), positive bcl-2 gene and PS2 protein were associated with better outcomes [63–67], whereas mutant P53, epidermal growth factor receptors (EGFR), and HER-2/neu oncogene were associated with poor outcome in ER(+) patients treated with tamoxifen [68–75]. Although these genetic markers are important in predicting the therapeutic response of tamoxifen, multiple genes need to be identified before prediction. Therefore, developing an imaging technique to predict the responsiveness of tumors to tamoxifen therapy would be helpful.

Radiolabeling of tumor survival factors as a target would be a way to achieve better therapeutic index. These factors are oncogene (BRCA-1, HER-2/neu), hypoxia (<10 mmHg), metastasis (proteases), and cell detachment (signaling). Labeling theses factors may be a more accurate way to follow up treatment response. Application of genetic testing for cancer susceptibility as a predictor has been reported. The findings are outlined in Table 19.3. The biochemical mechanism and

TABLE 19.3. Predictive genetic testing for cancer susceptibility.

	Level	RR/DFS
ER	↑	↑
PR	↑	↑
bcl-2	↑	↑
m-P53	↑	↓
EGFR	↑	↓
HER-2/neu	↑	↓

pharmacological response could be assessed by correlating these genetic results and imaging findings, and this could serve as a basis for prediction of treatment response.

In summary, a folate receptor-imaging ligand was developed. ^{99m}Tc-EC-folate is a promising ligand to assess folate receptors. A hydrophilic ER+ ligand, DTPA-tamoxifen, is useful in the diagnosis of ER (+) diseases by SPECT.

The tumor suppressor gene p53 encodes a nuclear phosphoprotein, which is critical for cell-cycle control and prevention of uncontrolled cell proliferation that can lead to cancer. The p53 accumulation is known to be useful for the clinical management of cancer. Numerous reports have indicated that p53 mutations may be linked to the tyrosine kinase protein and hypoxia signaling pathway. Correlation of the level of P53 expression pre- and post treatment of tumors with ^{99m}Tc-EC-NIM uptake may explain the success or failure of chemotherapy. Although further studies with different tumor and animal models would obviously be required to better define the value of these ligands, our results suggest that these ligands could be a good candidate to characterize tumors.

Antisense Imaging

Over the past 25 years, the molecular aspects of carcinogenesis have been increasingly well defined. The role of genetic alterations in triggering cancer has been highlighted by the activated growth-promoting genes or oncogenes and tumor suppressor genes or anti-oncogenes, and the imbalance between oncogenes and anti-oncogenes is responsible for derailing cellular growth controls. Both structural and regulatory alterations may account for the activation of cellular proto-oncogenes and determine a cell to grow autonomous mutation, which consists of a modification of a single nucleotide in the gene and results in a change of one amino acid in the encoded protein with compromised function.

Regulatory changes are produced by translocation or amplification of a chromosomal segment carrying a proto-oncogene. The translocation mechanism juxtaposes a proto-oncogene and an unrelated regulatory region and determines the deregulated synthesis of a normal protein. The amplification mechanism leads to a deregulated replication of a proto-oncogene, and multiple copies of the gene appear either as tandemly duplicated segments within the chromosome or as extrachromosomal particles. In both instances, an increased amount of the messenger RNA produced by the oncogene ensues, representing a potential target for radiolabeled antisense DNA sequences [76]. The idea of utilizing antisense deoxyoligonucleotides was proposed in 1967 to specifically inhibit gene expression through the formation of mRNA–DNA duplex suppressing or preventing the translation of the targeted message into protein [77]. At that time, no automated method was available to produce oligomers of more than four bases and in sufficient amount. During the past 15 years, the progress in nucleotide chemistry and the automation of the synthetic process have made DNA antisense molecules readily available and a true explosion of antisense research has been witnessed.

It is estimated that an oligonucleotide (oligo) of 15 to 17 nucleotides in length would have a unique sequence relative to the entire human genome. Watson–Crick base pair formation confers an extremely high degree of specificity to the deoxynucleic acid structure. This specificity has been the driving force to develop oligodeoxynucleotides for diagnosis and therapy of cancer and viral disease. The antisense oligonucleotide can be used to target any known sense RNA, the beginning of the poly A

chain, or even some segments of RNA. Antisense reagents are believed to block the expression of targeted proteins by hybridizing with their mRNA and preventing its translation. Other targets for antisense oligos include donor-acceptor sites for splicing pre-mRNA to inhibit replication of the human immunodeficiency HIV-1 virus [78]. Rather than interfering with physiological processes, diagnostic applications view these intracellular sites as high-affinity receptors, amenable to binding a radiolabeled antisense oligo with high specificity for imaging mRNA content of the lesion.

For successful antisense imaging, six criteria have been emphasized [79].

1. Easy and bulky synthesis of oligos. Phosphoramidite chemistry and its automated development allow routine synthesis and purification of gram quantities of antisense oligos [80]. Radiolabeling the oligos typically requires construction of a conjugate molecule using linkers such as 5'-alkyl primary amine or poly-(L)-lysine with potential complications [81,82]. Kit formation is important for routine clinical imaging.

2. Stable oligos in vivo. The human body is rich in serum and intracellular endo- and exo-nucleases, which degrade the phosphodiester backbone of naturally occurring oligo [83]. Phosphate, sugar, and pyrimidine modifications into the oligos have significantly reduced nuclease activity; however, changes in membrane permeability, binding affinity of the oligos to the target mRNA, and ability to activate ribonuclease are simultaneously altered. Phosphorothioate and methylphosphonate were readily prepared and utilized [82]. Lu et al. [81] reported 30% dissociation of glycoprotein-poly (L) lysine–DNA complex after 7 min under chromatographic conditions and up to 85% dissociation by preincubation in phosphate buffer or media plus serum for 1 h. Dewanjee et al. [82] also showed 15% to 35% degradation of oligo complexes after 2 h incubation in human plasma. The radiolabel must remain bound to the antisense oligochelate by minimizing transmetallation or demetallation.

3. Entering of the oligos into the target cells. Naturally occurring phosphodiester and synthetic phosphorothioate oligos are polyanionic and cannot passively diffuse across cell membranes. However, internalization of polyanionic drugs has been found in most cells by receptor-mediated fluid-phase pinocytosis and adsorptive endocytosis [80]. Cells pinch off surface membrane and engulf bulk extracellular medium into plasma membrane-derived vesicular structures in the cytosol. The mechanism of vesicular transport is not known, and 5′-terminus modifications of polyanionic oligos with poly (L)-lysine may mask the negative charge of the oligo, thus enhancing the transit of the oligo from vesicular compartments into the cytoplasm [84].

4. Retention of radiolabeled oligos by the target cells. In cells such as HL60, more than 90% of the exocytosis occurs in oligos with half-times of 30 min or less and consists of full-length or truncated forms [79]. If the rates of exocytosis are equal to or greater than the rates of hybridization to target mRNA, then antisense cell-targeting efficiency will be compromised [79]. In addition, if cytosolic metabolism of the oligo–radiolabel complex were to occur, the free oligo would be transported out of the cell while the radioactive metal–chelate complex is trapped in cytosolic compartments.

5. Interaction of the oligos with their cell targets. Intracellular antisense targets such as mRNA, pre-mRNA, and genomic DNA are often protein bound, and two of the most common targets for antisense approaches have been the 5′-cap and initiation codon regions. The 3′-untranslated region of the mRNA of the intercellular adhesion molecule was reported to be a better target than the initiation region [85]. Tumor homogenates in vivo indicated a disappointing 20% to 39% of total radiolabeled antisense bound to mRNA, while HPLC of mRNA extracts of cell lysates in vitro showed 70% to 80% of radiolabeled antisense probe was bound to mRNA.

6. No interaction of the oligos with other macromolecules in a nonsequential-specific manner. It has been shown that longer oligos, rather than increasing specificity, may actually decrease specificity through nonsequential-specific and length-dependent increases in the number of potential hybridization sites [86]. In addition, during experimental validation, many control therapeutic oligos have been found to produce biological effects that are indistinguishable from the antisense oligos [87]. It has been suggested that the oligo complex was bound to target mRNA with 2.5-fold increase of cellular accumulation in vitro and 10-fold greater localization in tumor-bearing Balb/c mice of radiolabeled antisense oligos in vivo.

Oncogenes amplified by cancer were targeted so that multiple copies of mRNAs and hybridization sites would be available for binding and retention of radiolabeled antisense probes for noninvasive imaging. The c-*myc* oncogene works in cooperation with other oncogenes in a variety of cancers and encodes a nuclear phosphoprotein, a transcription factor, that may be involved in regulating transcription and replication. The 15-mer oligonucleotide sequence was synthesized, amino linked (sense and antisense phosphodiester and monothioester), and coupled with DTPA-isothiocyanate and aliquots were lyophilized to make a DTPAAHON kit. ^{111}In was separated by gel filtration. The radiolabeled antisense and sense probes were injected intravenously in mammary tumor-bearing Balb/c mice. The highest uptake was observed at 2 h with both thio and oxo derivatives, and small tumors could be imaged. Tumor uptake and tumor/blood and tumor/muscle count density ratios for sense probe (control) were significantly lower than those of the antisense probe [82]. A 23-mer oligonucleotide sequence was synthesized and grafted in 5′ with a tyramine group (complementary to the translation initiation site of transforming growth factor-α), which was radioiodinated. The 5′-tyramine group allowed specific and stable radiolabeling of the antisense with ^{125}I. The radiolabeled antisense was injected intratumorally in mammary tumor-bearing mice. The ^{125}I antisense oligonucleotide was rapidly cleared from the tumor by intestine and kidneys. Four hours later, $6.5\% \pm 1.5\%$ of the dose was retained in the tumor (Figure 19.6) as nondegraded ^{125}I antisense [88].

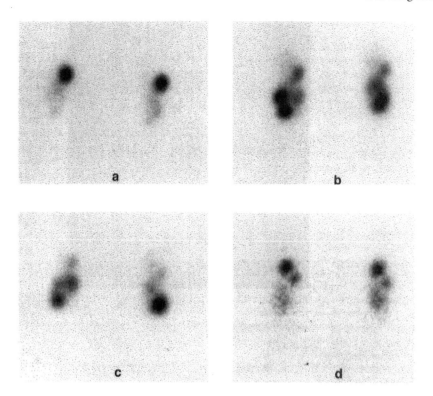

FIGURE 19.6. Serial ^{125}I-Tyr-ON23 antisense scintis-cans (2 mice per field). Immediately after intratu-moral injection (**a**) only breast tumor was visualized. Images at 1 h (**b**) and 2 h (**c**) showed increased ac-tivities in the abdomen. Image at 24 h (**d**) shows that tumor radioactivity remained. (From Cammilleri et al. Eur J Nucl Med 23:450, 1996, with permission.)

Conclusion

Advances in determining the genetic basis of diseases has made the concept of gene replace-ment to treat tumors increasingly attractive. For instance, P53, which is a key tumor suppressor gene, has proven to be an attractive target for detecting cancer cell mutation. P53 has been implicated in numerous cancers including breast, colon, and small-cell lung carcinoma. Viral-based gene delivery is the most effective way to transfer genes to cells. However, concerns about immunogenic and long-term oncological effects have increased the need to develop a nonviral gene delivery system.

References

1. Jordan VC. The role of tamoxifen in the treat-ment and prevention of breast cancer. Curr Probl Cancer 1992;16:129–176.

2. Neijt JP. New therapy for ovarian cancer. New Engl J Med 1996;334:50–51.

3. Feehery K, Benjamin I. NIH Consensus Confer-ence. Ovarian cancer: screening, treatment and follow-up. JAMA 1995;273:491–497.

4. Brock CS, Meikle SR, Price P. Does ^{18}F-fluorodeoxyglucose metabolic imaging of tumors benefit oncology? Eur J Nucl Med 1997;24: 691–705.

5. Verbruggen AM, Nosco DL, Van Nerom CG, et al. ^{99m}Tc-L,L-ethylenedicysteine: a renal imaging agent. Labeling and evaluation in animals. J Nucl Med 1992;33:551–557.

6. Van Nerom CG, Bormans GM, De Roo MJ, et al. First experience in healthy volunteers with ^{99m}Tc-L,L-ethylenedicysteine, a new renal imaging agent. Eur J Nucl Med 1993;20:738–746.

7. Surma MJ, Wiewiora J, Liniecki J. Usefulness of ^{99m}Tc-N,N'-ethylene-1-dicysteine complex for dynamic kidney investigations. Nucl Med Commun 1994;15: 628–635.

8. Wang J, Maziarz K, Ratnam M. Recognition of the carboxyl-terminal signal for GPI modification requires translocation of its hydrophobic domain across the ER membrane. J Mol Biol 1999;286:1303–1310.

9. Wang J, Shen F, Yan W. Proteolysis of the carboxyl-terminal GPI signal independent of GPI modification as a mechanism for selective protein secretion. Biochemistry 1997;36(47): 14583–14592.

10. Chung KN, Roberts S, Kim CH, et al. Rapid turnover and impaired cell-surface expression of the human folate receptor in mouse L(tk-) fibroblasts, a cell line defective in glycosylphosphatidylinositol tail synthesis. Arch Biochem Biophys 1995;322:228–234.

11. Blusch J, Alexander S, Nellen W. Multiple signal transduction pathways regulate discoidin I gene expression in *Dictyostelium discoideum*. Differentiation 1995;58:253–260.

12. Janssens PM, Van Haastert PJ. Molecular basis of transmembrane signal transduction in *Dictyostelium discoideum*. Microbiol Rev 1987; 51:396–418.

13. Bernstein RL, Rossier C, van Driel R, et al. Folate deaminase and cyclic AMP phosphodiesterase in *Dictyostelium discoideum*: their regulation by extracellular cyclic AMP and folic acid. Cell Differ 1981;10:79–86.

14. Lewis CM, Smith AK, Nguyen C, et al. PMA alters folate receptor distribution in the plasma membrane and increases the rate of 5-methyltetrahydrofolate delivery in mature MA104 cells. Biochim Biophys Acta 1998;1401: 157–169.

15. Orr RB, Kreisler AR, Kamen BA. Similarity of folate receptor expression in UMSCC 38 cells to squamous cell carcinoma differentiation markers. J Natl Cancer Inst 1995;87:299–303.

16. Hsueh CT, Dolnick BJ. Altered folate-binding protein mRNA stability in KB cells grown in folate-deficient medium. Biochem Pharmacol 1993;45:2537–2545.

17. Weitman SD, Lark RH, Coney LR, et al. Distribution of folate GP38 in normal and malignant cell lines and tissues. Cancer Res 1992;52: 3396–3400.

18. Campbell IG, Jones TA, Foulkes WD, Trowsdale J. Folate-binding protein is a marker for ovarian cancer. Cancer Res 1991;51:5329–5338.

19. Holm J, Hansen SI, Hoier-Madsen M, Sondergaard K, Bzorek M. Folate receptor of human mammary adenocarcinoma. APMIS 1994;102: 413–419.

20. Ross JF, Chaudhuri PK, Ratnam M. Differential regulation of folate receptor isoforms in normal and malignant tissue in vivo and in established cell lines. Cancer (Phila) 1994;73:2432–2443.

21. Franklin WA, Waintrub M, Edwards D, et al. New anti-lung-cancer antibody cluster 12 reacts with human folate receptors present on adenocarcinoma. Int J Cancer (Suppl) 1994;8:89–95.

22. Weitman SD, Frazier KM, Kamen BA. The folate receptor in central nervous system malignancies of childhood. J Neuro-Oncol 1994;21:107–112.

23. Fernandez MD, Burn JI, Sauven PD, et al. Activated estrogen receptors in breast cancer and response to endocrine therapy. Eur J Cancer Clin Oncol 1984;20:41–46.

24. Vering A, Vockel A, Stegmuller M, et al. Immuno-biochemical assay for determination of nuclear steroid receptors during tamoxifen therapy. Cancer Res Clin Oncol 1993;119: 415–420.

25. Creasman WT, McCarty KS, Barton TK. Clinical correlates of estrogen- and progesterone-binding proteins in human endometrial adenocarcinoma. Obstet Gynecol 1980;55:363–368.

26. Quinn MA, Pearce P, Fortune DW. Correlation between cytoplasmic steroid receptors and tumour differentiation and invasion in endometrial carcinoma. Br J Obstet Gynaecol 1985;92: 399–405.

27. Martin JD, Hahnel R, McCartney T. The effect of estrogen receptor status on survival in patients with endometrial cancer. Am J Obstet Gynecol 1983;147:322–327.

28. Schutze N, Kraft V, Deerberg F, et al. Functions of estrogens and antiestrogens in the rat endometrial adenocarcinoma cell lines RUCA-1 and RUCA-II. Int J Cancer 1992;52:941–949.

29. Hamm JT, Allegra JC. Hormonal therapy for cancer. In: Witts RE, ed. Manual of Oncologic Therapeutics. New York: Lippincott, 1991:122–126.

30. Yang DJ, Cherif A, Tansey W, et al. *N,N*-Diethylfluoromethyltamoxifen: synthesis, assignment of ^{1}H and ^{13}C spectra and receptor assay. Eur J Med Chem 1992;27:919–924.

31. Wittliff JL. Steroid-hormone receptor in breast cancer. Cancer Res 1984;53:630–643.

32. Lum SS, Woltering EA, Fletcher WS, et al. Changes in serum estrogen levels in women during tamoxifen therapy. Excerpta Med 1997; 173:399–402.

33. Barakat RR. The effect of tamoxifen on the endometrium. Oncology 1995;9:129–142.

34. Uziely B, Lewin A, Brufman G, et al. The effect of tamoxifen on the endometrium. Breast Cancer Res Treat 1993;26:101–105.

35. Fisher B, Costantino JP, Redmond CK, et al. Endometrial cancer in tamoxifen-treated breast cancer patients: findings from the national surgical adjuvant breast and bowel project (NSABP) B-14. J Natl Cancer Inst 1994;86:527–537.

36. Gishizky ML. Tyrosine kinase induced mitogenesis breaking the link with cancer. In: Bristol JA, ed. Annual Reports in Medicinal Chemistry, Vol. 30. New York: Academic Press, 1995:247–253.

37. Moasser MM, Sepp-Lorenzino L, Kohl NE, et al. Farnesyl transferase inhibitors cause enhanced mitotic sensitivity to taxol and epothilones. Proc Natl Acad Sci USA 1998;95:1369–1374.

38. Gibbs JB, Kohl NE, Koblan KS, et al. Farnesyl-transferase inhibitors and anti-Ras therapy. Breast Cancer Res Treat 1996;38:75–83.

39. Sepp-Lorenzino L, Ma Z, Rands E, et al. A peptidomimetic inhibitor of farnesyl: protein transferase blocks the anchorage-dependent and -independent growth of human tumor cell lines. Cancer Res 1995;55:5302–5309.

40. Sepp-Lorenzino L, Rosen N. A farnesyl-protein transferase inhibitor induces p21 expression and G1 block in p53 wild type tumor cells. J Biol Chem 1998;273:243–251.

41. Riva C, Chauvin C, Pison C, et al. Cellular physiology and molecular events in hypoxia-induced apoptosis. Anticancer Res 1998;18:4729–4736.

42. Shizukuda Y, Helisch A, Yokota R, et al. Downregulation of protein kinase c delta activity enhances endothelial cell adaptation to hypoxia. Circulation 1999;100:1909–1916.

43. Tomasevic G, Shamloo M, Israeli D, et al. Activation of p53 and its target genes p21(WAF1/Cip1) and PAG608/Wig-1 in ischemic preconditioning. Brain Res Mol Brain Res 1999;70:304–313.

44. Rupnow BA, Alarcon RM, Giaccia AJ, et al. p53 mediates apoptosis induced by c-Myc activation in hypoxic or gamma irradiated fibroblasts. Cell Death Differ 1998;5:141–147.

45. Stempien-Otero A, Karsan A, Cornejo CJ, et al. Mechanisms of hypoxia-induced endothelial cell death. Role of p53 in apoptosis. J Biol Chem 1999;274:8039–8045.

46. Yang DJ, Ilgan S, Higuchi T, et al. Noninvasive assessment of tumor hypoxia with ^{99m}Tc-labeled metronidazole. Pharm Res 1999;16:743–750.

47. Ratner S, Clarke HT. The action of formaldehyde upon cysteine. J Am Chem Soc 1937;59:200–206.

48. Blondeau P, Berse C, Gravel D. Dimerization of an intermediate during the sodium in liquid ammonia reduction of L-thiazolidine-4-carboxylic acid. Can J Chem 1967;45:49–52.

49. Yang DJ, Tewson T, Tansey, W, et al. Halogenated analogs of tamoxifen: synthesis, receptor assay and inhibition of MCF7 cells. J Pharm Sci 1992;81:622–625.

50. Yang DJ, Li C, Kuang L-R, et al. Imaging, biodistribution and therapy potential of halogenated tamoxifen analogues. Life Sci 1994;55:53–67.

51. Paik CH, Quadri SM, Reba RC. Interposition of different chemical linkages between antibody and ^{111}In-DTPA to accelerate clearance from non-target organs and blood. Nucl Med Biol 1989;16:475–481.

52. Delpassand ES, Yang DJ, Wallace S, et al. Synthesis, biodistribution and estrogen receptor scintigraphy of an ^{111}In-DTPA-tamoxifen analogue. J Pharm Sci 1996;85:553–559.

53. Yang DJ, Wallace S, Delpassand ES, et al. DTPA-tamoxifen and DTPA-retinal: a new combined radiotracer to target breast tumors. Radiology 1995;197:320 (abstract).

54. Chung KN, Saiwaka Y, Paik TH, et al. Stable transfectants of human MCF-7 breast cancer cells with increased levels of the human folate receptor exhibit an increased sensitivity to antifolates. J Clin Invest 1993;91:1289–1294.

55. Jordan VC. A current view of tamoxifen for the treatment and prevention of breast cancer. Br J Pharmacol 1993;110:507–517.

56. Green S. Modulations of estrogen receptor activity by estrogens and antiestrogens. J Steroid Biochem Mol Biol 1990;37:747–751.

57. O'Brian CA, Liskamp RM, Solomon DH, et al. Inhibition of protein kinase C by tamoxifen. Cancer Res 1985;45:2462–2465.

58. Edashige K, Sato E, Akimaru K, et al. Nonsteroidal antiestrogen suppresses protein kinase C: its inhibitory effect on interaction of substrate protein with membrane. Cell Struct Funct 1991;16:273–281.

59. Lam HY. Tamoxifen is a calmodulin antagonist in the activation of cAMP phosphodiesterase. Biochem Biophys Res Commun 1984;118:27–32.

60. Pollak MN, Huynh HT, Lefevre SP. Tamoxifen reduces serum insulin-like growth factor 1 (IGF-1). Breast Cancer Res Treat 1992;22:91–95.

61. Rose DP, Chlebowski RT, Connolly JM, et al. Effects of tamoxifen adjuvant therapy and a low-fat diet or serum binding proteins and estradiol

bioavailability in postmenopausal breast cancer patients. Cancer Res 1992;52:5386–5390.

62. Vogel CL, East DR, Vogt W, et al. Response to tamoxifen in estrogen receptor-poor metastatic breast cancer. Cancer (Phila) 1987;60:1184–1189.

63. Gasparini G, Barbareschi M, Doglioni C, et al. Expression of *bcl-2* protein predicts efficacy of adjuvant treatments in operable node-positive breast cancer. Clin Cancer Res 1995;1:189–198.

64. Soubeyran I, Quenel N, Coindre J-M, et al. pS2 protein: a marker improving prediction of response to neoadjuvant tamoxifen in post-menopausal breast cancer patients. Br J Cancer 1996;74:1120–1125.

65. Ravdin PM, Green S, Dorr TM, et al. Prognostic significance of progesterone receptor levels in estrogen receptor-positive patients with metastatic breast cancer treated with tamoxifen: results of a prospective southwest oncology group study. J Clin Oncol 1992;10:1284–1291.

66. Elledge RM, Green S, Howes L et al. *bcl-2*, p53, and response to tamoxifen in estrogen receptor-positive metastatic breast cancer: a southwest oncology group study. J Clin Oncol 1997;15: 1916–1922.

67. Foekens JA, Portengen H, Look MP, et al. Relationship of PS2 with response to tamoxifen therapy in patients with recurrent breast cancer. Br J Cancer 1994;70:1217–1223.

68. Borg A, Baldetorp B, Ferno M, et al. *ERBB2* amplification is associated with tamoxifen resistance in steroid-receptor positive breast cancer. Cancer Lett 1994;81:137–144.

69. Laitzel K, Teramoto Y, Konrad K, et al. Elevated serum c-*erb*B-2 antigen levels and decreased response to hormone therapy of breast cancer. J Clin Oncol 1995;13:1129–1135.

70. Berns EMJ, Foekens JA, Van Staveren IL, et al. Oncogene amplification and prognosis in breast cancer: relationship with systemic treatment. Gene (Amst) 1995;159:11–18.

71. Nicholson RI, McClelland RA, Gee JMW, et al. Epidermal growth factor receptor expression in breast cancer: association with response to endocrine therapy. Br Cancer Res Treat 1994; 29:117–125.

72. Silvestrini R, Benini E, Veneroni S, et al. p53 and *bcl-2* expression correlates with clinical outcome in a series of node-positive breast cancer patients. J Clin Oncol 1996;114:1604–1610.

73. Wright C, Nicholson S, Angus B, et al. Relationship between c-erbB-2 protein product expression and response to endocrine therapy in advanced breast cancer. Br J Cancer 1992;65: 118–121.

74. Yamauchi H, O'Neill A, Gelman R, et al. Prediction of response to antiestrogen therapy in advanced breast cancer patients by pretreatment circulating levels of extracellular domain of the HER-2/c-*neu* protein. J Clin Oncol 1997;15: 2518–2525.

75. Carlomagno C, Perrone F, Gallo C, et al. c-*erb*B2 overexpression decreases the benefit of adjuvant tamoxifen in early-stage breast cancer without axillary lymph node metastases. J Clin Oncol 1996;14:2702–2708.

76. Weinberg RA. Oncogenes and tumor suppressor genes. CA Cancer J Clin 1994;44:160–170.

77. Urbain JLC, Shore SK, Vekemans MC, et al. Scintigraphic imaging of oncogenes with antisense probes: does it make sense? Eur J Nucl Med 1995;22:499–504.

78. Agrawal S, Temsamani J, Tang JY. Pharmacokinetics, biodistribution and stability of oligodeoxyribonucleotide phosphorothioates. Proc Natl Acad Sci USA 1991;88:7595–7599.

79. Stein CA, Cheng Y-C. Antisense oligonucleotides as therapeutic agents—is the bullet really magical? Science 1993;261:1004–1012.

80. Pianica-Worms D. Making sense out of antisense: challenges of imaging gene translation with radiolabeled oligonucleotides. J Nucl Med 1994;35:1064–1066.

81. Lu X-M, Fischman AJ, Jyawook SL, et al. Antisense DNA delivery in vivo: targetting to liver by receptor-mediated uptake. J Nucl Med 1994;35: 269–275.

82. Dewanjee MK, Ghafournipour AK, Iapadvanjwala M, et al. Noninvasive imaging of c-*myc* oncogene mRNA with In-111 labeled antisense probes in a mammary tumor-bearing mouse model. J Nucl Med 1994;35:1054–1063.

83. Elder PS, deVine RJ, Dogle JM. Substrate specificity and kinetics of degradation of antisense oligonucleotides by a 3′ exonuclease in plasma. Antisense Res Dev 1991;1:141–151.

84. Leonetti J, Degols G, LeBlue B. Biological activity of oligonucleotide-poly-(L-lysine) conjugates: mechanism of cell uptake. Bioconjugate Chem 1990;1:149–153.

85. Chiang MY, Chan H, Zounes MA, et al. Antisense oligonucleotides inhibit intercellular adhesion molecule 1 expression by two distinct mechanisms. J Biol Chem 1991;266:18162–18172.

86. Rittner K, Burmester C, Sczakiel G. In vitro selection of fast-hybridizing and effective antisense RNAs directed against the human immu-

nodeficiency virus type 1. Nucleic Acids Res 1993;21:1381–1387.

87. Wagner RW, Matteucci MD, Lewis JG, et al. Antisense gene inhibition by oligonucleotides containing C-5 propyne pyimidines. Science 1993;260:1510–1513.

88. Cammiller S, Sangrajrang S, Perdercan B, et al. Biodistribution of I-125 tyramine transforming growth factor-β antisense oligonucleotide in athymic mice with a human mammary tumor xenograft following intratumoral injection. Eur J Nucl Med 1996;23:448–452.

20
Imaging of Gene Delivery and Expression

Carolyn Nichol and E. Edmund Kim

Recent advances in cell biology and genetic engineering have led to the identification of genes that control many disease states, including cancer, cystic fibrosis, sickle cell anemia, AIDS, and Parkinson's disease. These discoveries have led to an increased understanding of the fundamental mechanisms of disease and to the development of genetically based therapies. Although new genes are being identified at the rate of approximately one new gene per day and progress is being made in the use of new gene therapies in animal studies and clinical trials, the primary method to test for gene expression involves tissue analysis. Tissue analysis is expensive, time consuming, painful, and subject to sampling errors. Only recently it has been possible to determine noninvasively if exogenous genes are being delivered to the diseased sites and if the exogenous protein is being expressed. The modalities that have been used to image gene expression include single photon emission computed tomography (SPECT), position emission tomography (PET), magnetic resonances (MR), and optical imaging. To date, the imaging of gene expression has been exclusively in the realm of in vitro and preliminary animal studies. However, translation to the clinical setting will probably be rapid because most of the marker genes that are being imaged have previously been used in the clinic.

Imaging endogenous gene expression is somewhat more difficult because there are no obvious differentiating characteristics to exploit, but immunofluorescent labeling and confocal microscopy have advanced the in vitro imaging of gene expression. Immunofluorescent labeling has been used to characterize reporter genes, the *myc* gene, apoptosis, and receptor status. Confocal microscopy is a powerful tool to image these fluorescent probes and obtain detailed information about cellular processes. These studies are usually performed on lysed cells. This technology has recently begun to transfer to in vivo imaging systems with the use of genes that overexpress surface markers, for example, to target gene expression and optical imaging systems based on green fluorescent protein (GFP) or luciferase imaging.

Gene Therapy

The goal of gene therapy is to supplement or replace the function of mutated genes with the correct genetic code. Rather than altering the disease phenotype by using agents that interact with gene products, or are themselves gene products, gene therapy can theoretically modify specific genes that will correct the underlying cause of the disease. Initially gene therapy was envisioned for the treatment of inherited genetic disorders, but it is currently being studied in a wide range of diseases including cancer, peripheral vascular disease, arthritis, neurodegenerative disorders, and other acquired diseases.

One of the impediments to successful gene therapy is the inefficient delivery of genes because of short in vivo half lives, degradation by protein serum or lysosome, lack of cell-specific targeting, and low transfection efficiencies. A variety of gene transfer systems have been developed to penetrate the cell and deliver DNA to the nucleus where a therapeutic or marker protein can be expressed. These technologies include (1) replicant-deficient viral vectors such as adenovirus [1,2], adeno-associated virus [3], retrovirus [4,5], and herpes simplex virus [6–8]; (2) synthetic non-viral systems [9–15] such as liposomes, polylysine, dendrimers, and molecular conjugates [16]; (3) physical methods such as the gene gun and electroporation [17]; (4) naked DNA [18]; and (5) combinations of these various technologies [19,20].

Both ex vivo and in vivo protocols have been developed. For ex vivo gene therapy, the patient's cells are extracted and the gene is inserted into the cells in vitro. The cultured cells are then readministered to the patient. For in vivo delivery, the gene is transferred directly to the site of interest. Typically, marker or reporter genes that do not naturally occur in the host are used to develop the vectors and to characterize their transfection efficiency or their ability to produce a foreign protein. For example, the protein produced by the beta-galactosidase marker gene can be identified through enzymatic staining, the luciferase gene by a chemiluminescent reaction, and green fluorescent protein via fluorometric analysis.

Adenoviral, adeno-associated, and retroviral-based systems currently account for approximately 85% of gene therapy research because these agents are efficient carriers of the gene into the cell. Retroviral vectors are often a replication-deficient Moloney murine lukemia virus (MoMLV), which is small and permits long-term expression. However, retroviral vectors replicate only in dividing cells and are expensive to manufacture because of the potential for recombination and activation. Adenoviral vectors are large (38 kb) and transduce nondividing cells. Adenoviral systems are limited by a brief persistence of protein expression (usually 2 weeks or less) and by the ability of the human immune system to recognize and render these viral invaders less effective upon subsequent administration. There are also limitations to the size of the gene that can be inserted into the virus and to the large-scale manufacturing of viral vectors. Adeno-associated vectors have also been developed based on a small single-stranded DNA virus and may have a lower immune response. They have the ability to transduce nondividing cells and elicit long-term expression, but have a small insert size (4 kb) and are difficult to manufacture.

Nonviral gene therapy techniques are also being developed based on naked plasmid DNA and a variety of synthetic systems to enhance gene transfer [9–15]. Although less efficient than viral vectors in terms of the amount of gene required for cell transfection, nonviral vectors have the advantage of a lower risk of eliciting an immune response and are simple systems. Naked DNA has been used in vivo and can transduce muscle tissue, but it has low transfection efficiency and is subject to nucleic hydrolysis. The nonviral gene transfection agents currently available include molecular conjugates (ligand attached to polylysine), cationic liposomes, polymers, and dendrimers. Most nonviral systems are cationic, have high amine ratios, form ionic complexes with negatively charged DNA, and can bind to the cell surface. Receptor-targeting ligands and endomolyic proteins have been added to these systems in attempts to increase transfection and specificity.

More than 1000 patients in the United States have undergone human gene transfer in clinical trials, the majority of which have been for cancer. Many gene therapy protocols to date have concentrated upon treatments for cancer. Although many cancers have a genetic predisposition, they all involve acquired mutations, and as they progress their cells become less differentiated and more heterogeneous with respect to the mutations they carry. In general, cancers have at least one mutation to a proto-oncogene (yielding an oncogene) and mutations of at least one to a tumor suppressor gene, allowing the cancer to proliferate. The range of different cancers encountered and the mutations they carry have led to a variety of strategies for gene therapy, namely genetic immunization, oncogene inactivation, tumor suppressor gene replacement, molecular chemotherapy, and drug resistance genes. The aim of immunopotentiation, or cancer vaccines, is to enhance the response of the immune system to cancers by expressing cytokines such as IL-2 and TNF-α. Onocogene inactivation may be designed to target the promotor regions of oncogenes such as *erb-2* or *bcl-2*, or to use antisense techniques that prevent transport and translation of the oncogenes.

Many cancers result from the abnormal function of the protein product from the p53 tumor suppressor gene. The p53 gene is one of the most commonly mutated genes identified in human cancers, and its function is critical to cell-cycle regulation and DNA repair. For example, mutant p53 protein may be unable to activate the transcription of molecules that control cell growth, leading to uncontrolled cell proliferation. If DNA damage has occurred, mutant p53 may not be able to arrest cell growth at the G_1 checkpoint phase of the cell cycle. Augmenting the function of the p53 gene in cells that express insufficient levels of functional p53 protein could restore normal cell-cycle arrest or apoptosis (programmed cell death), which may be clinically important to treating cancer.

An alternative means of killing a tumor cell is to transduce a gene coding for a toxic product, known as molecular chemotherapy or suicide gene therapy. The gene of choice is usually herpes simplex virus thymidine kinase (HSV/tk), which converts the prodrug ganciclovir and its derivatives into toxic metabolites [7,21]. Transfection of the tumor cells with the HSV-tk gene creates a biochemical difference between normal and tumor tissue that can be a target for the antiherpetic agent [22].

Imaging Gene Expression

Cell biology provides many means for identification of gene expression. These techniques include (1) Northern blot for RNA; (2) Southern blot for DNA; (3) Western blot testing for protein expression; (4) luminometer marker gene detection using luciferase; (5) enzyme staining for beta-galactosidase expression; (6) fluorescent imaging of green fluorescent protein; and (7) immunostaining for CAT and HSV-tk expression. In addition, polymerase chain reaction (PCR), which makes copies of a DNA segment, and RFLP mapping (restriction fragment-length polymorphism) can be used for DNA fingerprinting. There also exist many peptide, antibody, and enzyme probes that are exploited by confocal and fluorescent microscopic techniques to image biological processes including mitosis, apoptosis, and necrosis.

To qualitatively or quantitatively image gene expression noninvasively, these techniques could be adapted to in vivo systems. So far, the most promising gene imaging system is based on the HSV-1-tk marker gene expression. However, optical imaging systems are also being developed to potentially image many of the biological processes that can be observed microscopically.

Nuclear Imaging

Nuclear medicine has the power to image functional and metabolic processes as well as structural morphology. Nuclear medicine has been used to characterize tumor receptor status and oncological staging and to monitor therapeutic efficacy. For these reasons, it holds promise for imaging the emerging clinical applications in gene therapy by monitoring gene delivery and identifying protein expression. Recent studies have shown that scintigraphic imaging can offer unique information on biodistribution of the genetic vector and the extent and location of gene expression.

Radiolabeling can be used to trace the biodistribution of both viral [23] and nonviral genetic vectors [24,25] and exogenous protein expression [6,26–32]. Radiolabeling of the vector does not show that the protein of interest is being expressed, but rather shows the dynamic location of the genetic delivery system. It is known that the route of DNA administration can have a marked effect on the efficacy of the gene expression [33,34]; this could result from several factors including vector instability in the bloodstream, immunological responses, and tissue biodistribution

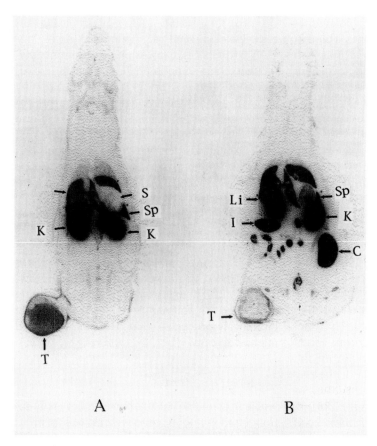

FIGURE 20.1. Whole-body autoradiograms (coronal section) obtained at (**A**) 2 h and (**B**) 24 h after intravenous injection of ^{111}In-DTPA-PEI; 13762 cells (10^6) were implanted s.c. in the thigh approximately 2 weeks before imaging study. T, tumor; K, kidney; Li, liver; L, lung; I, intestine; Sp, spleen; S, stomach; C, colon. (From Nichol et al. [25], with permission.)

effects. For example, a majority of the adenoviral vector accumulates in the liver following intravenous administration expression [33,34]. Nuclear medicine can be used to ensure that the genetic vector is reaching the tissue of interest and to assist in the development of new genetic delivery systems with enhanced biological effectiveness. Zinn et al. [23] have radiolabeled the recombinant trimeric adenovirus vector of serotype (Ad5K) with technetium-99m (^{99m}Tc). They used an Anger gamma camera to follow the biodistribution following intravenous administration in mice. Using nuclear medicine dynamic imaging techniques, these authors showed the Ad5K-^{99m}Tc initially in the caudal vena cava, then the heart, then rapidly binding in the liver. A neutralizing antibody was also employed to block liver uptake. They found that the Ad5K had a high affinity for its cellular receptor, which leads to high liver uptake. From these nuclear medicine images, information was obtained about re-

ceptor binding, nonspecific vector uptake, and the future directions for adenoviral vector development, that is, the need to disrupt the adenoviral knob domain of the trimeric fiber capsid protein.

Nonviral vectors also have tissue targeting and biodistribution challenges. Figure 20.1 shows gamma scintigraphic images of the nonviral vector polyethlyeneimine that has been conjugated to DTPA and labeled with indium-111 [25]. These images show that polymer was rapidly eliminated from the bloodstream, with high uptake in the liver. Radiolabeling of the vector does not show that the protein of interest is being expressed, but rather shows the location of the genetic delivery system.

HSV-1-tk

One of the most exciting developments in imaging has been the use of nuclear medicine for noninvasive transgene expression imaging using herpes simplex virus type 1 thymidine kinase (HSV-1-tk) as a marker gene. The HSV-1-tk gene transfer followed by gancylovir treatment has been investigated as a potential gene therapy [7,21]. Tjuvajev et al. [27,35,36] have developed a system in which the HSV-1-tk marker gene enzyme product reacts with a radiolabeled marker substrate and converts it to a metabolite that is selectively trapped in the transduced cell. HSV-1-tk is an enzyme that is encoded in the virus. HSV-1-tk has been used as a target for nucleoside prodrug activation of treatments for herpes infection. The enzyme that is produced via the HSV-1-tk gene can phosphorylate antiherpetic agents such as gancylovir (GCV) to its monophosphate form. Once it is phosphorated, the substrate cannot be transported out of the cell, so it accumulates in the transduced cell. Therefore, cells in which successful gene transfer has occurred can be distinguished from nontransfected cells.

In 1995, Tjuvajev et al. [36] found that imaging of HSV-1-tk gene expression was possible. They used the rat RG2 glioblastoma cell line that was transfected in culture using the STK retrovirus containing the HSV-1-tk gene. Several marker substrates including GCV, 5-iodo-2-deoxyuridine (IUDR), and 5-iodo-2-fluoro-2-deoxy-beta-D-arabinofuranosyl uracil (FIAU), were evaluated as radiotracers. Both the sensitivity and selectivity of the marker substrates were tested. Sensitivity was as defined by the change in substrate accumulation divided by the change in HSV-1-tk expression in transduced cells. Selectivity was defined as the sensitivity divided by the substrate accumulation due to endogenous thymidine kinase. They determined that IUDR did not exhibit adequate selectivity and that gancylovir had low sensitivity. From studies on relative cellular accumulation of these three radiolabeled antiherpetic agents in RG2 cells transduced with the HSV-1-tk and wild-type RG2 cells, FIAU was selected for imagining HSV-1-tk-positive RG2 intracerabral rat tumors. Quantitative autoradiographic images (QAR) of intercerebral tumors were obtained using [14C]FIAU (Figure 20.2). The transduced tumor was clearly identified in the left hemisphere whereas the control RG2 tumor on the right was negative. This was the first publication showing the potential use of nuclear imaging technology for gene expression in vivo.

Several researchers [27,29,30] have since used biodistribution, autoradiography, clinical gamma cameras, and single photon emission tomography (SPECT) to image the HSV-1-tk expression. Administering ^{131}I labeled FIAV,

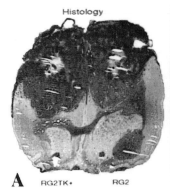
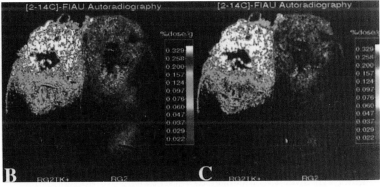

FIGURE 20.2. Imaging HSV-1-tk gene expression in RGTk+ intracerebral tumors. (A) Toluidine blue-stained histological section (macro-view). (B) Quantitative autoradiographic image of 2-[14C]FIAU accumulation 24 h after administration expressed as percentage of administered dose per gram tissue. (C) Images of section adjacent to that in (B) that was rinsed in 10% TCA for 4 h before autoradiographic exposure. The RG2TK-positive tumor is located in the left hemisphere and the nontransduced RG2 tumor is in the right hemisphere. (From Tjuvajev et al. [36], with permission.)

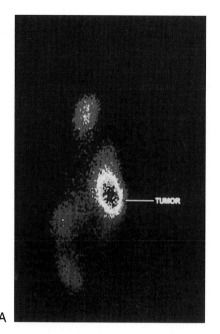
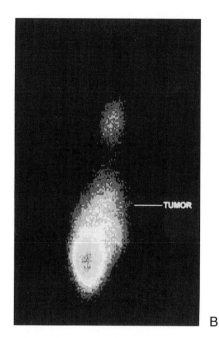

A   B

FIGURE 20.3. Scintigraphic images of KBALB-STK tumors showing (**A**) scintigram of a mouse bearing a subcutaneous KBALB-STK tumor before ganciclovir treatment illustrates the selective uptake of [^{131}I]IVFRU in KBALB-STK tumors expressing HSV-1-tk and (**B**) scintigram of the same animal after reinjection of [^{131}I]IVFRU and 4 days of ganciclovir treatment. Most of the activity present in the scan was present in the bladder, whereas the region of the shrinking tumor was devoid of activity. (From Morin et al. [30], with permission.)

Tjuvajev et al. [27] used rats bearing subcutaneous tumors RG2 glioma or W256 mammary carcinoma cells transfected with HSV-1-tk to image gene expression. Gambhir et al. [29] showed that [8-^{14}C]gancyclovir could accumulate in C6 rat glioma cells that were transfected with the HSV-1-tk gene using autoradiography and biodistribution analysis. Morin et al. radioiodinated another nucleoside analogue (E)-5-(2-iodovinyl)-2′-fluoro-2′-deoxyuridine (IVFRU) [30] to image HSV-1-tk expression in KBALB, KBALB-LNL, and KBALB-STK murine tumor cells implanted on Balb/c mice (Figure 20.3). The dose of [^{131}I]IVFRU was 3.7 MBq via the tail vein. These images were obtained 8 h after i.v. injection to rats bearing tumors 10 mm in diameter using a Searl gamma camera. After the initial dose, the rats were treated with gancyclovir (100 mg/kg) daily to compete with the radiolabeled probe. Although there was still a palpable tumor mass following gancyclovir treatment, no tumor was evident in the image. This illustrated that gancyclovir treatment inhibited IVFRU uptake. In addition, the authors found that 7 days of gancyclovir treatment resulted in complete tumor regression.

Recently, positron emission tomography (PET) also has been used to image HSV-1-tk expression. Several groups have synthesized ^{18}F-labeled nucleoside analogues including acylcovir [37] and gancylovir [38,39] for PET imaging of HSV-tk expression. Alauddin et al. have prepared 9-[(3-^{18}F-fluoro-1-hydroxy-2-propoxy)methyl]-guanine ([^{18}F]-FHPG) for (PET) imaging of gene incorporation and expression in tumors [40–42]. They used human colon cancer cells, HT-29, transduced with the retroviral vector G1Tk1SvNa, which showed fourfold higher uptake of the radiolabeled substrate in 1 h and up to 15 times higher at 7 h than the control (wild-type) cells. In vivo studies in tumor-bearing nude mice demonstrated that the tumor uptake of the radiotracer is three-

and sixfold higher in 2 and 5 h, respectively, in transduced cells compared with the control cells. These results suggest that [^{18}F]-FHPG is a potential in vivo PET imaging agent for monitoring gene incorporation and expression in gene therapy of cancer.

Tjuvajev et al. [32] evaluated ^{124}I conjugated to FIAU. They have shown that HSV-1-tk expression can be imaged via PET. In addition, they obtained a high level of correspondence between ^{124}I-FIAU radioactivity and independently measured HSV-1-tk expression. Levels of HSV-1-tk mRNA in the cell lines correlated to their level of sensitivity to the antiviral drug, ganciclovir. In addition, Gambhir et al. [29] obtained coronal micro-PET images of HSV-tk expression (Figure 20.4). They used an adenoviral vector to deliver the HSV-1-tk gene to C6 rat glioma cells and [8-^{18}F]fluoroganciclovir as an imaging probe. It is clear from these studies that PET/HSV1-tk imaging is promising for clinical monitoring of gene incorporation and expression in gene therapy for cancer [6].

Receptor-Mediated Gene Imaging

Receptor-mediated imaging of gene expression utilizes genes to encode cell-surface receptors that can be then targeted with a ligand-labeled radiotracer. For example, Raben et al. [43] have used adenoviral gene transduction of human glioma D54 MG cells in vitro to increase the expression of human carcinoembryonic antigen (CEA). The transduced cells exhibited high binding to ^{125}I-labeled COL1 Mab. In addition, the efficiency of transduction of direct intratumor injection of the adenoviral CEA vector in D54MG xenographs was determined by measuring ^{131}I-labeled COL-1 uptake through external scintigraphic imaging (Figure 20.5).

Other reporter genes have also been investigated for use in imaging gene expression, such as the gene that produces the dopamine type 2 (D2R) receptor [44]. Several radioisotopes including ^{11}C-raclopride, ^{18}F-fluoroethylspiperone (FESP), and ^{123}I-iodobenzamine are substrates for D2R. In this study, MacLaren et al. [44] used an adenoviral viral delivery system to transfect

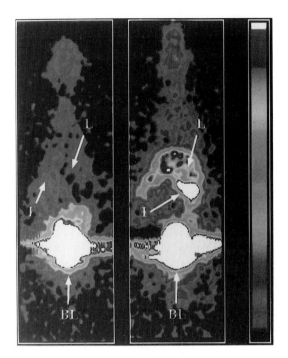

FIGURE 20.4. [^{18}F]FGCV coronal micro-PET images from mouse injected with control adenovirus (*left*) and adenovirus carrying HSV-1-tk gene (*right*). Each viral vector was injected 48 h before imaging. Images were obtained 1 h after injection of 150 μCi of [^{18}F]FGCV with 8 bed positions and 8 minutes/bed. Each image is normalized to common global maximum with *white* representing maximum counts. L, liver; I, intestine; BL, bladder. Reprinted by permission of the Society of Nuclear Medicine from Gambhir, et al. [29].

tumor cells with a D2R reporter gene. FESP was used as a probe to target the gene expression. PET was used to image gene expression in vivo (Figure 20.6).

Another novel approach to improve molecular imaging in oncology was developed by Mandell et al. [45]. They tranduced cancer cells with a rNIS^3 gene that facilitates iodide accumulation in follicular thyroid cells to mimic iodide uptake of the thyroid. Iodide is one of the few true "magic bullets" that allows for specific imaging of the thyroid with few side affects. In this study, the rNIS^3 gene was delivered via retrovirus to A375 human melanoma cells. Transduced and nontransduced A375 cells were then inoculated intradermally and grown

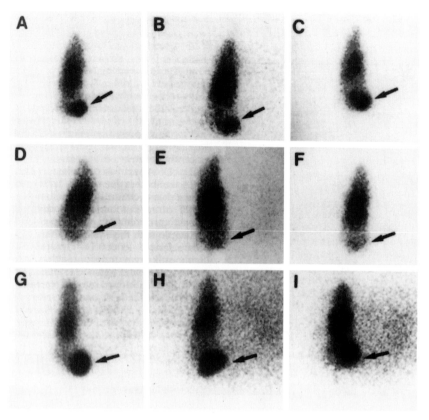

FIGURE 20.5. Whole-body scintigraphic images of athymic nude mice bearing (**A–C**) AdMCVCEA-transduced D54 MG subcutaneous tumors (*arrows*), (**D–F**) AdCMVlacZ-transduced D54 MG tumors (*arrows*), and (**G–I**) LS174T tumors (*arrows*) given an injection of 11.1 MBq ^{131}I-labeled COL-1 Mab. Dorsal images were taken at 5 days after intraperitoneal injection. Images were acquired for 50,000 c.p.m. The tumor weights at 5 days after injection were 0.3 to 1.1 g. (From Raben et al. [43], with permission.)

to 10 mm in nude mice. The rNIS-transduced tumors can be visualized in vivo using gamma scintigraphy (Figure 20.7). In addition, the authors investigated the use of iodide accumulation to selectively kill transfected cells with ^{131}I. They found that mice bearing rNIS^{3}-transfected tumors (including A375 human melanoma, BNL.1ME transformed mouse liver, CT26 mouse colon carcinoma, and IGROV human ovarian adenocarcinoma cells) had a highly significant improved survival rate over the nontransfected tumors.

MR Imaging of Gene Delivery

Magnetic resonance imaging (MRI) is a powerful technology for noninvasive imaging of disease conditions. Recently, MRI has been investigated as a tool to image gene delivery by conjugating paramagnetic contrast agents to the gene delivery vector. Kayyem et al. [46] conjugated diethylene triaminepetaacetic acid (DTPA) to the nonviral vector polylysine (PL) with and without a transferrin receptor ligand The vector was then chelated with the contrast agent gadolinium diethylene triaminepentaacetic acid (Gd-DTPA). They transfected K562 leukemia cells with the polymer–DNA complexes and found that MRI could be used to noninvasively track the delivery of the polymeric gene delivery system.

More recently de Marko et al. [47] have also used MRI to image gene delivery with a nonviral vector. In this study, dextran-

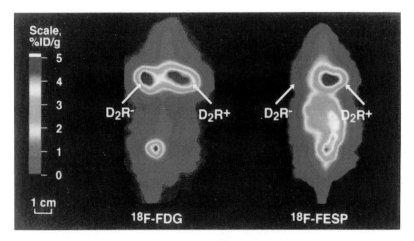

FIGURE 20.6. PET images of glucose metabolism and D2R reporter gene expression in a mouse with D_2R^- and D_2R^+ tumors. A nude mouse was injected subcutaneously with 1×10^6 D_2R^- cells and D_2R^+ on the left and right shoulders, respectively. Three weeks later, when the tumors were approximately 1 cm in diameter, the mouse was injected via tail vein with FDG (200 μCi) and imaged in the ACAT PET scanner after 1 h (*left image*). Two days later the same mouse was injected with FESP and then underwent a second PET scan. Each image represents the sum of the coronal images from the dorsal half of the same mouse. (From MacLaren et al. [44], with permission.)

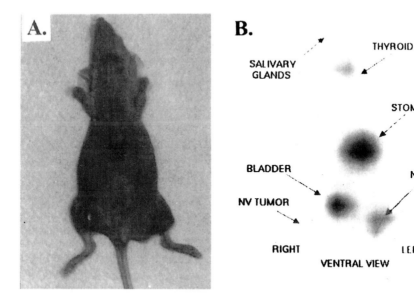

FIGURE 20.7. Imaging of rNIS-transduced compared with nontransduced A375 human melanoma tumors by a gamma camera. Tumors were established in vivo by intradermal injection of 5×10^6 cells into athymic nude mice. Mice (**A**) with established A275 xenographs, approximately 10 mm in diameter, were injected i.p. with 0.2 ml of saline solution containing 8.0 μCi [125]I. One hour after injection, a planar image (**B**) of the mouse was obtained using a Park Isocam II camera. Note the easily visualized rNIS-transduced tumor (*right side* of the image) compared with the nonvisualized NV tumor (*left side* of the image). (From Mandell et al. [45], with permission of *Cancer Research*.)

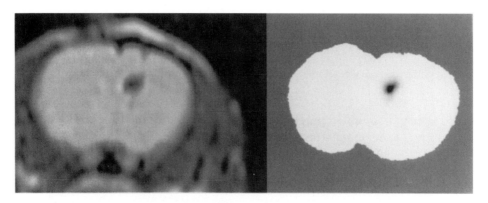

FIGURE 20.8. Cerebral DNA distribution in vivo using MR imaging. Correlation of spin-echo (1500/40) MR image (*left*) and autoradiograph (^{33}P-labeled contruct) superimposed on histological outline of corresponding brain section (*right*). There is good correlation between the in vivo imaging appearance of the construct and the autoradiographic distribution of the construct (section thickness for MR image, 300 μm; autoradiograph, 30 μm). (From de Marko et al. [47], with permission.)

polylysine-iron oxide–DNA particles were evaluated both in vitro using a 293 embryonic kidney cell line and in vivo using adult Sprague-Dawley rats. Figure 20.8 shows that MRI can be used to image gene delivery vectors. However, these studies do not actually image the expressed protein but rather the delivery system.

Initial studies have been performed to use MR technology to image gene expression. To assess gene expression using MRI, Weissleder et al. [48] developed a pcDNA3tyr plasmid that encodes for human tyrosinase. The tyrosinase enzyme is central in the formation of melanin that can bind with paramagnetic metals. The authors investigated whether tryosinase expression could induce melanin production, and, in turn, if this could be imaged using gamma scintigraphy and MR imaging technology. They used a mouse fibroblast L929 cell line and a human embryonic kidney 293 cell line, each transduced with the tyrosinase gene using calcium phosphate transfection protocol. Both nontransfected and mock-transfected cells were used as controls. The melanin production capability of these transfected cells was established using a Fontana stain with silver nitrate. ^{111}In-binding studies were performed to determine the metal-binding capacity of the transfected cells. The transfected 929 cells were found to have a significantly higher binding affinity than either of the control cells, and this binding was dependent on the dose of DNA. MR studies were performed on 293 transfected and mock-transfected cells that were incubated in media with 5 mg sulfated iron/l for 3 days. Using a superconducting magnet system at 1.5 T, T_1-weighted images were obtained of the cells in culture (Figure 20.9). A higher signal intensity corresponded to higher expression of tyrosinase, which produced the iron-binding melanin. This study demonstrated the feasiblity of using MR for gene expression imaging, but the tyrosine induction levels are low for in vivo imaging and the gene insert size is quite large, making adenoviral vectors unsuitable for gene delivery.

Another approach to using MRI to image gene expression is to use gene therapy to overexpress a cell-surface receptor that can then be targeted with paramagnetic contrast agents containing a ligand for the expressed receptor. Moore et al. [49] used a gene that encoded for human transferrin receptor (hTfR) to transfect rat 9L gliosarcoma cells with three forms of hTfR. A sterically protected iron containing a magnetic hTfR probe was used to demonstrate that the receptor expression could be visualized using NMR imaging.

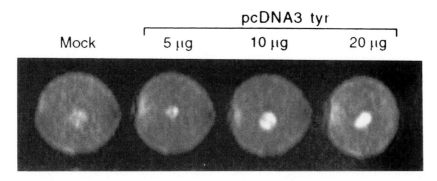

FIGURE 20.9. T_1-weighted, spoiled gradient-recalled acquisition in steady-state MR images (50/5, 60° flip angle) of human cells embedded in agarose. Cells were transfected with pcDNA3tyr (5, 10, or 20 μg) or were mock transfected (*far left*) 3 days before MR imaging and then grown in iron-containing cell culture medium. Note the higher signal intensity of cells after gene transfer; the higher signal intensity is caused by overexpression of tyrosinase-producing melanin, which scavenges iron. (From Weissleder et al. [48], with permission.)

Optical Imaging

Bioluminescent imaging is a potentially useful tool to image cellular and molecular processes. Contag et al. [50,51] have used the luciferase reporter gene from the firefly *Photinus pyralis* to indicate expression in vivo with bioluminescent imaging. A Hamamatsu charge-coupled device (CCD) camera was developed to detect photons that are emitted in vivo during the chemoluminescent reaction between the expressed luciferase and an injected or topically applied luciferin (D-(−)-2-(6′-hydroxy-2′-benzothiazolyl)thiazone-4-carboxylic acid) substrate. This system can be used to follow tumor progression, as shown in Figure 20.10. Melanoma cells (16-F10) were transfected with the luciferase reporter gene and implanted

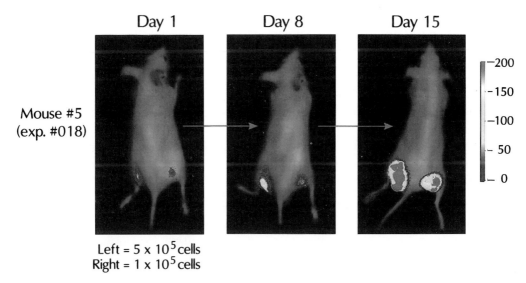

FIGURE 20.10. Tumor development over time in a mouse melanoma s.c. model (16-F10-luc) in nude mice; 10^6 cells were injected s.c. into the left flank, 10^5 cells s.c. into the right flank. (Courtesy of D. Jenkins, Xenogen Corporation, Alameda, CA, USA.)

subcutaneously into the left thigh of nude mice. For imaging, sedated mice were placed in a lighttight chamber. A gray-scale body surface image was collected with the chamber door slightly open. For the gene expression imaging, the door was closed tightly. Following the injection of luciferin substrate in dimethylsulfoxide (DMSO), the photons emitted were clearly visible by this noninvasive imaging system, and the tumor growth with time can be visualized. This imaging technology approaches real-time whole-body scanning with integration times of approximately 5 min/image.

Bioluminescent imaging has several advantages as well as disadvantages over conventional imaging modalities. One of the strengths of optical imaging is the ability to probe the cellular and molecular processes by labeling and monitoring cancer cells in vivo without disrupting the normal processes. This technology has also been used to demonstrate the process of cancer metastasis [52] using luciferase-labeled cells to image microcolony formation. In addition, bioluminescent imaging has been shown to be quite sensitive, detecting as few as 1000 luciferase-labeled cells distributed intraperitoneally in nude mice [52]. This technology may detect nonpalpable tumors and have applications in monitoring therapy response in minimal desease models. However, this technology is thus far limited to small animals because of transmission limitations of the luciferase emissions due to absorption and scattering of the light and limited tissue penetration.

In vivo microscopy has also been investigated by Kan et al. [53] as a tool to evaluate gene expression in living animals. Using rat 13762 NF breast cells stably transfected with green fluorescent protein (EGFP-N1), the cancer cells were observed in vivo directly using video microscopy (see Chapter 21, this volume).

The strength of this technology includes its ability to monitor gene expression under dynamic conditions and has the potential for monitoring the metastatic phenomena associated with these green fluorescent-labeled cells. With green fluorescent protein as a marker for tumor cells, in vivo microcopy could be used to monitor tumor cells in circulation, intravasalation, and cell segregation from the primary tumor. In vivo microscopy can visualize tissues only within a limited depth and for a limited time because this technique requires anesthesia and surgical manipulation of animals.

Imaging Endogenous Gene Expression

Contag et al. [50] have used bioluminescent technology to detect reporter gene activity as a means to monitor gene expression from xenographic tumors but also to study endogenous gene regulation. The luminescence could be produced when the gene transcription was activated. They used transgenic mice with a promotor of HIV-1 that was induced by DMSO. When HIV-1 transcription was activated, the photons emitted could be imaged on the CCD camera.

Imaging of endogenous genes could enhance early detection of cancer and aid in treatment decisions. For example, diagnosis of multidrug-resistance (MDR) development could directly affect the treatment protocols for patients with cancer. Multidrug resistance (MDR) is caused by several different mechanisms. The most extensively characterized mechanism is that associated with the MDR-1 gene and its protein product, P-glycoprotein (PgP), and the multidrug resistance-associated protein (MRP). PgP and MRP are members of the ATP-binding cassette transporter family. PGP is a 170-kDa membrane glycoprotein that acts as an ATP-dependent efflux pump reducing the intracellular accumulation of anthracyclines, *Vinca* alkaloids, epipodophyllotoxins, actinomycin D, taxol, and other anticancer agents. The overexpression of the multidrug-resistance (*mdr-1*) gene is responsible for many tumors being resistant or refractory to treatment after therapy.

[99m]Tc-Sestamibi was correlated to *mdr* gene expression by Cordobes et al. [54]. In addition, Cranshaw et al. [55] found that organotechnetium complexes, which are cationic and lipophilic, could be used to image PgP transport. Both ^{99m}Tc-sestamibi and ^{99m}Tc-tetrofosmin have been used as functional

probes of PgP transport activity. If these probes could be amplified and modified so that they were highly specific to one genetic protein, then imaging of gene expression could become a reality.

Conclusions

As gene therapy continues to evolve, so will the technology to image gene delivery and expression. The resolution of imaging systems and the specificity of contrast agents have improved significantly in the last decade. In addition, the development of tumor cell markers, molecular probes, and ligands for molecular biology have created specific and detailed in vitro analysis via flow cytometry and confocal and fluorescent microscopy. Potentially, imaging systems could be developed that would allow for the translation of tissue culture analysis systems into in vivo systems. In addition, the further development of new genetic markers that are readily targeted with our current imaging technologies will make genetic imaging a reality in the future.

References

1. Ko S-C, Gotoh A, Thalmann GN, et al. Molecular therapy with recombinant p53 adenovirus in an androgen-independent, metastatic human prostate cancer model. Hum Gene Ther 1996;7: 1683–1691.
2. Nguyen DM, Wiehle SA, Koch PE, et al. Delivery of the p53 tumor suppressor gene into lung cancer cells by an adenovirus/DNA complex. Can Gene Ther 1997;4:191–198.
3. Braun-Falco M, Doenecke A, Smola H, Hallek M. Efficient gene transfer into heman keratinocytes with recombinant adeno-associated virus vectors. Gene Ther 1999;6:432–441.
4. Wiznerowicz M, Fong AZC, Mackiewicz A, Hawley RG. Double-copy bicistronic retroviral vector platform for gene therapy and tissue engineering: application to melanoma vaccine development. Gene Ther 1997;4:1061–1068.
5. Hanania EG, Deisseroth AB. Serial transplantation shows that early hematopoietic precursor cells are transduced by MDR-1 retroviral vector in a mouse gene therapy model. Can Gene Ther 1994;1:21–25.
6. Blasberg R, Tjuvajev J. Herpes simplex virus thymidine kinase as a marker/reporter gene for PET imaging of gene therapy. Q J Nucl Med 1999;43:163–169.
7. Ross D, Kim B, Davidson B. Assessment of ganciclovir toxicity to experimental intracranial gliomas following recombinant adenoviral-mediated transfer of the herpes simplex virus thymidine kinase gene by magnetic resonance imaging and proton magnetic resonance imaging. Clin Cancer Res 1995;1:651–657.
8. Schellingerhout D, Bogdanov A, Marecos E, Spear M, Breakefield X, Weissleder R. Mapping the in vivo distribution of herpes simplex virions. Hum Gene Ther 1998;9:1543–1549.
9. Smaglik P. Viral vs. nonviral in gene therapy: which vector will prevail? Scientist 1998;12: 5–6.
10. Kuo PYP, Saltzman WM. Novel systems for controlled delivery of macromolecules. Crit Rev Eukaryotic Gene Expr 1996;6:59–73.
11. Abdallah B, Sachs L, Demeneix BA. Non-viral gene transfer: applications in developmental biology and gene therapy. Biol Cell 1995;85:1–7.
12. Felgner PL. Nonviral strategies for gene therapy. Sci Am 1997;276:102–110.
13. Crystal RG. Gene as the drug. Nat Med 1995; 1:15–17.
14. Ledely F. Nonviral gene therapy: the promise of genes as pharmaceutical products. Hum Gene Ther 1995;6:1129–1144.
15. Sochanik A, Szala S. On the strategy of using nonviral carriers in cancer gene therapy. Acta Biochim Pol 1996;43:295–300.
16. Zenke M, Steinlein P, Wagner E, Cotten M, Beug H, Birnstiel ML. Receptor-mediated endocytosis of transferrin-polycation conjugates: an efficient way to introduce DNA into hematopoietic cells. Proc NY Acad Sci 1990;87:3655–3659.
17. Suzuki T, Shin B-C, Fujikura K, Matsuzaki T, Takata K. Direct gene transfer into rat liver cells by in vivo electroporation. FEBS Lett 1998;425:436–440.
18. Yang J-P, Huang L. Direct gene transfer to mouse melanoma by intratumor injection of free DNA. Gene Ther 1996;3:542–548.
19. Wagner E, Zatloukal K, Cotten M, et al. Coupling of adenovirus to transferrin-polylysine/DNA complexes greatly enhances receptor-mediated gene delivery and expression of transfected genes. Proc Natl Acad Sci USA 1992;89:6099–6103.

20. Bonnekoh B, Greenhalgh D, Bundman D, et al. Adenoviral-mediated herpes simplex virus-thymidine kinase gene transfer in vivo for treatment of experimental human melanoma. J Invest Dermatol 1996;106:1163–1168.

21. Haberkorn U, Altmann A, Morr I, et al. Monitoring gene therapy with herpes simplex virus thymidine kinase in hepatoma cells: uptake of specific substrates. J Nucl Med 1997;38:287–294.

22. Moolten FL. Drug senstivity ("suicide genes") for selective cancer chemotherapy. Cancer Gene Ther 1994;1:279–287.

23. Zinn K, Douglas J, Smyth C, et al. Imaging and tissue biodistribution of ^{99m}Tc-labeled adenovirus knob. Gene Ther 1998;5:798–808.

24. Harrington KJ, Peters AM, Mohammadtaghi S, Glass D, Epenetos AA, Stewart JSW. Biodistribution and pharmacokinetics of In-111-labels Stealth liposomes in patients with solid tumours. J Nucl Med 1996;37:54P.

25. Nichol CA, Yang D, Humphrey W, et al. Biodistribution and imaging of polyethyleneimine—a gene delivery agent. Drug Delivery 1999;6:187–194.

26. Weibe L, Knaus E, Morin K. Radiolabelled pyrimidine nucleosides to monitor the expression of HSV-1 thymidine kinase in gene therapy. Nucleosides Nucleotides 1999;18:1065–1066.

27. Tjuvajev J, Joshi R, Kennedy J, et al. Gamma camera imaging of HSV-tk gene expression with [^{131}I]-FIAU: clinical applications in gene therapy. J Nucl Med 1996;37:53P.

28. Urbain JLC, Shore SK, Vekemans MC, et al. Scintigraphic imaging of oncogenes with antisense probes: does it make sense? Eur J Nucl Med 1995;22:499–504.

29. Gambhir S, Barrio J, Wu L, et al. Imaging of adenoviral-directed herpes simplex virus type 1 thymidine kinase reporter gene expression in mice with radiolabled gancyclovir. J Nucl Med 1998;39:2003–2011.

30. Morin K, Knaus E, Wiebe L. Non-invasive scintigraphic monitoring of gene expression in a HSV-1 thymidine kinase gene therapy. Nucl Med Commun 1997;18:599–605.

31. Poptani H, Puumalainen A, Grohn O, et al. Monitoring thymidine kinase and ganciclovir-induced changes in rat malignant glioma in vivo by nuclear magnetic resonance imaging. Cancer Gene Ther 1998;5:101–109.

32. Tjuvajev J, Avril N, Oku T, et al. Imaging herpes virus thymidine kinase gene transfer and expression by positron emission tomography. Cancer Res 1998;58:4333–4341.

33. Huard J, Lochmuller H, Acsadi G, Jani A, Massie B, Karpati G. The route of administration is a major determinant of the transduction efficiency of rat tissues by adenoviral recombinants. Gene Ther 1995;2:107–115.

34. Kass-Eisler A, Falck-Pederson E, Elfenbein DH, Alvira M, Buttrick PM, Leinwand LA. The impact of developmental stage, route of administration and the immune system on adenovirus-mediated gene transfer. Gene Ther 1994;1:395–402.

35. Timmermans J, Moes AJ. Factors controlling the buoyancy and gastric retention capabilities of floating matrix capsules: new data for reconsidering the controversy. J Pharm Sci 1994;83:18–24.

36. Tjuvajev JG, Stockhammer G, Desai R, et al. Imaging the expression of transfected gene in vivo. Cancer Res 1995;55:6126–6132.

37. Srinivasan A, Gambhi S, Green LA, et al. A PET reporter gene (PRG)/PET reporter probe (PRP) technology for repeatedly imaging gene expression in living animals. J Nucl Med 1996;37:107P.

38. Green LA, Gambhir SS, Barrio JR, et al. Tracer kinetic modeling of 8-(F-18)-fluoro-ganciclovir PET data: a new tracer for measuring reporter gene expression. J Nucl Med 1998;39:10p.

39. Goldman S, Monclus M, Cool V, et al. A novel PET tracer for evaluation of gene therapy. J Nucl Med 1996;37:53P.

40. Alauddin M, Conti P, Mazza S, Hamzeh F, Lever J. 9-[(3-[^{18}F]-Fluoro-1-hydroxy-2-propoxy)methyl]guanine ([^{18}F]-FHPG): a potential imaging agent of viral infection and gene therapy using PET. Nucl Med Biol 1996;23:787–792.

41. Alauddin M, Conti P. Synthesis and preliminary evaluation of 9-(4-[^{18}F]-fluoro-3-hydroxymethyl-butyl)guanine ([^{18}F]FHBG): a new potential imaging agent for viral infection and gene therapy using PET. Nucl Med Biol 1998;23:175–180.

42. Alauddin M, Shahinian A, Kundu R, Gordon E, Conti P. Evaluation of 9-[(3-^{18}F-fluoro-1-hydroxy-2-propoxy)methyl]guanine ([^{18}F]-FHPG) in vitro and in vivo as a probe for PET imaging of gene incorporation and expression in tumors. Nucl Med Biol 1999;26:371–376.

43. Raben D, Buchsbaum DJ, Khazaeli MB, et al. Enhancement of radiolabeled antibody binding and tumor localization through adenoviral transduction of the human carcinoembryonic antigen gene. Gene Ther 1996;3:567–580.

44. MacLaren DC, Gambhir SS, Satyamurthy N, et al. Repetitive, non-invasive imaging of the

dopamine D-2 receptor as a reporter gene in living animals. Gene Ther 1999;6:785–791.

45. Mandell R, Mandell L, Link C. Radioisotope concentrator gene therapy using the sodium/iodide symporter gene. Cancer Res 1999;59:661–668.

46. Kayyem J, Kumar R, Fraser S, Meade T. Receptor-targeted co-transport of DNA and magnetic resonance contrast agents. Chem Biol 1995;2:615–620.

47. de Marko G, Bogdanov A, Marecos E, Moore A, Simonova M, Weissleder R. MR imaging of gene delivery to the central nervous system with an artificial vector. Radiology 1998;208:65–71.

48. Weissleder R, Simonova M, Bogdanova A, Bredow S, Enochs W, Bogdanov A. MR imaging and scintigraphy of gene expression through melanin induction. Radiology 1997;204:425–429.

49. Moore A, Basilion JP, Chiocca EA, Weissleder R. Measuring transferrin receptor gene expression by NMR imaging. Biochim Biophys Acta 1998;1402:236–249.

50. Contag PR, Olomu IN, Stevenson DK, Contag CH. Bioluminescent indicators in living animals. Nat Med 1998;4:245–247.

51. Beraron D, Contag P, Contag C. Imaging brain structure and function, infection and gene expression in the body using light. Philos Trans R Soc Lond Ser B Biol Sci 1997;352:755–761.

52. Edinger M, Sweeny TJ, Tucker AA, et al. Non-invasive assessment of tumor cell proliferation in animal models. Neoplasia 1999;1:303–310.

53. Kan X, Liu T-J. Video microscopy of tumor metastasis: using the green fluorescent protein (GFP) gene as a cancer-cell-labeling system. Clin Exp Metastas 1999;17:49–55.

54. Cordobes M, Starzec A, Delmon-Moingeon L, et al. Technetium-99m-sestamibi uptake by human benign and malignant breast tumor cells: correlation with mdr gene expression. J Nucl Med 1996;37:286–289.

55. Crankshaw CL, Marmion M, Luker GD, et al. Novel technetium(III)-Q complexes for functional imaging of multidrug resistance (MDR1) P-glycoprotein. J Nucl Med 1998;39:77–86.

21
Optical Imaging and In Vivo Microscopy

Zuxing Kan and E. Edmund Kim

Useful images of hidden structures or pathological lesions can be created with X-rays, ultrasound, radioactive tracer, and magnetic resonance. However, there are many biological processes that cannot be easily or directly monitored by using computed tomography (CT), magnetic resonance imaging (MRI), or nuclear imaging because key molecules in these processes are not distinguishable from each other with these imaging techniques. Light penetrates tissue and is reflected at the surface. Whatever light does penetrate tissue is scattered widely so that shadows of internal structures are blurred beyond recognition. Light has been used in all the varieties of endoscopic imaging, where rigid or flexible tubes are inserted through incisions or natural body openings. Conventional endoscopies use only visible light and look only at the surface of internal structures, while the new techniques may use other wavelengths and look below the surface.

A variety of techniques are being explored, and they are quite distinct although they all use light. Optical coherence tomography (OCT) uses infrared light and forms images of subsurface boundaries from signals reflected at the boundaries. Optical tomography uses light to create cross-sectional images. Induced fluorescence devices use light from lasers or incandescent sources to stimulate tissue. Different tissues fluoresce differently, and thus cancerous lesions may fluoresce differently than normal tissues. A variety of other responses induced by light include electrophysiological potentials and elastic light scattering. In vivo microscopy also uses ultraviolet light for illuminating organs that depict microvasculature at the cellular level.

Optical Tomography

In CT, X-ray photons follow a nearly straight path along which they are differently absorbed by various tissues through which they pass, and the mathematics used in CT to reconstruct an image assumes a straight-line path. By contrast, in optical tomography, light photons generally follow a random path and are refracted and scattered by the tissues through which they pass. Optical coherence tomography (OCT) focuses light on a very small area and uses the reflected light as the signal. The light reflections occur not only from the outside surface, but also from interior surfaces. One could measure the depth of an internal reflector by measuring the time for a light pulse to travel from the source to the reflector and back to a sensor. It is difficult to generate such short pulses and measure such brief time intervals. In OCT, the depth of a reflection is measured by the interference between the reflected signal and the original reference signal. The OCT system uses a filtered broadband light source that creates two beams. One beam is focused on the site of interest and the other on a corner reflector. To form an image, the corner reflector is physically moved back and forth, generating signals derived from reflections at different depths while the beam focused on the tissue of interest is scanned back and forth, generating reflections along a line or an arc. To generate a series of slices, the focusing apparatus is moved laterally after the data along a line or arc have been accumulated.

Because the wavelengths of light in OCT are very short, the system produces images with spatial resolution of $10\mu m$, roughly two orders of magnitude better than typical CT and MR images. The depth of OCT is about 4 mm, but this is enough to characterize cells in a zone of suspected cancer. An OCT system with a diameter of 1 mm can be placed at the end of a catheter, which provides a possible role in noninvasive histology and cytology because individual cells making up a tissue are visible without staining. OCT should also have a role in developmental biology such that it will no longer be necessary to kill an animal to examine the cells in its tissues. OCT is ideally suited for the rapid acquisition of micrometer-scale-resolution two-dimensional (2-D) and three-dimensional (3-D) images of biological tissues such as small vessels and nerves. It permits rapid feedback for assessment of microsurgical procedures [1]. Future work will focus on methods to increase the rate of data acquisition, to increase the resolution, and to combine structural imaging with OCT Doppler techniques. Use of a high-speed optical delay line, decreasing the number of pixels, and high-speed volume acquisition will improve the acquisition time. Resolution as high as 2 to $5\mu m$ may be achieved by using broader-bandwidth laser sources.

A number of companies are developing products based on induced fluorescence to illuminate the surfaces of certain organs with visible or ultraviolet light from a laser or a filtered broadband source to stimulate autofluorescence. Cancerous and precancerous tissues fluoresce differently than normal tissues. The FDA-approved LIFE (lung imaging fluorescence endoscope) Lung system uses a modified bronchoscope. Blue light (442 nm) from a laser illuminates the walls of the bronchi, and cancerous regions are seen as reddish-brown while normal tissues are visualized as green. These images increase the sensitivity and specificity of bronchoscopic examinations by making cancer far more conspicuous than it is in white-light images. The system can reveal areas of incipient cancer that appear normal under white light. It is likely that the fluorescent signatures of cancers in different regions of the body are different, and therefore the signal processing part for these newer systems is not the same as for the LIFE-Lung system. The MediSpectra system makes point-by-point measurements by illuminating each point with a light beam about 1 mm in diameter, producing about 100 samples in a 10×10 raster in 15 s. Early trial results indicate higher sensitivity and specificity of the light test than those of the Pap test in the examination of the uterine cervix [2,3]. Fonet uses broadband light from an arc lamp that covers the visible spectrum and a bit more in the infrared and ultraviolet spectrums. It measures elastic light scattering instead of measuring induced fluorescence. The system is said to be useful for the detection of genitourinary and colon cancers [3].

The near-infrared region (700–1000 nm) offers unique advantages for the imaging of pathophysiological states. Water and most naturally occurring fluorochromes do not absorb substantial amounts of energy in this region. Thus, near-infrared radiation penetrates tissues more efficiently than does visible light or photons in the infrared region [4,5]. Exogenously added contrast agents would aid in the sensitivity and specificity of tumor detection, but they accentuate nonspecific differences such as differences in perfusion or permeability, which results in relatively low target-to-background ratios (usually <4:1) [5].

A class of contrast agents that fluoresce only after interaction with specific enzymes expressed in tumors have been developed [6]. They become fluorescent after enzymatic conversion as the result of fluorochrome release and abatement of intramolecular optical fluorescence quenching. Using a biocompatible autoquenched near-infrared fluorescent compound that is activated by tumor-associated proteases for cathepsins B and H, tumors as small as 1 mm become detectable with the imaging system using the source that delivered 610- to 650-nm excitation light with a 700-nm longpass filter (Figure 21.1) [5]. Molecular

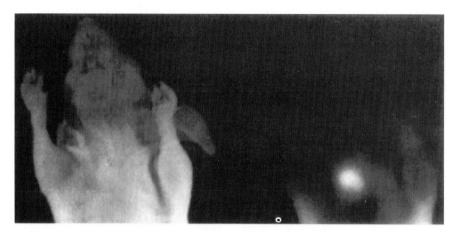

FIGURE 21.1. Light image (*left*) and near-infrared fluorescence image (*right*) in a mouse at 24 h after injection of protease-sensitive polylysine methoxy-polyethyleneglycol shows an implanted 2-mm breast tumor. Near-infrared fluorescence signal is scaled linearly and shows the high target-to-background ratio. (From Mahmood et al. [5], with permission.)

events may be imaged by near-infrared fluorescence imaging, which will allow the detection and localization of disease states before anatomical changes become apparent.

In Vivo Microscopy

In vivo microscopy allows the direct observation of various living organs, including measurements of the rate, direction, and magnitude of the microcirculation of the organs. High resolution in vivo microscopy depicts well the microvasculature at the cellular level, and this makes it a unique technique for probing cell activities that occur in the microcirculation [7]. In our laboratory, in vivo microscopy has been used in a series of experiments to study blood supply to the normal liver and to liver cancers and to monitor the distribution and effects of intravascular embolic or target delivery agents, of host reactions to the therapies, and of the fate of metastatic tumors in response to interventional radiological therapies.

The in vivo microscope used in our laboratory is one that was modified from a standard compound binocular microscope (Carl Zeiss, Thornwood, NY, USA) and is equipped for both transillumination and epiillumination of the organ to be studied. A tray has been designed for placement of the animal on the stage. The organ or tissue to be examined, such as the liver of a rat, is exposed and gently exteriorized through a midline abdominal incision and then placed over the observing window on the tray. After this, the organ is covered with a piece of thin transparent plastic wrap and separated from the other organs to limit movement caused by respiration, heartbeats, and intestinal peristalsis. The organ surface is constantly irrigated with Ringer's solution at body temperature. Organs are transilluminated with selected wavelengths of light from a monochromator that are projected through a focusable condenser with a long working distance under the stage. Organs are epiilluminated with light, for example, the ultraviolet light used for fluorescein isothiocyanate fluorescence excitation, projected through the objective lens from above. Epiillumination produces images with less resolution than transillumination does, but there is no thickness limitation to the organ to be studied. The power of the objective lenses used in our equipment ranges from 2.5× to 80×. The higher-power objective lenses (40× and higher) are water immersion lenses, which achieve better resolution images than dry lenses and yield pictures free from blurring caused by moist live tissue.

Hepatic Microcirculation and Blood Supply to Hepatic Tumors

A thorough understanding of the hemodynamics of the liver and of hepatic tumors is essential for both the diagnosis and the treatment of these tumors. The liver derives its blood supply from the portal vein (70%–80%) and the hepatic artery (20%–30%), whereas hepatic tumors are primarily nourished by the hepatic artery (>90%), with minimal supply from the portal vein. This characteristic allows specific therapies such as embolization and chemoembolization to be carried out via the hepatic artery while preserving adequate liver function.

At the microcirculation level in normal liver, the sinusoids are the direct continuation of the portal vessels; however, the termination of the hepatic arterioles is complex. Anatomically, hepatic arterioles communicate with the peribiliary plexus, the terminal arterioportal anastomosis, the vasa vasorum of the portal vein, and the direct arterioportal connections [8]. Aided by fluorescent tracer injection via a catheter placed in the hepatic artery, in vivo microscopy has shown that hepatic arterial blood appears in the terminal portal venules before entering the sinusoids (see Figure 21.2), which indicates that arterioportal communications play an important role in hepatic microcirculation.

In vivo microscopy confirmed that both hypervascular and hypovascular hepatic tumors are predominantly supplied by the hepatic artery (Figure 21.3). The portal venous blood flow is impeded at the periphery of the tumor, and only a small amount enters the tumors. Further in vivo microscopy studies of the blood circulation in tumors have demonstrated that the hepatic artery and the portal vein are closely interrelated in supplying blood to hepatic tumors. Interruption of either the hepatic arterial or the portal venous flow by ligation or embolization does not eliminate the blood circulation through the tumors. In fact, the average reduction in the flow rates of blood in either vessel is statistically insignificant. Fluorescent tracer injected into the hepatic artery has revealed that hepatic arterial blood enters tumors via the portal venules and the sinusoids surrounding the tumor, and no obvious dilatation of the terminal hepatic arterioles was observed. Histological studies have also shown that the dense vascular network surrounding hepatic tumors is formed by dilated portal veins and not hepatic arteries. As the arterial blood shunts into the portal venules at the tumor border, the high arterial pressure created within these vessels impedes the portal flow entering the tumors. As soon as the arterial flow is interrupted, the high pressure is released and the portal flow increases to supply the tumor. As the tumors grows larger, more arteries and veins become involved and pressure increases in the vasculature surrounding the tumors, which explains the changes in blood supply during tumor growth and the formation of portal hypertension in the late stage of tumor-bearing livers [9].

Distribution, Clearance, and Effect of Embolic Agents in Chemoembolization Therapy

Hepatic arterial embolization and chemoembolization, which combines embolization with chemotherapy, are the alternative therapies for inoperable liver cancers. The roles of the embolic agents used in chemoembolization are to interrupt the blood supply to hepatic tumors and to carry and deliver the anticancer drugs to the tumor [10].

The iodized poppyseed oil, Lipiodol (Laboratoires Andre Guerbet, Aulnay-sous-Bois, France), has been the most commonly used embolic agent for more than 20 years and is used for both the treatment and diagnosis of hepatic tumors [11]. However, until the advent of in vivo microscopy, the fate of this oily embolic agent in hepatic circulation was little understood.

In vivo microscopy showed that, when injected into the portal vein, Lipiodol instantly filled the terminal portal venules. When injected into the hepatic artery, Lipiodol also appeared in the terminal portal venules, but in this instance in the form of a series of small droplets (Figure 21.4). In addition, arterially injected Lipiodol entered the portal system in

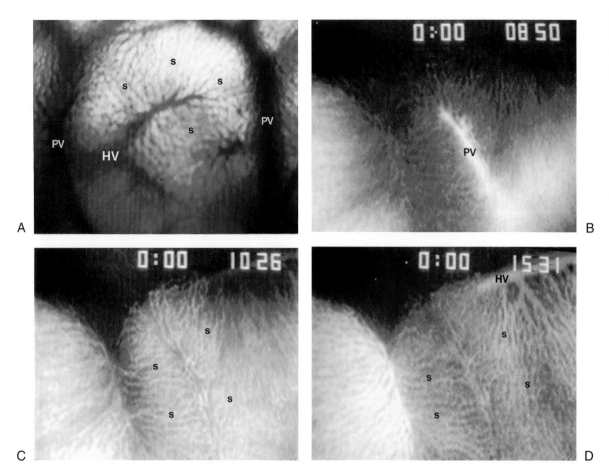

FIGURE 21.2. In vivo micrographs of normal hepatic microcirculation in rat. **A**. Hepatic lobule shows blood flow from portal venule (PV) through the sinusoids (s) to the hepatic venules (HV). ×125.

B–D. Fluorescent dextran solution injected into the hepatic artery shows the arterial flow entering the portal venules (PV) before entering the sinusoids (S) and subsequently the hepatic venules (HV). ×50.

all rats, mice, rabbits, and swine [12,13]. Further study demonstrated that arterially injected Lipiodol passed through the peribiliary plexus to enter the portal vein [14]. The amount of the oil appearing in the portal vein was dose dependent. Lipiodol distributed unevenly in the liver, with certain segments or lobes containing more oil than others. Changing the position of the animal and injecting the oil in a pulsative manner did not improve the oil distribution. Some time after the injection, from minutes to hours depending on the dose used, when the portal venules were filled with the oil and the sinusoidal circulation was obstructed, blood flow to irrigate the sinusoids resumed in the

hepatic arterioles. Ligation or reembolization of the hepatic artery stopped the arteriolar flow immediately. In vivo microscopy further demonstrated that Lipiodol traverses the sinusoids and enters the hepatic veins and subsequently the systemic circulation. Solid particulate materials, such as degradable starch microspheres (40 μm), plastic microspheres (25–100 μm), and Gelfoam powder (75–200 μm), never appeared in the portal vein when injected into the hepatic artery. The blood flow in the portal system and the sinusoids was not significantly affected.

The sinusoidal congestion occurred as soon as Lipiodol accumulated in the portal venules.

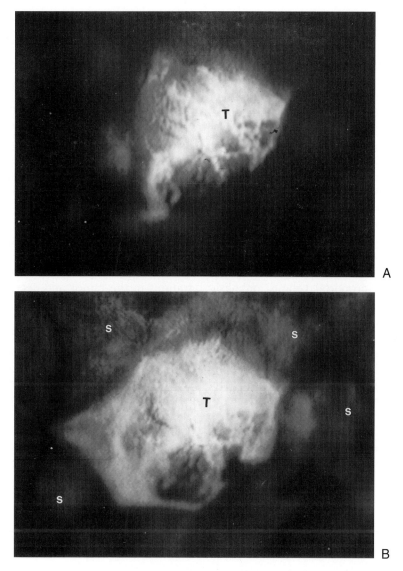

FIGURE 21.3. Tumor blood supply. Fluorescent dextran solution injected into the hepatic artery of a rat with liver tumor shows that arterial blood enters the tumor (T) earlier (**A**) and in larger amounts than it enters the sinusoids (s) in normal liver (**B**). ×50.

The oil that accumulated in the portal venules slowly entered the sinusoids over hours to days, depending on the dose. The resumed hepatic arterial flow plays an important role in clearing the oil from the liver [9]. Although hemorrhagic necrosis of the hepatic parenchyma could occur 1 day after Lipiodol administration, liver regeneration was observed to occur in 5 to 7 days after injection. Reembolization of the hepatic artery with particulate embolic agents, which prevents resumption of the arterial circulation, caused more severe damage to the liver than Lipiodol embolization alone.

On the basis of the finding that the iodized oil enters the portal vein almost immediately after being injected into the hepatic artery, we conjectured that it should be possible to create a dual hepatic arteroportal venous embolization with a single arterial catheterization procedure [15,16]. To test this, absolute ethanol was added to iodized oil in a proper ratio to reinforce the embolic effect. A 3:1 and 4:1 ratio of Lipiodol to ethanol mixture was optimal in pigs and rats, respectively. In both rats and pigs, segmental atrophy and diffuse hypertrophy of residual liver was accomplished by selective infusion of the hepatic artery. Subsequent use of this technique in patients showed that Lipiodol/ethanol embolization is a safe and efficacious method for the treatment of hepatocellular carcinoma. It effectively shrank the tumor, caused hepatic hypertrophy, and improved liver function and tumor resection with a better survival rate [17].

In Vivo Microscopy of Lipiodol Emulsion in Hepatic Circulation

In chemoembolization for the treatment of liver cancers, the anticancer drugs are dissolved in water or water-soluble contrast medium and the solution is then mixed with iodized oil to form an emulsion for intrahepatic arterial injection. The anticancer drug is intended to be delivered by the oil into the tumor and released in a controlled manner. Pharmacokinetic studies confirmed that the use of emulsion has the dual advantage of increasing drug concentrations in the tumor and decreasing systemic exposure [18]. In vivo microscopy has additionally helped to define the physical phase characteristics of emulsions consisting of different ratios of drug solution to iodized oil, to determine the stability of the emulsion in hepatic circulation, and to compare the delivery capacity of the different types of emulsions in liver chemoembolization [19].

In elucidating the physical characteristics of the emulsion, in vivo microscopy has shown that the emulsion phase is determined by the proportion of aqueous solution to the oil. Specifically, the smaller part of the mixture always splits and disperses as the internal phase

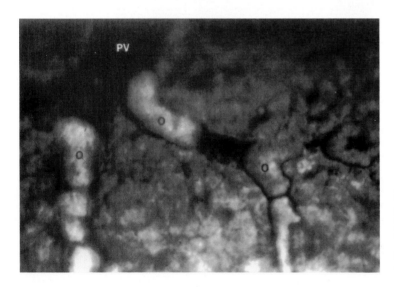

Figure 21.4. In vivo micrograph of rat liver 4 min after injection of Lipiodol into the hepatic artery. The oil droplets (O) reached and accumulated in a terminal portal venule (PV). ×400.

in the larger part, which forms the continuous external phase. It has also shown that both water-in-oil (w/o) and oil-in-water (o/w) phase emulsions are stable in the hepatic circulation and that the iodized oil in the emulsions carries the aqueous drug solution to its destination. In both hypervascular and hypovascular tumors, the emulsions enter the tumor vessels following hepatic arterial administration, the w/o emulsions having a higher capacity of drug delivery than the o/w emulsions.

In Vivo Microscopy of Hepatic Metastases

Tumor metastasis is a complex process that includes separation of the tumor cells from the original tumor, intravasation, circulation, arrest, extravasation, migration, and new tumor formation [20]. High resolution in vivo microscopy has been useful in elucidating the details of the invasion process in the microcirculation, an insight unobtainable using other techniques [21].

The arrest and lodgment of tumor cells in the blood vessels is an important step in tumor invasion. In vivo microscopy has demonstrated the adhesive nature of tumor cells, in particular, that the tumor cells tend to escape from the bloodstream and adhere to the endothelial lining. Later, they flatten and merge with the sinusoidal wall and eventually extravasate and migrate in the parenchyma (Figure 21.5). Electron microscopy confirmed that tumor cells extravasate through the widened fenestrae of the endothelial cells. The tumor cells then divide in the hepatic parenchyma, compress, and displace the hepatocytes. The endogenously generated tumor cells exhibited great deformability as they moved through the lumen of the sinusoids. However, the narrowness of the vascular lumen caused by swollen endothelial cells, adherent leukocytes, and aggregated thrombocytes did facilitate tumor cell arrest.

Kupffer cells are the fixed macrophages in the liver that have a nonspecific tumoricidal ability. Activation of the Kupffer cells enhances their tumoricidal function, resulting in slowed tumor growth and prolonged patient survival.

In vivo microscopy has shown that Kupffer cells are actively involved in the host defense mounted against tumor cell invasion [21]. In particular, Kupffer cells in tumor-bearing livers were activated, as evidenced by the markedly increased number of Kupffer cells and the increase in their ability to phagocytose. This increase was most prominent in the sinusoids surrounding tumors, probably because Kupffer cells combat the tumor cells at the active margin of invasion. In normal liver, centrilobular areas have fewer Kupffer cells and the function of these Kupffer cells is reduced compared with the function of Kupffer cells in periportal areas. In tumor-bearing livers, Kupffer cells in centrilobular areas were also increased in number and activity.

In Vivo Microscopy of Tumor Cells Labeled with the Green Fluorescent Protein Gene

To better detect and track tumor cells in the circulation of living animals, tumor cells are labeled to distinguish them from background tissues. The technique currently used is to stain the tumor cells with fluorescent dyes in vitro and then to introduce the labeled cells into the animal circulation. The cell labeling produced by this technique is temporary because the fluorescence is lost quickly through fading, quenching, and cell division [22]. In addition, the fluorescent dyes are toxic and may alter the function of tumor cells, causing unreliable and controversial results in experiments. With this technique that the tumor cells are labeled in vitro and then introduced into the animals, the behavior of the cells does not necessarily represent that of the endogenously generated metastatic cells because of the differences between the two in terms of the origin, the route of access, and the number of cells.

These difficulties appear to have been overcome with the advent of GFP labeling of tumor cells. The green fluorescent protein, GFP, gene was cloned from the genome of the jellyfish *Aequorea victoria* [23]. GFP yields a bright, stable green fluorescence, which is species independent and can be detected in the tissues of live animals. Because the GFP gene is integrated into the chromosome, cell division will pass the GFP gene on to subsequent generations of cells, which enables cancer growth, invasion, and metastasis to be tracked on a real-time basis [24]. In addition, the cancer cells labeled with GFP maintain their fluorescence intensity not only when the cells are alive but also when they are fixed, making reciprocal comparison of in vivo microscopy and histological studies practicable [25].

To study the long-term tracking of tumor cells in the living animals using the GFP method, we transfected EGFP-N1 (Clontech Laboratories, Palo Alto, CA, USA), an expression vector containing one of the GFP gene variants, into 13762NF murine mammary adenocarcinoma tumor cells using CLONfectin (Clontech). Twenty-four hours after transfection, cells were placed in selection medium containing 600 g/ml G418 and cultured for 2 weeks. G418-resistant clones were then isolated, expanded, and analyzed. Clonal cells were visualized under the fluorescence microscope to identify green fluorescence and Western blot analysis performed using the GFP monoclonal antibody to confirm GFP gene expression. The fluorescence exhibited by the tumor cells has

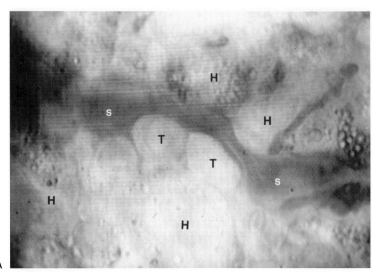

A

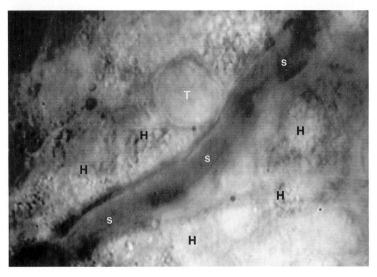

B

FIGURE 21.5. **A**. In vivo hepatic micrograph of the sinusoids close to a tumor in a mouse liver. Tumor cells (T) have arrested and adhered to the endothelial wall. The sinusoids (s) have become irregular in shape. **B**. In another area, a tumor cell (T) has extravasated into the sinusoid and lodged in the liver parenchyma. H, hepatocytes. ×1000.

FIGURE 21.6. Fluorescent micrograph of metastases in the lung in a Fischer-344 rat that received an orthotopic inoculation of tumor cells in the mammary gland fat pad. The metastatic nodules (T) exhibit strong green fluorescence, which is easily discernible against the background of nonfluorescent host tissue and blood vessels (v). ×40.

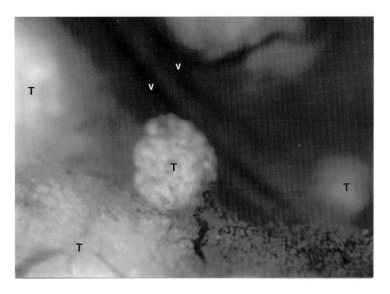

been proved to be stable and efficient for in vivo microscopy in living animals. There was no perceivable fading or reduction in the intensity of fluorescence [26].

In all the animals inoculated with GFP-labeled cancer cells in thigh muscle, liver, or mammary gland fat pad, tumors grew in the original site, and the metastases in the remote organs both showed an intensity of fluorescence. The location, size, shape, and invasion pattern of the tumors were well delineated. Tiny metastases or daughter nodules, which

are sometimes undetectable macroscopically, were easily located because of the fluorescence (Figure 21.6). Early small colonies of tumor metastases formed by a cluster of tumor cells were usually next to or very close to the blood vessels, an indication of their bloodborne origin (Figure 21.7). In early stages, the small tumors were supplied with no new vessels, while the larger metastases always had a new vascular plexus at their periphery. All the animals that received the GFP-labeled tumor cell inoculation had individual, arrested cancer cells in the

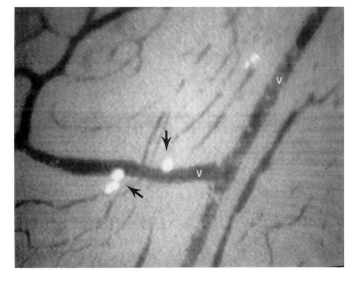

FIGURE 21.7. Fluorescent video micrograph of the mesentery in a Fischer-344 rat that received an orthotopic inoculation of tumor cells in the mammary gland fat pad 25 days earlier. Cancer cells (*arrows*) that have extravasated the blood vessel (v) are detected by their intense fluorescence. ×400.

capillaries or in the vicinity of the blood vessels in the liver, mesentery, intestine wall, spleen, kidneys, and lungs. The majority of these cells were dead, as evidenced by their irregular contours and disintegrated membrane. Viable metastatic cells existed, although these were much fewer than the dead cells. The viable cell exhibited a normal size, regular configuration, and clear internal structure, and some appeared to be in the process of division.

With the development of in vivo microscopic technology that eliminates limitations such as those imposed by observation time, image quality, and illumination, direct observation of each step in tumor metastasis, such as cell segregation from the original tumor, cell migration in extravascular tissues, intravasation, distribution, extravasation, and micrometastasis formation, is possible [27]. The technique could also be extended to investigation of the mechanisms and factors involved in provoking and prohibiting tumor growth and metastasis and hence to the development of new strategies of tumor treatments.

Acknowledgment. This work was supported by Radiological Society of North America Seed Grant 1998, PRS and BRS grants of The University of Texas M.D. Anderson Cancer Center, and the John S. Dunn Research Foundation.

References

1. Boppart SA, Bouma BE, Pitris C, et al. Intraoperative assessment of microsurgery with three-dimensional optical coherence tomography. Radiology 1998;208:81–86.
2. Tearney G, Brezinski M, Bouma B, et al. In vivo endoscopic optical biopsy with optical coherence tomography. Science 1997;277:2037–2039.
3. Hebden JC, Delpy DT. Diagnostic imaging with light. Br J Radiol 1997;70:S206–S214.
4. Benaron D, Stevenson D. Optical time-of-flight and absorbance imaging of biologic media. Science 1993;259:1463–1466.
5. Mahmood U, Tung C-H, Bogdanov A Jr, Weissleder R. Near-infrared optical imaging of protease activity for tumor detection. Radiology 1999;213:866–870.
6. Rao JS, Steck PA, Mohanam S, et al. Elevated levels of M(r) 92,000 type IV collagenase in human brain tumors. Cancer Res 1993;53:2208–2211.
7. McCuskey RS. Microscopic methods for studying the microvasculature of internal organs. In: Baker CH, Nastuk WF, eds. Physical Techniques in Biology and Medicine: Microvascular Technology. New York: Academic Press, 1986:247–264.
8. Grisham JW, Nopanitaya W. Scanning electron microscopy of casts of hepatic microvessels. Review of methods and results. In: Lautt WW, ed. Hepatic Circulation in Health and Disease. New York: Raven Press, 1981:87–109.
9. Kan Z, Ivancev K, Lunderquist A, et al. In vivo microscopy of hepatic tumors in animal models: a dynamic investigation of blood supply to hepatic metastases. Radiology 1993;187:621–626.
10. Charnsangavej C, Wallace S. Interventional radiologic techniques in the diagnosis and treatment of hepatobiliary malignancy. In: Wanebo H, ed. Surgery for Gastrointestinal Cancer: A Multidisciplinary Approach. Philadelphia: Lippincott-Raven, 1997:597–606.
11. Nakakuma K, Uemura K, Kono T, et al. Studies on anticancer treatment with anticancer drug injected into the ligated hepatic artery for liver cancer (preliminary report). Nichidoku Iho 1979; 24:675–682.
12. Kan Z, Ivancev K, Hagerstrabd I, et al. In vivo microscopy of the liver after injection of Lipiodol into the hepatic artery and portal vein in the rat. Acta Radiol Diagn 1989;30:419–425.
13. Kan Z, Sato M, Ivancev K, et al. Distribution and effect of iodized poppyseed oil in the liver after hepatic artery embolization: experimental study in several animal species. Radiology 1993;186:861–866.
14. Kan Z, Ivancev K, Lunderquist A. Peribiliary plexus: an important pathway to the portal vein for Lipiodol and Microfil when injected into the hepatic artery. Invest Radiol 1994;29:671–675.
15. Kan Z, Wallace S. Sinusoidal embolization: impact of iodized oil on hepatic microcirculation. J Vasc Intervent Radiol 1994;5:881–886.
16. Kan Z, Wallace S. Transcatheter liver lobar ablation: an experimental trial in an animal model. Eur Radiol 1997;7:1071–1075.
17. Cheng YF, Kan Z, Chen CL, et al. The efficacy and safety of preoperative lobar or segmental ablation via transarterial administration of ethiodol and ethanol mixture in the treatment of hepatocellular carcinoma: a clinical study. World J Surg 2000, in press.

18. Lin SY, Wu WH. Physical parameters and release behaviors of w/o/w multiple emulsions containing cosurfactants and different specific gravity of oil. Pharm Acta Helv 1991;66:342–347.

19. Kan Z, Wright K, Wallace S. Ethiodol oil emulsion in hepatic microcirculation: in vivo microscopy in animal models. Acad Radiol 1997;4:275–282.

20. Evans CW. The invasion and metastatic behaviour of malignant cells. In: Evans CW, ed. The Metastatic Cell: Behavior and Biochemistry. London: Chapman & Hall, 1991:137–214.

21. Kan Z, Ivancev K, Lunderquist A, et al. In vivo microscopy of hepatic metastases: dynamic observations of tumor cell invasion and interaction with Kupffer cells. Hepatology 1995;21:487–494.

22. Rost FD. Principles of fluorescence microscopy. Fluorochrometry. In: Rost FD, ed. Fluorescence Microscopy. Cambridge: Cambridge University Press, 1992;1–10:80–107.

23. Steams T. Green fluorescent protein: the green revolution. Curr Biol 1995;5:262–264.

24. Heim R, Cubitt AB, Tsien RY. Improved green fluorescence. Nature (Lond) 1995;373:663–664.

25. Chishima T, Miyagi Y, Wang X, et al. Cancer invasion and micrometastasis visualization in liver tissue by green fluorescent protein expression. Cancer Res 1997;57:2042–2047.

26. Kan Z, Liu TJ. Video microscopy of tumor metastasis: using the green fluorescent protein (GFP) gene as a cancer-cell-labeling system. Clin Exp Metastasis 1999;17:49–55.

27. Naumov GN, Wilson SM, MacDonald IC, et al. Cellular expression of green fluorescent protein, coupled with high-resolution in vivo videomicroscopy, to monitor steps in tumor metastasis. J Cell Sci 1999;112:1835–1842.

Index

ISBN 0-387-95028-1